"This book is certainly a treasure for marathoners of all levels. I know that I picked up some tricks from its pages. I found myself nodding along with each page I read. This book is overflowing with good, sound, sage advice."

—RYAN HALL, 2-time US Olympic marathoner

"I hate this book. For years now, I've been pretending running marathons is impossibly difficult, incredibly painful, and completely outside the reach of normal humans. But if people read this book, they'll find out that almost anyone can complete a marathon or half-marathon, and my achievements will seem much less impressive. DAMN YOU ALL."

—PETER SAGAL, host of NPR's *Wait, Wait . . . Don't Tell Me!*
and *Runner's World's* "Road Scholar" columnist

"I had a running goal. I wanted to run a half-marathon in under 2 hours—and the *Runner's World* Challenge team and training plan got me to the finish line victorious. The support, motivation, and direct and personalized feedback from *Runner's World* experts was invaluable to me as a participant in the program's online forum. *The Runner's World Big Book of Marathon and Half-Marathon Training* offers that same sense of community in the form of a book you can carry anywhere. It's conversational, it's inspirational, it's chock-full of tips from running gurus Bart Yasso, Amby Burfoot, and Jennifer Van Allen. It's a recipe for success. The first step is believing you can do it—whatever "it" is. Follow the plan and you'll get there."

—LAUREN JOHNSTON, deputy managing editor for NYDailyNews.com
and creator of the *Running Dialogue* running blog

"Make room on your bookshelf for the latest comprehensive marathoning how-to: *The Runner's World Big Book of Marathon and Half-Marathon Training*. What sets this guide apart from the rest is the accumulated wisdom of the *Runner's World* authors and the infectious passion of the magazine's readers, who share stories of triumph that will get you off your couch and out on the road.

—LENNY BERNSTEIN, "MisFits" columnist, *The Washington Post*

Winning strategies, inspiring stories, and the ultimate training tools

THE RUNNER'S WORLD

BIG BOOK

OF

MARATHON
and Half-Marathon
TRAINING

Jennifer Van Allen, Bart Yasso, and Amby Burfoot, with Pamela Nisevich Bede, RD, CSSD

RODALE.

To Noah

Direct online and Trade paperback are being published simltaneously in 2012.

© 2012 by Rodale Inc.
Exercise Photographs © 2012 Rodale Inc.

Rodale books may be purchased for business or promotional use or for special sales. For information, please write to:
Special Markets Department, Rodale, Inc., 733 Third Avenue, New York, NY 10017

Runner's World is a registered trademark of Rodale Inc.

Printed in the United States of America
Rodale Inc. makes every effort to use acid-free ♾, recycled paper ♻.

Exercise Photographs by Mitch Mandel/Rodale Images
Book design by Christopher Rhoads

Library of Congress Cataloging-in-Publication Data

Van Allen, Jennifer.
    Runner's world big book of marathon and half-marathon training : winning strategies, inspiring stories, and the ultimate training tools / Jennifer Van Allen . . . [et.al.].
        p.   cm.
    Includes bibliographical references.
    ISBN 978–1–60961–684–7   trade paperback
    ISBN 978–1–60961–915–2   direct hardcover
    1. Marathon running—Training.   I. Title.
    GV1065.17.T73V36   2012
    796.42⸱2—dc23   2012010217

Distributed to the trade by Macmillan

2   4   6   8   10   9   7   5   3   1   trade paperback
2   4   6   8   10   9   7   5   3   1   direct hardcover

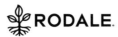

RODALE.

We inspire and enable people to improve their lives and the world around them.

rodalebooks.com

Contents

PART IV: PUTTING IT ALL TOGETHER

Introduction

Anyone can run a marathon. Oprah Winfrey did it. Senators, presidents, and movie stars do it all the time. The hit reality show *The Biggest Loser* even culminated in a marathon for the contestants who have lost the most weight—as if to make the point that anyone, even the morbidly obese, can become an athlete with enough grit and determination.

It's been said that the marathon has become the "everyman's Everest." There is a mystique about it, but even nonrunners know what a marathon is. They may not know the exact distance, but everyone knows that it's a mighty long way and requires months of preparation.

Indeed, the training is an all-guts-for-little-glory proposition. It involves achy knees, gallons of sweat, chafed skin, and blisters the size of silver dollars. It requires waking at the crack of dawn to run in weather conditions that most people won't drive in, as well as running solo for hours at a time. It means fending off accusations that you're crazy—not to mention tackling self-doubt and repeatedly asking yourself why you're doing this at all.

That's where we come in.

Here at *Runner's World,* we pride ourselves on being the experts when it comes to preparing for marathons. After all, we've been telling people how for more than 40 years.

In 2009, we decided to try something new. Rather than just champion the time-tested principles of long-distance running from the pages of our magazine, we decided to hit the road and test it for ourselves. A dozen *Runner's World* editors decided to train for a marathon together, and we invited readers to join us.

Bart Yasso, the man hailed as the "Mayor of Running," developed a 16-week program for the *Runner's World* editors. We then offered the plan to our readers, along with all of the tools they'd need to get from the starting line to the finish. We created an online community on runnersworld.com, and we put ourselves on call 24/7 to answer everyone's questions about training, nutrition, motivation, and injury prevention. The *Runner's World* Challenge was born.

To be honest, we had no idea what would happen. I remember staring at my computer screen on the day we opened registration, waiting for the first sign-up. *Please,* I begged the machine, *we just need one person.*

Thankfully, a 50-year-old postal worker finally signed up, and others soon followed. Since then, more than 3,000 people have taken the *Runner's World* Challenge while preparing for marathons and half-marathons (which we later added to the program) all over the world. More than 1,600 of them have raced alongside us at marathons in Richmond, Cincinnati, San Francisco, Toronto, Big Sur, and Philadelphia. They have hailed from more than 50 locales, stretching from Wisconsin to Guatemala; they have been first-timers and 2:40 hopefuls; college kids and grandparents. Some have been shooting for their fastest times ever. Some were celebrating milestone birthdays or anniversaries. Others had reached get-up-or-give-up moments, and the Challenge was the call to action they needed to start turning their lives around. A few were in the throes of chemotherapy, trying to survive the hardest times of their lives.

In *Runner's World*'s online community, the Challengers formed a global running club, bonded by the breakthroughs and bonks they shared during hundreds of days of training. There were wild-animal sightings, 2:30 a.m. long runs, and an infinite number of tweaked hamstrings and IT bands. There were assorted exclamations of Ouch!, Doh!, and Oof! There was at least one treadmill casualty. Along the way, the Challengers became friends and one another's support systems.

"The online community became my family and my cheerleading section," says Nancy Kissak, 60, an accountant from Merced, California. "I just needed someone to tell me that

I could do this. And *Runner's World* provided that."

And the Challengers accomplished way more than they'd imagined or that we could have promised. Jonathan Steckel finished his first marathon in 2:57. After struggling to break 5:30 for six marathons, Christopher Sanford of Newport News, Virginia, nabbed a 4:51 finish, and 17 months later he went on to run a 4:08 marathon. Dan Kovacevic, a 41-year-old home builder from Cleveland, Ohio, shed 80 pounds from his 6-foot frame, became a 3:57 marathoner, and grew into a person that others turn to for inspiration and advice.

"I went from feeling indolent," he says, "to feeling like an athlete."

Ultimately, the Challengers found that the most enduring benefits of the marathon amounted to way more than anything that could be measured on a clock at the finish line.

"Getting through the training and completing the race has given me incredible confidence that I never had before," says Stephanie Russell, 28, of Oakton, Virginia. "And it has made me think that maybe this whole time I have been a lot stronger than I ever realized."

David Jones, 58, an elementary school principal from Edmonds, Washington, discovered that strength 3 miles from the finish of the 2009 Richmond Marathon. As the spring left his stride and his energy plummeted, he came across a runner wearing a *Runner's World* Challenge T-shirt just like his. They pushed on together, helping each other to gut out the last bone-weary steps to the finish.

"His encouragement kept me loose and brought me in much stronger than I would have finished on my own," says Jones.

It wasn't until after they got their medals that Jones realized that the other runner was David Willey, editor-in-chief of *Runner's World.*

"Those last miles illustrated what I experienced in the Challenge," says Jones. "Nice folks learning and working together to accomplish something bigger than they could have by themselves."

In this book, we'll be sharing the *Runner's World* Challenge experience with you.

You'll find all the tools you need to run your first or your fastest marathon or half-marathon. You'll find some of the marathon and half-marathon plans that the *Runner's World* Challengers used to achieve their race-day goals (see page 260), plus more than two dozen different workouts recommended by elite runners (see page 251). You'll get answers to the most enduring questions

Challengers asked about training and injury prevention, many of which were first addressed in the pages of *Runner's World,* in the *Runner's World* Challenge forums, over e-mail, and on race weekends. Sports dietitian Pamela Nisevich Bede, answers all of the burning (and uncomfortable) questions about nutrition and weight loss that may come up during the Challenge. You'll find a glossary to help you sort through all the mystifying running jargon (see page 233), plus suggestions for the most nutritious, easy-to-make meals and snacks for runners (see page 242). You'll also hear some of the most valuable (and, okay, embarrassing) lessons that the *Runner's World* editors learned during their training.

And what's more, you'll find the moving stories of the runners who took the Challenge. They taught us all here at *Runner's World* what it really takes to go the distance. If you have ever thought that you are too old, too busy, or too out of shape to run a marathon or half-marathon, these people will convince you otherwise.

— *Jennifer Van Allen*

About the *Runner's World* Challenge

The *Runner's World* Challenge is the magazine's online marathon and half-marathon training program. Since it was launched in 2009, more than 3,300 runners from all over the world—from first-timers to seasoned veterans—have taken the Challenge to finish their first races, and their fastest.

The *Runner's World* Challenge includes:

- A training plan
- Online access to the *Runner's World* experts on training, nutrition, and injury prevention
- A 4-month free trial to *Runner's World*'s premium interactive training log
- Daily e-mails with reminders about your workouts
- Weekly motivational e-mails from *Runner's World*'s chief running officer Bart Yasso
- A *Runner's World* book
- A *Runner's World* Challenge technical T-shirt
- Online access to the *Runner's World* Challenge community, where you can connect with other runners who are training for marathons and half-marathons

Runners can also choose to come run with Bart Yasso and the *Runner's World* editors at one of our select special events. They receive all of the benefits described above, plus VIP treatment on race weekend. That includes:

- Entry to the race
- Private bib pickup
- Exclusive training run and strategy session with Bart Yasso and the *Runner's World* editors
- Starting line amenities, including private bathrooms and bag check
- Postrace massage
- Exclusive postrace party at the finish

For more information, go to runnersworldchallenge.com or you can e-mail us directly at challenge@runnersworld.com.

About the Authors

We assure you, you are in good hands.

Amby Burfoot, who won the 1968 Boston Marathon, has run more than 75 marathons and has a personal best of 2:14. He has logged more than 105,000 lifetime miles and has written and edited four books about running, including the *Runner's World Complete Book of Running* and *The Runner's Guide to the Meaning of Life*. He has been at *Runner's World* for 34 years, and in the 18 years that he served as its editor, he helped guide *Runner's World* into being the leading running magazine in the world.

Bart Yasso is a veteran of more than 1,000 races and more than 100 marathons, with a personal best of 2:40. He invented the Yasso 800s, a workout that has become legendary for predicting marathon finishing times. His victories include the 1998 Smoky Mountain Marathon and the 1987 National Biathlon Championship. He has run races on every continent, finished the Ironman five times, run the Badwater 146 through Death Valley, and cycled solo and unsupported across the country. He chronicled those adventures in his book *My Life on the Run*. Now, as *Runner's World*'s chief running officer, Bart is on the road 50 weekends a year, dispensing the wisdom and inspiration runners need as they dash off to the starting line and handing out high-fives at the finish line.

Over the past 30 years, Amby and Bart have become gurus of running. Even as elites have risen into the spotlight and faded back into obscurity, as trends like barefoot running have gone in and out of popularity, Amby and Bart have remained. They have rubbed elbows with running royalty like Haile Gebrselassie and Joan Benoit Samuelson, and they are just as at ease with Olympians and elites as they are with newbies heading from the couch to their first 5-K. And whenever running makes the mainstream news, they are the go-to guys for reporters seeking sage advice. Celebrities, politicians, elites, and Fortune 500 CEOs—including Mike Huckabee and Bill Rodgers—have sought out Amby and Bart for training advice. At race expos, crowds mob them for autographs, photos, or just an opportunity to thank them for their inspiration and their guidance.

Both Amby and Bart claim that they have the best jobs in the world, but I'd arm wrestle them for that claim. Getting to work with these two icons has been the highlight of my career, and it's been a lot of fun. No matter how busy they are, they're happy to stop what they're doing to share their wisdom with anyone who asks, whether it's about proper pacing or how to get over a disappointing race. And they approach their work with the same kind of endurance and passion that they do their own running lives.

Pamela Nisevich Bede, a 3:09 marathoner and Ironman in her own right, co-owns Swim, Bike, Run, Eat! LLC, a Dayton, Ohio-based nutrition consulting firm. As a Certified Specialist in Sports Dietetics (CSSD), she counsels athletes of all ages and abilities, developing meal plans for individuals and teams, developing event-day nutrition strategies, and lecturing on acute and chronic diseases that affect different sports.

Throughout the Challenge, she has been the ultimate resource for anyone needing a little nutrition RX. She helped scores of runners figure out how to fuel up properly, stay hydrated, shed pounds, and avoid awkward midrace trips to the port-o-let. She has generously shared all of that expertise—and so much more—for this book.

As for me (Jennifer Van Allen), I just bumbled my way into running. I grew up chubby in a suburban community in Indiana—the only training I did happened with my butt planted firmly on a piano bench.

My running life began with a walk around the block in high school and continued in college with a 3-mile jog in a vain attempt to foil the freshman 15. In 1998, a friend convinced me to throw my name into the lottery for the New York City Marathon, and to my shock and dismay, I got in. I had never run more than 6 miles in my life. I finished the race in 4:51, wailing "never again!" as I lumbered over the final hilly miles in Central Park.

Fourteen years and a lot of blisters later, I have finished 36 marathons and ultras, with a 3:08 personal best at the 2009 Boston Marathon. I love running so much that I started going beyond 26.2. I won the 2008 Lone Ranger 24-hour ultramarathon, and I went on to win the 24-Hour National Championship a few months later. The next spring, I competed in the 24-hour World Championships in Italy as a member of Team USA.

How the heck did that happen?

I certainly never could have imagined any of it. The courage to start and the stubbornness to finish always seemed like enough of a miracle to hope for.

Two years after my "never again" moment in Central Park, I ran the Vancouver Marathon to raise money for the Arthritis Foundation, and I cut 40 minutes off my previous time. Two years after that, after moving to a new town, I joined a marathon-training program as a way to meet people. I sliced nearly 40 minutes off my time at the 2003 Philadelphia Marathon, and I qualified for Boston.

My training partners quickly became friends, and I kept signing up for marathons. The experience of running distances that seemed impossible—whether it was a 3-mile run in a summer squall or a 20-miler at 3 a.m. on a 10-degree January morning—transformed me. I fell deeply in love with the feeling that I got from being outside and the utterly spent sensation I got after a long run left me buzzed all day long.

It didn't matter that most of my races weren't personal best times (most were personal worsts) or that I got frustrated, injured, and so burnt out that I wanted to throw my running shoes out the window. Even the most awful days on the road—when my quads felt like lead weights and I was sucking wind at an easy pace—were better than days when I didn't run. I fell a lot, most of the time flat on my face. But my black toenails and bruises became badges of honor. I gained an appetite for adventures, plus the courage to actually get off my butt and make them happen.

I started doing homegrown excursions, including a 100-K run through Maryland, Delaware, and Pennsylvania to celebrate the longest day of the year. I ran 35 miles to celebrate my 35th birthday, spontaneously and self-supported.

This is how running transforms a person from the outside in. We hear it all the time from people like you who write to us at *Runner's World*. You go from assuming that things are impossible to having the burning desire to find out what's possible. You go from believing that you cannot to wondering if you can.

Whatever blood, sweat, and tears I've shed in marathons and half-marathons is chump change compared to all the ways that running has made my life so much fuller.

It is our hope that your investment in this book—and in your long-distance dreams—gives back just as much to you.

PART I

TRAINING

Running 13.1 or 26.2 miles is no small task, to be sure. But anyone who has done it will tell you that getting to the finish line isn't the tough part—getting to the starting line is.

After all, at most events there are aid stations with food and drink every few miles, scores of cheering spectators offering encouragement, plus the camaraderie of thousands of fellow runners. And at the end, everyone earns a medal for his or her effort.

Ah . . . if only training was that luxurious.

Indeed, race preparation is where the biggest challenge lies. It entails figuring out how to drive your body and mind further than they've ever gone before, without burning out either in the process. It demands pushing yourself through hours on the road, often solo, fueled only by your own determination to cover the miles for the day and the faith that you can do it. It requires figuring out which discomforts you can grit your teeth through and which pains demand surrender. It involves committing to the goal every day for hundreds of days before the event, even when the chaos of your own life, or your own self-doubt, makes it extremely tempting to give up.

To be sure, it's on this long, sweaty journey to the starting line that the true personal transformation takes place. This is where individuals morph into athletes, with the gear, training logs, and war wounds that go along with that; it's where dreamers become doers.

In this section, you'll find everything you need to kick off your training on the right foot and to successfully make it to the starting line. You'll learn how to find a race that's appropriate for you, pick a goal that's realistic, and determine the best strategy to follow to accomplish that goal. You'll learn the basic principles of training, find out what to wear, and get tips on how to juggle the demands of training with the work, family, and social commitments of everyday life.

Master the techniques we give you here, and the race itself will become a victory lap for all of the hundreds of miles you logged, the countless sacrifices you made, and the physical and emotional transformation that took place along the way.

CHAPTER 1

GETTING STARTED

Ready or Not? Before you jump into marathon or half-marathon training, it's important to honestly assess whether you're ready. If you've never run a step before or you're just starting out, jumping into a 25-mile-a-week training program is a surefire way to end up hurt and burned-out.

That is not to say that you have to wait until you reach some ideal weight, or you get perfect running weather, or you get some stress-free 4-month chunk of time at work, the kids are self-sufficient, and you have so much free time that you can train whenever you want, as much as you want. (That day will likely *never* arrive.)

But by taking a few critical steps before you start training for a big race, you'll save yourself a lot of time, hurt, and heartache down the road. Here's what to do before you get started.

Build a base. As long as you've been running at least four times a week for about 6 months and you're in the habit of exercising regularly, you should be able to complete a marathon or half-marathon training program without a problem. Many training plans begin with a minimum of 4 days a week of running and a total of about 25 miles a week for a marathon or about 15 miles a week for a half-marathon. If you've been running only sporadically and have to give your weekly routine an extreme makeover to start training, it's going to be tough to stick with it. Plus, you're bound to end up with any variety of overuse injuries that come from doing too much too soon, such as iliotibial (IT) band syndrome or plantar fasciitis. If you haven't been training that consistently, don't fret. You can still run a marathon or half-marathon in the near future. Pick a date one year away, and work your way up to it.

Time it right. Marathon and half-marathon training are time-consuming, there's no question about it. At a minimum, it will require 30 minutes to 1 hour a day during the week, and on weekends you'll need up to 3 hours for long runs. That's not counting the extra time you'll need to cool down, stretch, and refuel, as well as regale your family and friends with the news of what you managed to accomplish before they even got out of bed. Training will take even more time—up to 10 hours a week in the 3 to 6 weeks before the race—as the long runs and weekly mileage peak. Examine the entire 16-week marathon program or 10-week half-marathon plan next to a schedule of your family and work commitments, and figure out if it's doable right now. You won't enjoy running if you constantly feel rushed, stressed, and guilty that you're not doing something else. Plan ahead for any conflicts; figure out which workouts need to be rearranged and which parts of your usual routine will need to be adjusted. Make childcare arrangements before your long runs, swap your car pool shifts, and arrange to come in an hour late to the office if you need to. Set these plans in motion before you start training. That way, as the runs get longer and the race draws near, you won't have the added pressure of figuring out how you'll fit it all in.

Assess your stress. While running can be a great stress relief, trying to train for a race—especially your first—while contending with other big life changes, like a new baby or a cross-country move, can be a bit much. Some people welcome the structure and the distraction that training brings to an otherwise chaotic time of life. For others, it is just too overwhelming. Only *you* can decide whether training would reduce or increase your stress.

Amby's Advice

Most experts think you should work up to marathons and half-marathons slowly and gradually. Run a few 5-Ks first, then a few 10-Ks, and so on. So naturally that's what I think you should do, too. Except for this difference: I'm willing to acknowledge the power of the marathon and half-marathon to "grab" runners and motivate them to jump into the unknown. So if it grabs you hard, I say: What the heck, go for it! But remember this: You have to be very realistic about your expectations. Unless you're young and fit, you'll have to do most of your training on a run-walk pattern. You might have to pick a run-walk ratio as conservative as run 2 minutes, walk 1 minute. It will likely take you 5 hours or more to cover the marathon course or 3 hours to finish a half-marathon. Both events are doable. Don't be afraid—just have reasonable expectations. And follow a solid training program that builds up your miles. They can be slow miles, but you gotta do them.

See the doctor. It's best to get a checkup before you start training, especially if you're coping with injuries or you have a family history of heart attack, diabetes, or other chronic illnesses. If you're over 40 or your doctor recommends it, get a stress test. Go to the doctor right away if you experience chest pain, pressure, shortness of breath, or some other abnormal feeling while exercising.

Choosing a Race

Once you decide that you're ready to train for a marathon or a half-marathon, it's best to pick a race and sign up for it as soon as possible. Most races offer early bird discounts, and if you sign up early you won't have to worry about getting shut out if the race fills up. But there are other benefits, too. Once you fork over the cash for an entry fee—not cheap, these days—you shift from running to training. You progress out of casual exercise. You have a mission to accomplish and a road map to help you accomplish it. Knowing that you've registered for the race can get you out of bed on those subzero-degree days when it might be tempting to hit the snooze button. But which race to choose? It pays to be picky. Here are some factors to consider.

Plan ahead. Most marathon plans last for 4 months; many half-marathon plans last for 2½ months. But if you're just starting out, it's best to pick a race that is at least 6 months away. That way, you'll have extra time to build up your base of fitness, develop a consistent exercise routine, and allow for any unexpected hitches, injuries, or false starts. Also, when you compare your work and family calendars, make sure that the most intense parts of training and the race itself don't conflict with other major life events.

Location, location, location. Races can be a passport to adventure and an excuse to see a new place that you haven't been to before. On the other hand, travel can add a whole new layer of stress to your race experience. There are pros and cons to running in your hometown and to traveling to a far-off place. If you're a first-timer, you might want to consider going local. On race weekend, being able to eat what you trained with on long runs, race on a course you've run on millions of times, and go through the same prerun rituals you did during training will help you stay calm as you step to the line. Not having to worry about getting to the airport or whether you packed your shoes or your favorite brand of energy gel will be a big load off your shoulders. On the other hand, seeing 13.1 or 26.2 miles of a new place—and seeing it in a way that you can't from a tour bus or a car—might be a welcome distraction from the pressures of the race itself. If you turn race weekend into a getaway with family and friends, it can feel like a vacation with a big catered run at the end!

Consider the conditions. You want to make sure that you'll be able to prepare for the race in conditions that are similar to what you'll be racing in. A spring race might sound nice, but it means you're going to be training in the snowy, icy, dark depths of winter. If you're training for an early fall marathon or half-marathon, you'll be training in the heat of summer, which means 90-degree long runs. A late fall race is ideal. You'll start training in late July and August, when the days are long and you can run early, while it's light. And as your runs get longer, the weather will get cooler and much more hospitable for those hours-long long runs.

What's more, on race day, you're more likely to get those perfect running conditions. Studies have shown that 50° to 54°F (10° to 12°C) is the ideal temperature range for running marathons and that performance slows by 3 percent for every 7.2°F (4°C) above that. And the slower you are, the more affected you are by the heat.[1] (Read more about this in "Beating the Heat" on page 139.) Matthew Ely, coauthor of the study, has not examined half-marathon runners, but he said he believes the results would be applicable to those going 13.1 miles, since many tend to finish between 2:15 and 3 hours. Of course, there's no accounting for a freak storm or a heat wave. No one could have predicted that 85-degree April day at the 2004 Boston Marathon or the nor'easter with 40-mile-per-hour wind gusts that hit 3 years later. But most races post an "average temperature" for race day on their Web sites. If they don't, you can look it up on a site like weatherunderground.com.

Find the right size. There's a big difference between racing shoulder to shoulder with 30,000 other people while millions of people on the sidelines cheer you on and doing a smaller event where you'll run for miles without seeing another competitor or spectator. Some people find that they thrive on the energy of the screaming spectators on the sidelines and the constant company of other runners. Others find the crowds stressful; they don't like jostling with others at the water stops, and they like the simplicity of a smaller race.

Go with a known quantity. There's nothing wrong with running a race in its inaugural year, but if this is your first time racing, you might want to go with an established race. Look for experienced race direc-

BART SAYS...

I think that if you're going for a personal best or you want to run all-out, the perfect size marathon or half-marathon is 5,000 runners. That's big enough so that you have lots of runners to pace with, but it's small enough to ensure that you can get on pace right away, and you'll have plenty of room for you to run.

tors, sponsors, and running clubs; ask people at your local running store for recommendations. A poorly marked course or too few water stops can ruin your whole day. You want the confidence of knowing that the aid stations are going to be where you're expecting them: at least every 2 to 3 miles. If you have questions, e-mail the race director.

Choose your terrain. Check out the course map and elevation chart on the race Web site. Do you want a course that's fast and flat, even if that means running through some not-so-great parts of town? Or would you rather run through pretty scenery even if that means doing some climbing? If you're looking to set a personal best or want to qualify for the Boston Marathon, look for a course that advertises that. (See "Fastest Races Around" on page 8.) A word of warning about courses that brag about being "pancake flat" or "all downhill": They can be deceptively tough. On a flat course, you'll pound the same muscles over and over again, and this can zap your strength. A course that's all downhill can exact a much bigger beating on your leg muscles than a flat or uphill course. Your best option is a course that offers some variation. A few rolling hills will work different muscle groups and keep you from getting bored. The most important factor is that you're able to practice running on terrain that mimics the elevation change that you'll face during the race. If you're training for a marathon in Colorado and you live in Indiana, you're going to have to make some time to train in areas where you can practice that

Race Checklist

Use this checklist when you're comparing different races. Consider each of these factors to figure out which marathon or half-marathon is right for you.

RACE	RACE DATE	WEEKS TO TRAIN	LOCA-TION	NUMBER OF RUNNERS	TYPICAL WEATHER CONDITIONS (AVERAGE TEMPERATURE ON RACE DAY)	HILLY OR FLAT?	COURSE TIME LIMIT	MUSIC FRIENDLY
1								
2								
3								

Fastest Races Around

The marathons* below had the fastest median finishing times in 2011. These courses will undoubtedly be among those ranked the fastest of all courses—but for a point-to-point course, a tailwind or headwind might make the difference from one year to the next. Some races (such as the Boston Marathon) simply attract faster runners. But you can be sure that any marathon on this list is not slow.

Boston Marathon	3:44:58
Eugene Marathon	3:59:17
Lincoln National Guard Marathon	4:01:44
Wineglass Marathon	4:04:05
Steamtown Marathon	4:05:27

*Among marathons with more than 1,000 finishers
Source: RunningUSA.org

hillwork. (You'll find out how in Chapter 3, Integrating Training into Your Everyday Life, starting on page 46.)

Course cutoffs. Many races have strict time limits, but others have extended times and advertise that they are walker friendly. If you're a walker or worry that you won't be able to finish before the course closes, it's a good idea to pick a race with a more liberal time limit. You will have enough to think about on race day without adding the stress of worrying whether you'll have to be pulled off the course or whether there will be any

water or medals left at the finish line. In most cases, the course time limit refers to the amount of time that the aid stations will stay up and operating and the amount of time that the roads will be closed to car traffic.

Music friendly. It is no longer against the rules to wear an iPod or a music player during a marathon. USA Track and Field, the governing body of running, briefly banned music players in 2007, but that ban was lifted in 2009. That said, some races do prohibit the use of headphones, while other races brand themselves as iPod friendly. If you're used to training with music and you can't race without it, make sure that the race you choose allows it. Even if it does, it's a good idea to run with just one earbud in or to keep the volume low enough that you can hear other runners approaching or directions from course officials. You don't want to cause a collision at a water stop or miss hearing another runner call out a warning about a pothole or a curb.

Picking a Training Plan

There are a million different flavors of training plans that you can use to prepare for a marathon or half-marathon: 4-days-per-week plans, walk/run plans, and break-3-hours plans. You'll find people who have succeeded and failed with each of them. There is no one

What it takes to . . .
Become a marathoner at age 64

Bowen Tucker, 73, Chicago, IL
Retired attorney, father of two, grandfather of six
Experience: 3 marathons; 4:30 PR
Runner's World Challenge Race: 2010 Chicago Marathon

I started running when I retired. A career that included travel and rich meals was enjoyable, but about 50 pounds too much remained around my waist. I realized that less weight might provide me with a longer and more enjoyable retirement. At the time, I weighed 195; in high school, I weighed 145. I went on a diet, and within 6 months most of the weight was gone. I knew diet wasn't enough, and I needed to exercise. So I started running. Each day I ran I tried to better my time. I retained a trainer at an athletic club and started using the treadmill. One day she timed me running 1 mile on an indoor track. I finished the mile in 6:30. She suggested I run the Shamrock Shuffle 8-K and gave me a training plan. I finished 16th out of 91 in my age group with an 8:06 pace. This encouraged me to keep going, and I ran the Chicago Marathon in 2002. I anticipated being last, but I found that there were thousands behind me. The training was easy and it was fun running in a pace group. Spectators cheered me on; children wanted to touch my hand because I was a marathoner. My pace was slow, but there was a tremendous sense of accomplishment. Now that I'm a marathoner, I feel healthier, and I'm in better shape than I have been in since high school. My body got stronger and it works better. They say it can't happen in your 60s, but I'm convinced it did. And running feels great. Some people just sit on the couch and rust. But I don't want to live that way. You've got to make sure your body is in shape if you want to be around for a few years longer. And if I can get more out of it while I'm here, I want to do that, too.

right kind of plan, there is only the one plan that is the best fit for you right now.

The most important factor above anything else is that your plan feels doable. The first few weeks should be a natural extension of the running routine that you've already been maintaining. If the plan is a good fit, you'll finish most workouts feeling challenged and exhilarated—like you put in a good, honest effort—but not demolished. But if the plan is too hard for your current level of fitness, you'll go home feeling frustrated and possibly hurt. And if it requires more time than you can spare, you'll have relentless guilt and stress, and you'll feel like you're constantly giving short shrift to something or someone. "You end up feeling like you're cheating on your marathon with your spouse," says Harvard psychologist Jeff Brown, author of *The Winner's Brain.*

Each runner has a unique threshold for what he or she can tolerate without getting hurt, and that threshold is determined by genetics, injury history, and level of fitness. Some people can't run more than 50 miles a week without getting injured; for others, one night at the track will put them out for weeks.

If you're a beginner, pick a plan that includes rest days and running days. That plan will give you the most opportunity to practice running and develop the endurance you need with the least risk of injury. If you get through your first race and you enjoyed it enough to do another, then you can focus on getting faster by adding speed sessions and other different kinds of workouts to your training.

Amby's Advice

The hardest thing for first-timers is usually not the mileage and long runs, it's the summer weather and the lack of confidence all first-timers feel. I can assure you of two things: First, if you manage to get through training in relatively good health, you can do the race. Second, and even more unbelievable, is that the race won't be as bad as you're imagining today.

Here are the factors to consider when picking a training plan. Read about each of them, and then choose from one of our training plans (see pages 260–272).

Weekly mileage. How many miles per week did you run on average for the past 6 weeks? You don't want to start a routine that is a huge jump in mileage from what you've been doing. The first few weeks should be no more than 10 percent more than what you've been doing for the past 6 weeks.

Days of running. Ideally, you'll have 4 to 6 days each week to run. That said, it is possible to train for a marathon or a half-marathon on 3 days of running each week, as long as you cross-train on the other days to maintain your cardiovascular fitness. Reserve at least 1 day each week for complete rest, with no cross-training or easy running, to allow for full recovery. That day will help you steer clear of injury and will also allow you to catch up on all the little details of your everyday life, like cleaning and errands, that you might not have time for on your running days.

Room for other activities. The best way to train for a marathon or a half-marathon is to run. But cross-training and strength training can help you stay injury free and keep you feeling mentally fresh. If you want to incorporate strength training or classes like yoga or Pilates into your schedule, pick a plan with lower mileage, which gives you the flexibility to do that.

Setting Smart Race Goals

Like a lot of runners, when *Runner's World* Challenger Pete Githens signed up for his first marathon, he had a time goal in mind. He'd heard that you should just enjoy your rookie run and focus on finishing, but the 45-year-old computer analyst from Reading, Pennsylvania, had done his first 5-K in August of 2009 and went on to finish the 2010 Lehigh Valley Half-Marathon in 1:38—an impressive pace of 7:28 minutes per mile. After reading and talking to other runners, he set his sights on a 3:30 marathon, the time he'd need to qualify for the Boston Marathon. Even though he'd never run 26.2 miles before, "based on my past, shorter races, and never actually missing any of my goals, I felt I could do better than just finishing," he says.

Githens got a rude awakening on race day. He missed gels that were being handed out at an aid station and got all the way to mile 17 on just one gel and water. At mile 18 he was battling cramps, light-headedness, and the overwhelming urge to quit. "I had hit the wall," Githens said, "and the wall had fallen on top of me. I spent most of the second half of the race feeling sorry for myself and feeling like I'd lost. It wasn't until I was near the end that I again began to feel like I was accomplishing something." He finished in 3:53, just ecstatic to call himself a marathoner.

"As it turns out, it was pretty arrogant to feel I could go out and run my first 26.2 that well," he says. "'Respect the distance' is the mantra of marathoners. I did not, and the distance came up and gave me a big ol' slap of reality."

Runners tend to measure success by the minute. But focusing your sights only on a single time can set you up for failure. Miss your mark after all your hard training, and it's such a downer that you may end up quitting. That is not to say that it's impossible to qualify for Boston or break 4:00 on your first try. But setting multiple goals—and making sure that at least one is not defined by the clock—will guarantee a sense of accomplishment come race day, no matter what happens. "If you set a variety of goals that include some you know you can achieve," says Patti Finke, an exercise physiologist and coach of Team Oregon, "you'll always be successful and hungry for the next challenge."

Here's a guide to setting good race goals.

Make it to the finish. No matter how long you've been running, how good your genes are, or how dedicated you are to training, if you're a first-timer, we urge you to just focus on getting to the starting line injury-free and reaching the finish feeling strong and healthy, having enjoyed the experience enough to want to do it again. This sounds like an easy goal, but most people don't realize how tough a mission this is to accomplish until they're staring down 20-milers or, like

Githens, until they reach the halfway point of the race. Just covering the distance is a key goal—especially for those attempting a new distance and veterans coming back from a layoff. Even if you finish far off your PR (personal record), you still accomplished this huge thing of covering 13.1 or 26.2 miles, and that's something to feel good about.

Make it personal. Most runners say they're not competitive and are only trying to beat their previous times. But the temptation to compare ourselves to others is intense. We're conditioned to do it when it comes to grades, appearances, and wealth. And in running, age-group rankings and finishing places only encourage that. Try to forget everyone else. How any one individual performs on any given race day depends on his or her training, level of fitness, injury history, biomechanics, genetics, psychological preparation, and the weather. In fact, the only common denominators between you and any

What it takes to . . .
Train for a marathon while undergoing cancer treatment

Jeremy Dobrick, 38, New York
Finance IT, and father of Kaylia Zoe, age 2
Experience: 2 marathons; 5:10 PR
Runner's World Challenge Race: 2010 Toronto Half-Marathon

I was diagnosed with lymphoma in late 2009. I know it is cliché, but once I started chemotherapy, I started taking my doctor's admonitions to diet and exercise seriously. In my fourth week of chemotherapy, I started the 8-week Couch-to-5-K program. I think I covered just over 1 mile in 20 minutes of jogging and walking on the first day. By the time I started radiation, I was getting pretty serious and had signed up for my first half-marathon—the GoodLife Fitness Toronto Half-Marathon.

I was lucky: My cancer was caught early, and the prognosis was positive. Still, it was hard to deal with the fact that there are no guarantees. I didn't know what was going to happen. I knew I wanted to be around to see my daughter grow up. Treatments were somewhat depressing. Going for chemotherapy once a week, knowing I was going to feel lousy, and getting on a train at 6:00 a.m. to get to the hospital for radiation every day would wear me out. Cancer can be rough, but that doesn't mean you are powerless and that whatever the fates have written is what will come to pass. For me, one of the best ways to fight the battle was to get out and run.

other runner are the distance you have to cover on race day and the conditions you're running in. "Comparing yourself to others can really cause undue stress, plus it's a waste of time," Brown says. "Don't give up control over your experience by defining 'success' in terms of factors that aren't relevant to your personal life. Your goal should be a very personal thing between you and the road."

Make it flexible. Ten or 16 weeks is a long time to train, and a lot of life happens in that time. Don't be afraid to change your goals if you miss big chunks of training or if, say, it's 90 degrees on race day. Go into the race with three acceptable outcomes, says Brown. One might be, "At least I finished." Another might be, "A pretty good time." And another might be, "Wow, a PR!" If you're particularly anxious, don't tell people your goal times, as it will only amplify the stress if you don't make them.

Make training goals. You don't have to

I was often tired, but I would run and be energized. I was depressed sometimes, but I would run and have time to think about the future and what I had to live for. Of course there were days when I didn't want to run, but getting out to run anyways was such a powerful motivator and gave me a way to measure progress beyond just how many weeks of radiation I had left. There were also many great mornings when I would feel like I could run forever and that I was part of an amazing world.

Getting out to run is not physically as hard as you might think. A lot of success is mental. It is the mental benefit that running provides that will carry you through the tough days. We all are capable of more than we think. My wife, Tamara, who has finished 30 marathons, always helped me to understand the importance of having the right mind-set. She made me feel good every time I would come home to announce my most recent triumph—regardless of how small it was.

One day I had an appointment with an oncologist who has an office near the park. I wore my running clothes to see him, and I went for a run afterward. It was raining pretty hard, but I ran anyway. When I told my wife I had run in the rain, she replied, "That's what I would have done. You won't melt." That's when I really felt like a runner. And it felt great.

How Fast Can You Go?

You can use the finishing time of shorter races to predict your pace for a longer distance.

5-K	10-K	HALF-MARATHON	MARATHON
17:13	35:54	1:19	2:45
17:44	36:59	1:21	2:50
18:16	38:04	1:24	2:55
18:47	39:10	1:26	3:00
19:18	40:15	1:28	3:05
19:50	41:20	1:31	3:10
20:21	42:25	1:33	3:15
20:52	43:31	1:36	3:20
21:23	44:36	1:38	3:25
21:55	45:41	1:40	3:30
22:26	46:46	1:43	3:35
22:57	47:52	1:45	3:40
23:29	48:57	1:48	3:45
24:31	51:08	1:52	3:55
25:03	52:13	1:55	4:00
26:05	54:23	2:00	4:10
26:37	55:29	2:02	4:15
27:39	57:39	2:07	4:25
28:10	58:44	2:09	4:30
29:13	1:01	2:14	4:40
29:44	1:02	2:16	4:45
30:47	1:04	2:21	4:55
31:18	1:05	2:24	5:00
32:32	1:07	2:28	5:10
32:52	1:08	2:31	5:15
33:55	1:10	2:35	5:25
34:26	1:11	2:38	5:30

Source: Runnersworld.com/trainingcalculator

wait for a finisher's medal to reap the rewards of your hard work. Set goals for training, like completing your long runs, finishing the plan, or making it to the track every Wednesday. Write down your goals in your training log, and note when you accomplish them. On days when workouts feel hard or you doubt that you can go the full race distance, having this list of all that you've accomplished so far will be evidence that *yes you can.*

Set performance goals. You can't PR every time you race, and once you've completed a certain distance, you know that you can finish. That's where having goals that are not tied to a finishing time comes in. These targets reflect the effort you put in to do your best given the circumstances. Make sure your performance goals are measurable, so you can tell if you've accomplished them, says Brown. An injury-prone runner might aim to get to the starting line healthy; a newer runner might try to run the hills instead of walking them.

Set realistic time targets. You may be aiming for your personal record or the fastest you've run in years, but these targets require consistent training, ideal race-day conditions, and perfect health.

To set an achievable time target, plug the results of your shorter races into a pace calculator (like the one at runnersworld.com /trainingcalculator). This can give you an idea of a realistic finish for your goal race based on your current fitness level. Use the calculator as a guide, but don't treat it as gospel. Realize that the calculator isn't computing your level of stress, your time to train, your injury history, or a snowstorm that blows in halfway through training. Each of these factors can have a big impact on how well you perform in your training and on race day.

What to Wear

The great thing about running is that it doesn't require any fancy equipment. But if you've ever run in a cotton T-shirt on a hot summer day, you know what a difference good gear can make. The money you invest in a few bare essentials to keep you comfortable and injury free will pay off for hundreds of happy miles.

— [WHAT WORKS]

Retail therapy

Mary-Pat Cormier, 40; Boston attorney, mother of four; 2 marathons; 3:59 PR

Researching, shopping for, and buying a new pair of shoes can be a powerful motivator. (Not to mention *fun*.) Once you spend $90 to $140, you'll want to wear them so that you squeeze every moment of utility out of them. Ask for a new piece of gear at least once a year. This Christmas, my mother-in-law gave me a North Face running jacket that I would have never had the guts to buy for myself. I love it. Even though we have had a month of absurd weather, I have run outside every weekend without fail—all so that I can wear my jacket.

Shoes

You don't absolutely need a new pair of running shoes, but getting the right pair will help prevent injuries. Shoes should be replaced every 300 to 500 miles. If you're heavier, or if you're a heel striker, you may need to replace them sooner. It's best to go to a specialty running shop (to find one, go to runnersworld.com /storefinder), where a salesperson can evaluate your gait and help you select a pair that offers your feet the support they need. It may feel like a lot to spend $90 to $140 on a pair of running shoes, but it costs less than visits to the doctor or time off of work because you got injured. Be sure to check out the *Runner's World* Shoe Finder to help you identify the right pair for you (runnersworld.com/shoeadvisor).

Here are some more shoe-shopping tips.

• **Size yourself up.** Be sure to get your feet measured each time you buy new shoes. Your feet change over time, and one model's fit can be drastically different from another's. You might also want to have your foot measured late in the day, when it's at its biggest. Many people end up getting a running shoe that's a half size larger than their street shoes. The extra room allows your foot to flex and your toes to

Make It Last

If you're going to invest money in high-quality running apparel, you want it to last for the long haul. Here are some tips to make sure it does.[2]

Use small loads and cold water. Wash technical T-shirts and shorts in cold water in small loads, and let everything air-dry. With most shirts, the wicking properties are a part of the fabric's construction and won't wash out. You don't need to separate your darks and brights—just toss everything in the washer and set it to cold. Don't fill the washer to the top, because small loads give your clothes more water to swish around in, which gets them cleaner.

Get the stink out. Washing your running duds with a sport wash such as Basewash by Nikwax, Granger's G-Wash Cleaner, or Penguin Sport-Wash can often get the stink out and restore your clothes to a more tolerable scent.

Slow dry your shirts. The synthetic fabrics used in technical tees are engineered to air-dry, with channels woven into them to draw sweat off your skin to the outer surface of the fabric, where it evaporates. If you want your shirts to last a long time, don't put them through the dryer, as the extra heat can bake odors into the fabric. And stay away from fabric softener; it can leave a coating that blocks your shirt's ability to wick away sweat.

Give 'em some breathing room. If you can't wash your shorts or skirts right away, don't wad them up—wait until they dry out a bit before tossing them into the hamper. Synthetic

move forward with each stride. When you're standing with both shoes on, make sure you have at least a thumbnail's space between the tip of the shoe and the end of your longest toe. Try shoes on both feet and take them for a test run around the shop, on a treadmill, or on the sidewalk.

• **Bring what you've been wearing.** When you go shopping, take along the shoes, socks, and any orthotics that you've been using. That way you can make a realistic evaluation of how well the new shoe will fit your feet.

• **Rotate your shoes.** Just like runners, shoes need to recover after a run; ideally, they should rest for about 24 hours. Though the loss of cushioning is extremely slight, if you run one evening and then the next day at noon, your shoes will not give you as much protection as shoes that have had a full day's rest. Because life is complicated enough without having to worry about whether or not your shoes are fully recovered, you might consider rotating in another pair. That way your shoes will always be ready when you are.

• **Break them in.** When you get a new pair of shoes, take them for a few short,

apparel loses its ability to breathe and wick moisture as dirt, oils, and bacteria from your sweaty skin permeate the materials. Since a sweaty shirt is a breeding ground for odor-causing bacteria, washing it immediately in cold water or spreading it out to dry stops the microbes from settling in.

Give your bra a break. By resting your bra for at least 24 hours between runs, you'll give the materials time to regain their original shape between washings.

Don't soften your wool. Unlike your old wool sweater, the Merino wool in socks can be tossed in with whatever load you're washing and go through the dryer without a thought about shrinkage. These socks can also sit in your bag for a few days postrun because wool doesn't hold on to bacteria or pick up odors like synthetic fabrics do. However, you shouldn't use liquid fabric softeners in the wash because they will coat the wool and make it less able to manage odor and moisture. And steer clear of dryer sheets for the same reason.

Keep your shoes out of the washer. With most traditional shoes, a trip through the washing machine will remove the shoe's bounce along with its dirt. That's because submersing the midsole in water for an extended period can break down the cell walls of the cushioning foam and firm up the sole.

easy test runs to make sure that the fit is good before you wear them to the track or on a long run. If the fit is slightly off and causes a blister or pain, you can easily head home and make a change. Make sure to do at least 8 to 10 runs or at least 20 miles in any new pair before race day.

• **Don't make any sudden switches.** In recent years, minimalist shoes have become wildly popular. Proponents say that the shoes can help runners strengthen their feet so that they can move in healthy ways. Others say that they lead to injuries. There's only one thing we know for sure: It's best not to make a quick switch. That could lead to a change in your biomechanics, and that can mean injuries. If you're going to make a change, ease into it. Wear your new shoes around the house or while you're out on a short jog before taking them on longer runs. Stick with your old shoes for long runs until you're used to training in the new pair.

Apparel and Gear

You don't have to break the bank on a closet full of new running outfits, but you won't regret what you spend on technical socks, shirts, pants, and shorts, all of which wick sweat away from your skin. They're lightweight, soft, and nonchafing. In the summer, they help you stay cooler. In the winter, you'll be warmer. They will make a huge difference in the quality of your running life. These are the basics any newbie needs.

INSIDE RUNNER'S WORLD®

BRIAN SABIN, 32, *RUNNER'S WORLD* SENIOR MULTIMEDIA EDITOR, BETHLEHEM, PA

LESSON LEARNED: RUNNING SHORTS ARE AMAZING.

Running + boxers and basketball shorts = pain. Like, fear-for-your-future-generations pain.

I was doing a 6-mile run on a treadmill at Rodale's Energy Center. The jarring was awful. And the chafing? Unbearable. Both set in slowly, starting with the feeling that something was slightly off. The sensation grew as the miles ran on, until my thighs were streaked with raw, red lines. I stepped off the treadmill slowly. That's when Rodale's senior director of employee fitness and health, Budd Coates, spotted me. He introduced me to the product that would save my life (and the lives of my potential children): running shorts with liners. The type of shorts I'd derided for so long. They spare you from chafing and red marks. And they have liners that keep those oh-so-important body parts from jostling around. I've been a short-shorts runner ever since.

Technical shirts and shorts. More style-conscious runners don't have to choose function over fashion. Clothing makers now provide running gear for women—and men—that performs well athletically and looks good, too.

Socks. Pick fabrics that are nylon, wool, Lycra, and Coolmax.

Hat. For the summer, get a hat that will keep the sun out of your eyes; a visor will keep you cooler than a hat on ultrahot days. For the winter, get a warm hat that covers your ears for cold and windy days.

Underwear. Stay away from cotton underwear; it absorbs a ton of sweat, which can trap cold and lead to uncomfortable chafing. If you're wearing shorts, it's okay to rely on the liner and go underwear-free—it's a matter of personal preference. If your shorts or pants don't have a liner, wool or synthetic underwear will offer the insulation and support you need.

Jog bra. Every female runner needs the right jog bra—one that fits well, offers adequate support, and wicks away sweat to minimize chafing. Your best bet is to try on a variety of different brands and styles to find the perfect bra for you.

Reflective gear. At some point during training, you're bound to run in the early morning before the sun comes up or in the evening after it goes down. It's important to wear gear that ensures that you can see and be seen. Your best bet is a handheld light or a headlamp. Drivers will see the light, but they'll also sense the movement and figure out that you're a runner. At the very least, wear a reflective vest or a blinking red light with a bright LED. (See "Vision Quest" on page 137.)

A watch. At first all you'll need to know is how long you've been running. Any watch with a timer will do. As you progress, you might invest in a heart rate monitor or a GPS watch, which can give you feedback on how fast and how far you're going, what your pace is, and what your heart rate is. There are dozens of gadgets out there that range from the simple to the elaborate. Some of these devices can help you track calorie burn, while others have foot pods that measure distance and cadence, which can improve your efficiency and form.

Some runners and coaches say that these devices are critical to training success; others log plenty of fast times without them. There certainly are some benefits for newbies and advanced runners alike: These devices provide feedback on how hard you're working, which can help you keep from training too hard on an easy day (which can lead to injury) or taking it too easy on a hard day (which can keep you from reaching your goal). These valuable insights can help you make breakthroughs or avoid making the same mistake over and over.

And the stats can provide motivation, too. Seeing the miles pile up on a 20-miler can keep you going when you're tempted to stop. Having a device that keeps track of your mileage frees you to run in unexplored territory, instead of sticking to the same old route. Many devices allow you to upload the data to a training log (like the one at runnersworld.com/personaltrainer) so you can track your progress over time and spot trends. Early on, for instance, a 12-minute pace might put you at 170 beats per minute. Later on in training, the same speed might let you run at 160 beats per minute, which would reveal that you have gotten fitter because you can maintain the same pace with less effort. Some say that these devices are ideal for beginners, who tend to run too hard, too soon, and get discouraged or injured.

Enduring Questions

Are marathons dangerous?

The last few years have been tough for those of us who believe that running makes us healthier. In 2007, 28-year-old Ryan Shay died while competing in the USA Men's Olympic Marathon Trials in Central Park. He was the first world-class marathoner to die from a heart attack while competing. And of course there is the classic story of Jim Fixx, whose bestselling *The Complete Book of Running*, which started the running boom in 1977, died of a heart attack in 1984 at age 52.

These stories often get more attention than those of the race winners. And they always raise the question: If running is so healthy, why do runners keep dropping dead?

Research has shown that the fittest people have heart disease death rates that are 30 to 50 percent lower than those of the least fit. They're also much less likely to have strokes or to develop diabetes, high blood pressure, and cancer, and they're at lower risk for diseases like Alzheimer's.

Notwithstanding all of the studies, there are no guarantees. Heart attack rates climb with age. Exercise is recommended, but it isn't a cure. In studies of more than 4.5 million marathoners over the last 30 years, 41 runners died of heart attacks—a rate of one in every 110,476 marathoners.

Dr. Paul Thompson, director of cardiology at Hartford Hospital in Connecticut, says that the runners who die when they're under 30 or 35 generally have structural defects in their hearts. When an over-35 exerciser dies on the run, the cause is almost always artery disease—that is, cholesterol deposits that rupture and provoke a heart attack.

Ultimately, an autopsy showed that Jim Fixx had significant blockage in all three coronary arteries. His heart muscle, strengthened by running, had probably extended his life by 8 to 10 years. (Before beginning to run, Fixx smoked and weighed over 200 pounds. His own father had suffered a heart attack at 37 and had died at 41.)

Running offers no sure protection from heart disease. "Exercise is not a savior," Thompson says. "The risks are very low, the benefits are real, and the benefits outweigh the risks. But there are no guarantees. If you want to live a long, vigorous life, you should do an hour of moderate exercise a day. "If your only goal is to survive the next hour of your life, you should get into bed."[3]

When in Doubt, Check It Out

The warning signals for a heart attack aren't always the classic chest tightness or pain down your left arm. You may feel:

- Pain in your right arm

- Indigestion

- A persistent sense of discomfort or breathlessness

- Fatigue beyond what's usual for the same level of activity

How much room for improvement do I have?

As nice as it would be to answer this question with a tidy little number, scientists haven't come up with a proven formula that applies to all people, all of the time. They do know a lot of different factors play roles in how much room for improvement all runners have.

Barring injuries and burnout, you are most likely to see the biggest gains in the first few years of training. If you train well and get a nice cool race day, you could set a 30- to 40-minute PR between your first few races. If you've never exercised regularly before, you could make even bigger gains.

"After genetics, the biggest factor is where your starting point is," says Jonathan Dugas, an exercise physiologist and coauthor of the popular *Science of Sport* blog. As you gain experience and endurance and you adapt to the specific demands of marathon training, you'll continue to see gains, although they might not be as big as they were at first. "Eventually, though, you'll approach your individual potential and hit a plateau."

But how many races do you have to run before you hit that plateau? It's different for each individual. The following factors each play a role in how much you'll be able to improve over time.

Level of fitness. When you start exercising on a regular basis, your body adapts in many ways that allow you to run faster with less effort. With regular aerobic exercise, your heart will get stronger, so it won't have to work as hard to get blood to the organs that need it. You will see this by a lower heart rate at the same running speed. Adding speedwork and race-pace runs to prepare your body for the specific demands of the marathon or half-marathon will help you run more comfortably at a faster pace for a longer distance.

Experience. As you run more and improve your biomechanics, you'll develop better running economy, so you can sustain the same pace with less energy. Plus, each time you step onto the road, you'll learn valuable lessons about what works best for you. You'll figure out which foods and drinks give you the most energy without upsetting your stomach and which clothes and shoes give you support without leaving you with blisters and chafing. Most important, you'll also learn how to pace yourself and keep yourself from going out too fast, thereby preventing a miserable last few miles of the race.

→RW CHALLENGER PROFILE:
Leslie Heywood, on becoming a real runner

Leslie Heywood's running career got off to a fast start. She won two state track titles in high school and even earned a scholarship to the University of Arizona. So when she started running again at the age of 45, she savored the feeling.

"It was like awakening," says Heywood, a mother of two and a professor at the University of Binghamton, New York. "My ear turned toward the familiar strains of some long-buried song."

She started with a 6-mile hilly loop 1 day a week, then added track work—ladders of 200s, 400s, and 800s. In early November of 2009, she signed up for the Lake Placid Marathon and set her sights on a sub-four finish.

"I ran all those years," she says. "I reasoned, 'How hard can it be?'"

She followed the *Runner's World* Challenge Intermediate Training Plan, always sneaking in some extra miles at the ends of long runs and some extra track meets midweek, ignoring urgings to focus on getting to the starting line injury free. Hard as she tried, she couldn't avoid comparing her current times to the times she logged when she was 18.

"I tend to feel like everything I do is pathetic because I was so much faster then," she says.

The training went smoothly until Monster Month arrived. That's when her body rebelled. Her hamstrings were so tight that she couldn't sit. She had chondromalacia in her left knee and the beginnings of it in her right. She was irritable, moody, and constantly exhausted. Her knee would crack like a gunshot every time she tried to straighten it. Stairs were out of the question, and she had to lower herself to the toilet slowly squatting on one leg, with her left leg

Aging. At some point, particularly after age 40, the forces of aging begin to kick in. Your aerobic capacity diminishes as your max heart rate declines by about one beat per year. Bone density starts to decrease, so you become more susceptible to stress fractures and other injuries. Muscle fibers shrink and the neurons supplying the muscles begin to die off, particularly after age 60. This affects the fast-twitch fibers first, which is why speed fades before endurance.

Your glycogen stores shrink and blood flow to your muscles is reduced. There's a decline in testosterone and growth hormone, which means that injured muscles don't repair themselves as quickly as they did before and you don't bounce back as quickly as you did when you were younger. It is not all doom and gloom, however, because maintaining your training with both regular resistance and cardiovascular exercise will slow the rate at which these things occur. We can't

extended. She had physical therapy three times a week.

Throughout training, she was haunted by a deep sense of shame, thinking of her 9-minute miles the way she and her teammates had when they were younger.

"Try as I might, I was no longer a real runner," she says. "I was old, I was slow, I was pathetic." She ran the Lake Placid in a knee brace, in pain the whole way. Most folks would have been pleased with a 4:13 for a first finish, but for Leslie, it was the final embarrassment. Exhausted, depleted, dragging her leg so stiffly behind her that it looked like it was set on a splint, it took her a full 2 months to recover.

She'd signed up for the Mount Lemmon Marathon, which bills itself as the toughest road marathon in the world. With 6,000 feet of ascent, the entire event is uphill.

This time, she knew she couldn't do the mileage the training plan asked for, and so she began to cross-train. She did core workouts, hillwork, and Yasso 800s, and she incorporated Ashtanga yoga, CrossFit, and some long bike rides. Because she was challenging her body in different ways, she was able to complete her long runs without pain. Her hamstrings were happy and her breathing was strong.

But the best part was that she gained valuable perspective.

"I am not 17 anymore," she says. "What I was and what I am are as different as frost and fire." She finished the marathon in 6 hours, sixth in her age group. She was tired, but pain free.

"Some may say that running that slowly, even uphill, isn't really running," she says. "But this time, I've learned I'm real."

reverse aging, but we can slow it down.

Genetics. The physiology you're born with determines how well you'll perform and how much room for improvement you have. All runners are limited, to a large extent, by the physiological characteristics that they inherit. With speed training, long runs, tempo work, and a little luck, however, you can make the most of whatever you were born with. "Everyone has their own personal ceiling on how well they can adapt

to training," says Dugas, "and trying to reach that potential is part of what makes running year after year so enjoyable and challenging."

I've had PRs when I was young, but now I'm older and can't train as much. How do I deal with finishing slower than I have in the past?

A lot of people start running when they're

young, single, and have few commitments, and they forget to adjust their expectations as their bodies and lifestyles change, says Brown. But the joy and contentment that come with a PR can also be found beyond the numbers on a clock. Don't give up control over your experience by defining "success" in terms of factors that aren't relevant to your personal life. Make a list of the reasons why you run. Maybe you enjoy the socializing time you get with your buddies, the meditative alone time, or the exhilaration that comes from pushing your body. Return to these reasons often, and do what you need to do to keep the training enjoyable: run with friends, explore new trails in your area, mentor a rookie to a first-marathon finish, or raise money for a charity. A marathon or half-marathon happens on one day; the journey to the starting line lasts for months.

How do I know whether my goal is realistic? I don't want to be disappointed, but I don't want to stop myself short of what I could accomplish.

If your goals are too easy or too difficult, it will be tempting to quit without giving it an honest effort. Your aims should be objective and measurable. If you're a first-timer, just focus on finishing. Don't base your goals on how your co-workers did in their first marathons. Just complete the training that's right for your fitness level, get to the starting line healthy, and focus on having a good race experience. Whatever your finishing time is, it's a personal best. If you're more experienced, set goals that are in line with your current level of fitness, and as you train for them, listen to your body for signs of

whether that goal is still realistic. If your workouts leave you tired, emotionally drained, fatigued, or injured, maybe your goals need a little readjustment. If you're feeling challenged but exhilarated and healthy, you're probably right on track.

I love the training, but I have a hard time getting motivated to get out the door. How can I get moving?

First, know that every runner goes through this, even elites. After days and days of running, training can feel like a grind. Get over the prerun dread by keeping reminders all around of why you do this—inspiring quotes, as well as race medals, numbers, and photos. Keep a training log, and total your lifetime mileage. Once you see that you've logged hundreds of miles, 5 more on a cold morning will seem like chump change. Refresh your runs by trying a new trail or a new route. Get a training watch or a GPS tracker, and make it a rule that you'll run on a new route every single week. Buy a new music player or download a new podcast. You'll be surprised by how that adds a whole new dimension to your runs. Or make a date with a friend; you won't want to stand him or her up early in the morning. And even if your friend can't run at your pace or your distance, a plan to link up for a few miles will be enough to get you out the door.

I'm not a beginner but I'm not intermediate, either. What kind of plan do I choose?

You can probably handle a tougher-than-you-anticipated program as long as you adjust your training pace. In other words, slow down. Don't push to hit a dictated speed in your workouts just because your plan says you should. Instead, learn to relax and run truly easy. We runners tend to be very tough on ourselves. For many workouts, however, it's the doing of them that's more important than the pace. This is particularly true for marathon training. After all, it's a 26.2-mile race. So the most important thing you can do is to log slow distance. Notice how much easier the running is; you can probably cover a lot more miles. And in the long run, this will pay dividends toward your marathon and your health.

CHAPTER 2

TRAINING BASICS

We hear from a lot of runners who decide to run a marathon or half-marathon and just go out and run as much as they can, as far as they can, and as fast as they can. You do have to push beyond your limits when you're preparing to run long distances, but there are time-tested methods of doing so that have worked for thousands of coaches and millions of runners—and that don't involve pain and anguish.

That's where a training plan comes in. Though there are an infinite number of marathon and half-marathon training programs, they all follow certain basic principles that have been proven to help a runner develop the endurance required to run 13.1 or 26.2 miles without getting injured. These programs systematically ramp up mileage and intensity so you gradually push yourself faster and farther than you've gone before. They follow hard efforts with rest days to stave off injury and burnout. There is as much payoff for your mind as there is for your body. Two to 4 months is a long time to train; the practice you get in training will help you develop the mental grit and the emotional toughness to gut it out on race day. You'll be much more confident stepping to the starting line knowing that you have gotten through 20-mile-long runs, speed sessions, and many, many days when you would have preferred to sleep in.

In this chapter you'll learn all about the fundamentals of preparation and why most training schedules—including those offered by *Runner's World*—are designed the way they are. If you're just starting out, understanding these principles will help you stick

20 percent of runners say they just winged it while training for their first marathon, according to a survey on runnersworld.com.

to your plan. If you're a seasoned runner, it's worth your time to brush up on these basics. They may help you break through performance barriers or overcome training frustrations. Follow these rules of the road, and you'll maximize your chances of reaching your goals and getting to the starting line fresh and ready to run your best.

Start slow and build gradually. The prospect of covering the race distance can be daunting, even for those who've done it before. Luckily, you don't have to do it all at once. Please don't try. The body needs time to adapt to training changes and jumps in mileage or intensity. Muscles and joints need recovery time so they can handle more training demands. If you rush that process, you could break down your body rather than building it up. Coaches have found that the best way to avoid injury is to follow the 10 percent rule: Increase your weekly mileage and the length of your long run by no more than 10 percent each week. It keeps you from getting injured, but it also makes the added mileage more manageable. Before you start training, the idea of running 13 miles might be intimidating. But after you've built up to it and run 10 miles the week before, the prospect of running just 3 more miles is not nearly as frightening. Stick to the plan as much as possible to stay injury free. If you do want to add miles, do it on an easy day, and don't add more than 1 to 2 miles at a time.

Run easy most of the time. About 80 percent of your runs are going to be done at an easy pace that's about 60 to 90 seconds slower than your goal race pace. The pace should feel comfortable enough for you to hold a conversation while you run. If you're using a heart-rate monitor, you want to be at 65 to 70 percent of your maximum heart rate. If you're huffing and puffing, you're going too fast. These miles strengthen muscles, build endurance, burn fat, and build blood volume. But the biggest benefit is that they allow you to get the most practice running without getting injured. After about 6 weeks of training, you may find that you're able to run the same pace and the same distance without as much effort. But try to run those same miles too fast, and you'll start to feel achy in your knees, shins, and feet. That's because your heart and lungs adapt and get stronger more quickly than your muscles, tendons, and bones do. Spend time running at an easy pace, and you'll give your musculoskeletal system a chance to get stronger and catch up with the cardiovascular gains you've already made.

Alternate between hard and easy efforts. Most training programs alternate between hard and easy efforts. In each week of training, you'll have a hard workout (like a speed session or a long run) followed by a rest day or an easy run. Similarly, every few weeks you'll cut back your mileage so you have time

What it takes to . . .
Lose 60 pounds and qualify for Boston in your first race

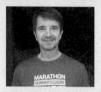

Michael Feldhaus, 47, Arlington, Virginia
Healthcare consultant, father of two
Experience: 2 marathons; 3:25 PR
Runner's World **Challenge Race: 2009 Richmond Marathon**

I had never run a step in my life before signing up for the Challenge. I had no idea what a PR or a split was. But I did know that I was carrying 215 pounds on my 6'1"frame. So I started walking and gradually building up to 3 miles a week. A friend had just given me a copy of *Runner's World,* and I saw the article about training for a marathon. I thought, "Why not?" I stuck to the plan religiously. There would be moments when I'd start to think I couldn't do it anymore, but then I would push myself a little further and find out, "Hey, wait a minute, I can do this!" By the time I finished the training plan, I'd lost 60 pounds. Old friends didn't recognize me; new people I met couldn't believe I'd ever been so heavy. I just wanted to finish the Richmond Marathon without hurting myself. I finished in 3:29. I didn't think it was that good, but then someone told me that I'd qualified for the Boston Marathon. I didn't know anything about qualifying for Boston. But when I ran it the next spring, I cut 3 minutes off my time and qualified for the next year, too. It was just an amazing sensation for me, at the age of 47, to realize that I could do this without any pain. I finally found this thing that I'm really good at.

to recover. Why is that? During the recovery periods that follow hard workouts, your body rebuilds and repairs the muscle tissue that's been damaged and broken down during the harder workouts. Through that rebuilding process, your body gets stronger and more resistant to fatigue at faster paces and longer distances. If you don't push your body far enough or fast enough, you'll never develop the ability to run farther or faster without tiring. If you overload your body too much or you don't rest enough, you'll get injured.

Run long every week. The long run is the cornerstone of marathon and half-marathon training. It helps you build endurance, get used to spending time on your feet, and practice the eating, drinking, gear, and bathroom logistics you'll need to get straightened out for race day. You'll also get emotionally and mentally prepared to spend hours at a time running, just as you'll have to do when you go 13.1 or 26.2. Beginners should take long runs at an easy pace and just focus on covering the distance feeling strong. These runs will help you get in the miles you need to prepare for the race without getting injured. If you're shooting for a PR, you can try other variations. Fast-finish long runs involve inserting a few miles at your goal race pace during the last 3 to 5 miles of a run. This helps you practice digging deep when you're most fatigued. Schedule one long run each week, on the day when you have the most time to get it done. Choose a time when you won't feel hampered or rushed to finish, and make sure you'll have plenty of time afterward to refuel, stretch, ice, and nap.

Hit the hills. During the first half of your training, you should include one day of running on the hilliest route you can find. Hills build leg and lung power, which will give you the muscle and stamina you need to run faster later in the program. They'll also help prepare you for hills you might face in the

Test Yourself

How "easy" should your easy runs be? How fast should you do your long runs? Whether you're a rookie or a seasoned runner, you have to assess your current level of fitness.

Do a time trial. A simple 1-mile time trial can give you a benchmark to determine which pace is appropriate for each daily run. Go to a track and jog an easy lap or two for a warmup. Walk for 3 to 4 minutes, then time yourself running four laps, which is about 1 mile. Record your time. By running on a track—which is flat and provides the most accurate measurement of distance—you'll get a solid indication of your top speed. Plug your "1-mile" time into the training calculator at runnersworld.com/trainingcalculator to get your training paces. Repeat the time trial every 2 weeks or so; try to beat your previous time and track your progress.

Do a tune-up. If you've been training for a while, race a 10-K, half-marathon, or a 10-miler and plug your time into a training calculator like the one you can find at runnersworld.com /trainingcalculator to determine the appropriate training paces for your race. Repeat that race at least 6 weeks before the marathon to determine how much you've improved.

Yasso 800s. Yasso 800s are renowned for helping gauge fitness and predict race performance. After a warmup, do 10 × 800 meters with a 400-meter recovery jog in between. You should be spent after the last repeat. The average of your 800 times is a good barometer of how fast you can run in a marathon—but in hours and minutes instead of minutes and seconds. (See "How the Yasso 800s Were Born" on page 40.) Plug that time into a training calculator to get your training paces.

BART SAYS...

More isn't always better. Don't be too quick to add miles to the plan, even if you can. Back in my younger days, I used to run 23 miles every weekend. I figured my body could handle it, but I paid for it later. In my 40s and 50s, I started getting aches and pains even after I didn't run that much. Trust me. Whatever miles you don't do this week, you'll be able to run 30 years from now.

race. You won't feel fast going up hills, but you'll feel strong. Even a small amount of hillwork can help you build leg strength, aerobic capacity, and running economy (how efficiently your body uses oxygen). Running up an incline places the same demand on your muscles as weight training—your glutes, quads, hamstrings, and calves have to lift you up the slope. And just as with plyometrics (jump drills), the "explosive" action of uphill sprints improves elasticity in your muscles and tendons, which allows you to quickly spring into action after landing, which is helpful no matter what kind of terrain you're negotiating. If you're a beginner, ease into it. Hills do put extra stress on muscles, knees, and Achilles tendons that may not be ready to handle the load. Here are some rules for hitting the hills.

• **Get some variety.** Incorporate a variety of steep short and long gradual inclines into your training. On the short, steep climbs,

you'll feel a quick cardiovascular boost. On the long, gradual inclines, you'll get more endurance training. Any incline will recruit different muscles than running on flat stretches will.

• **Mimic the course.** This is especially important on long runs, which are dress rehearsals for race day. Look at the course elevation map for the race, and plan your long runs so that they incorporate climbs at the same points that you'll face them during the race.

• **Don't neglect the downhills.** As fun as it can be to fly down a hill with the help of gravity's pull, if you've ever run a downhill race, you know that steep descents can zap the power you need to take on flat stretches and uphill climbs and leave your quads feeling trashed for days afterward. Running downhill requires the muscles to lengthen, or make eccentric muscle contractions. These contractions can cause microscopic tears in the muscle fibers and generate more force than when you're running uphill or on flat ground. To make matters worse, it's easy to hit top speed on a steep descent—and the faster you move, the harder each foot strikes the ground and the more pounding your muscles endure. But by incorporating downhills into your training, you can weather them better and bounce back from them sooner. Start with a short, gradual slope with a 2- to 3-percent grade, and move on to steeper and longer descents as you get more

This Way Up (and Down)

Run relaxed and maintain proper form when you're climbing and making descents to build your leg and lung power.

GOING UP	GOING DOWN
• Keep your head and chest up	• Keep your torso upright
• Look straight ahead	• Look straight ahead
• Visualize the road rising to meet you	• Visualize "controlled falling"
• Keep your shoulders back	• Keep your nose over your toes
• Push up and off the hill, springing from your toes	• Step softly; don't let your feet slap the pavement
• Don't bend at the waist and hunch over	
• Keep your hands and fists loose	

comfortable. To prevent injury, start by running on a gentler surface, such as grass, before moving onto the roads.

• **Run an even effort, not an even pace.** Your pace will slow when you're running uphill, but try to maintain the same level of effort—the same breathing rate and leg turnover—as when you've been running on flat ground. Why? If you try to charge up the hill, you'll end up spending all your energy and be zapped by the time you get to the top. You want to have something left at the end because there are likely to be plenty more hills where the one you just climbed came from. When you're running downhill, resist the urge to fly down, tempting as it is. Just enjoy the fact that the same pace feels easier. Use it as a chance to catch your breath for whatever challenges are up ahead.

Run at tempo pace. Tempo runs teach your body to run faster before fatiguing. How? They help you raise your lactate threshold pace, the speed you're able to run at before lactic acid begins accumulating in your leg muscles more rapidly than they can recycle it into usable fuel. When this happens, your muscles begin to perform less efficiently. The higher you push your lactate threshold through appropriate training, the farther and faster you can run before tiring. Tempo pace is typically about 35 seconds faster than your goal marathon pace, or slightly faster than half-marathon pace. Tempo runs should last for 20 to 35 minutes, and your effort level should be "comfortably hard." How can something be comfortable and hard at the same time? If you're on a tempo run with a training partner, you're able to say a few words here and there, but you can't deliver a lengthy diatribe. If you want to try out the tempo run, here's how: Find your tempo pace by plugging your race goal into the training calculator at runnersworld.com/trainingcalculator. Warm up with 10 to 15 minutes of easy running, then run 2 miles at tempo pace, then cool down. Every 2 weeks, add ½ mile of running at tempo pace until you're running 4 miles at that pace. Treat the tempo run as a hard workout, and follow it with a day of rest or easy running.

Run at race pace. Throughout the *Runner's World* training plans, you'll find lots of runs designated as marathon pace (MP) and half-marathon pace (HMP). It's important to get as much practice as possible running your race pace during training. That way, on the day of your big event, your body will just be able to dial into it, and it will feel like your body's natural rhythm. The workouts are as good for the body as they are for the mind. Knowing that you've run dozens of

---

— [WHAT WORKS] ———————————————————

Follow a training plan

Todd Pollock, 42, Sellersville, PA; IT business analyst, father of two; 9 marathons; 3:19 PR; *Runner's World* Challenge Race: 2009 Philadelphia Marathon

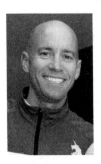

When I resolved to run my first marathon, I decided to wing it. I'd run track and cross-country in high school, and I'd finished the Philadelphia Half-Marathon in 1:39. So I Googled some suggested mileage, plugged the numbers into a spreadsheet, and hit the road. I figured, "It's running. It's simple. How hard could it be?" I bought the cheapest shoes I could find at Foot Locker and went out for 3- and 5-milers during the week. On weekends I'd run as far as 16 miles without any water, energy gel, or food. I couldn't figure out why I felt so tired. I thought I was just out of shape, and I just wasn't that good of a runner. Then one day my knee started hurting. I kept running, trying to stick it out, until my knee pain worsened and I couldn't run at all. Preparing on my own just got me an injury and a bib for a marathon I couldn't run. One year after my injury, I decided to take a second shot at a marathon, but this time I'd use a 16-week training plan from *Runner's World*. I followed it to the letter. I made it to the 2009 Philadelphia Marathon healthy, and I finished in 3:21. Five months later I went on to qualify for the Boston Marathon with a 3:19 finish at the Pocono Mountain Run for the Red Marathon. Training with a plan was a complete 180. I feel stronger and faster. I'm surprised at what I can do. I realized that if you have a solid training program and you listen to your body, there's no limit to how much you can excel.

miles at race pace will help you feel more confident when the starting gun goes off.

Run fast once a week. Even if you're not competitive, running faster once a week is a great way to improve your fitness and your race times. It will also build cardiovascular strength because your heart will be forced to pump harder to deliver oxygen to your leg muscles. Also, your leg muscles will get stronger and more efficient at extracting oxygen from your blood. And as your legs and feet turn over at a quicker rate, you'll shed sloppiness in your stride and run more efficiently. Speedwork also keeps your metabolism revved (and calories burning) even after your workout is over. And so with enough practice, this quicker stride becomes more natural, which means that it'll take less effort to move faster on any run. There's a mental benefit to speedwork, too: By running closer to maximum pace once a week, your race-pace and easy runs will feel truly "easy" by comparison. It's best to do speedwork on a track, which is flat and the distance is measured. But if you can't access a track, it's okay to do it on a flat stretch of road or a treadmill. Treadmills aren't ideal because the belt keeps you on pace even when your energy fades, but they do help you hit your target pace. If you're hitting the track for the first time, here are a few rules to help you get around:[1]

• **Stick with runners of the same fitness level.** If you start with faster runners and fall behind, you won't have time to recover before the next repeat.

• **Leave the headphones at home.** When you're in a large group of fatigued runners in a confined space trying to hit top speed, you'll want to tune in to what's going on around you.

• **Recover right.** When you finish fast bouts of running, walk or jog—don't stop abruptly or stand around. Gradually elevating and slowing your heart rate is healthier than suddenly hitting the brakes.

• **Clear lane one.** The innermost lane of the track is typically the place for the fastest runners. If you're warming up, cooling down, or running slower, move to an outside lane.

• **Lighten up.** You don't need track spikes, but it's a good idea to wear running shoes that weigh 10 ounces or less. Just knowing you've got your "fast shoes" on will give you a lift.

Taper. During the final weeks leading up to the marathon or half-marathon, drop your weekly mileage by 25 to 50 percent, but keep the intensity of the workouts high. The idea is to let your muscles recover from the buildup of mileage and intensity and adapt to the stresses of training so that you get to race day feeling fresh and ready to run your best. But don't put your feet up just yet. The idea is to rest, not rust. You're running fewer miles, but keep doing workouts like race-pace runs and speedwork.

Don't be surprised if you go a little nutty during the taper. Three weeks before a marathon and 2 weeks before a half-marathon, after all the buildup in training and all the anticipation about the race, most runners fret that they'll lose the fitness they worked so hard to build. As a result, many runners keep their mileage too high. Resist the urge to pile on the miles during the taper. Many runners tend to overcook themselves and end up reaching the starting line feeling mentally and physically fried. But trust the taper; research has proven that it works. A 2010 study[2] by researchers at Ball State University found that runners' race times improved when they dropped their weekly mileage by 25 percent 3 weeks before the race but kept running intervals and easy runs. They didn't lose any of their cardiovascular fitness, and they gained a lot of muscle strength.

Measure your effort. Training for a marathon or a half-marathon is all about running with purpose. Each workout has a goal—to build endurance, make you faster, or

— [WHAT WORKS]

Plan for the taper

Christine Orr, 36, Menlo Park, CA, mother of 2; 5 marathons: 3:29 PR; *Runner's World* Challenge Race: 2010 San Francisco Marathon

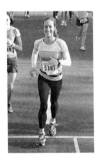

I'm very organized. I think you have to be in order to fit running into a busy schedule. So when I have no running on rest days—and no endorphins—I go batty. I plan ahead. Friday is usually an off day for me, so I plan adventures with my two young kids. I research the area for a new park, hike, or picnic. I try to stay outdoors as much as possible—it helps my mood and keeps me from coming unglued with pent-up energy. I try to stay active, just not running! We play soccer in the fields and walk the city. Not every day can be an adventure, so on those days I take the kids out for a bagel or to Starbucks during our normal running time. It's a way to fill the void, then get home and proceed as normal. The taper is particularly tough for me, since it is so many days of stillness. So I keep a list around the house of things that need to be done. When taper week comes, I attack. I do things like sort through all the clothes in the house for donation, steam the carpets, clean the garage, take the kids to their dental appointments, etc. On rainy days, we go to the local recreation center and play there. They have open swim, and I'm able to hop in with the kids.

help you recover. It's important to measure your effort while you're training to make sure that you're working out at the right intensity and you're reaping the benefit. Go too hard on the easy runs, and you won't have the energy to take on the speed sessions and long runs. Go too slow on your hard runs, and you won't push your fitness to the next level. There are a variety of ways to gauge your effort; pace, heart rate, and the talk test have all been proven to be effective. Choose which measure you want to use, and stick with it. Use the chart on page 36 as a guide.

• **Pace.** When you're doing speedwork on a measured stretch of road or a track, it's a good opportunity to let your watch do all the work and run strictly based on how many minutes it takes you to run each mile. At *Runner's World,* we like to discuss training paces relative to 5-K pace (simply because the 5-K is the most popular race distance around). If you don't know your 5-K pace, you can either go run a 5-K (check out runnersworld.com/racefinder to scout out an event near you) or do a 1-mile time trial and plug that time into a training calculator (like the one at runnersworld.com /trainingcalculator). Based on that pace, the calculator will tell you which paces to use for which workouts.

• **Heart rate.** Tracking your heart rate with a monitor (which reads your pulse via a sensor built into a chest strap) tells you precisely how hard—or easy—you're working. A heart rate monitor will track how many beats per minute your heart is taking so that you can make sure that you're working within a particular percentage of your maximum heart rate during every workout. For instance, you'll want to make sure that you're running within 65 to 70 percent of your maximum heart rate on easy days so that your body has a chance to recover from hard workouts. How do you find out your maximum heart rate? Most experts

INSIDE RUNNER'S WORLD®

CHRISTINE FENNESSY, *35, SENIOR EDITOR, EMMAUS, PA*

LESSON LEARNED: IF YOU'RE RUNNING A ROAD RACE, YOU HAVE TO TRAIN ON THE ROAD, AT LEAST SOMETIMES

I learned that in the last 4 miles of my first race, a half-marathon. Each step felt like it carved off a piece of my quads, hamstrings, and lower legs. I'd done virtually all of my training on a very forgiving, dirt bridle path. The whole time I thought, "Gee, I'm so smart, gradually ramping up my mileage, running on a soft surface, there's no way I'll get injured." And I was right. Training didn't hurt. But the race—with its 13.1 miles of tarmac—destroyed me. It ripped my trail-conditioned legs apart and it took far too long for them to recover.

Measure Your Effort

Here's a guide to using different methods to measure your effort during different kinds of workouts. Even when you're training for a marathon or a half-marathon, 5-K is a good reference pace because it's the most popular race distance. Also, keep in mind that it's best to use one variable to measure your effort—such as only pace or only heart rate—because trying to keep track of all of them at once might only confuse you.

TYPE OF RUN	PACE	HEART RATE	TALK TEST
EASY RUN	90–150 seconds/mile slower than 5-K pace	65–70% of max heart rate	Complete sentences
MARATHON-PACE RUN	45–100 seconds/mile slower than 5-K pace	88–92% of max heart rate	Short sentences
HALF-MARATHON-PACE RUN	25–50 seconds/mile slower than 5-K pace	92–94% of max heart rate	A few words at a time
SPEED WORK (800S, 1200S)	5–15 seconds/mile faster than 5-K pace	98–100% of max heart rate	Can't . . . talk . . . must . . . run . . .
TEMPO RUN	20–40 seconds/mile slower than 5-K pace	94–96% of max heart rate	A few words at a time
YASSO 800S*	See below	96–98% of max heart rate	A few words at a time
LONG RUN	90–150 seconds/mile slower than 5-K pace	65–70% of max heart rate	Complete sentences

*Yasso 800s are done at goal marathon pace in minutes and seconds. So if you're shooting for a 4-hour marathon, you'd aim to run each Yasso 800 in 4 minutes. If you want to finish a marathon in 3 hours and 30 minutes, you'd try to complete each Yasso 800 in 3 minutes and 30 seconds.

agree that a widely used formula—220 minus your age—may be inaccurate for many individuals. (That formula was derived from several different studies of men, some of whom were healthy, others of whom had coronary heart disease.) In 2010, researchers at Northwestern University found that a better formula for women ages 35 and older was 208 minus 88 percent of age.[3] A separate study[4] found that the best way to estimate maximum heart rate in healthy, active people is to do a 200-meter sprint time trial, and then repeat it a few days later. Take the highest heart rate you achieve in those trials as your maximum heart rate. If you want an exact number, says Martha Gulati, associate professor of medicine in the division of cardiology at the Ohio State University, go to an exercise physiologist and do a treadmill test. This test typically involves running on a treadmill while hooked up to machines that monitor your heart rate and blood pressure, as well as how much oxygen you're consuming. Every 3 minutes the treadmill gets faster and steeper, until you reach the maximum effort you can sustain. Your heart rate at that maximum effort is your max heart rate. That said, even with an accurate max heart rate, there are still going to be limitations when you're using it to guide how hard you're working out, Gulati cautions. If a heart-rate monitor accidentally gets wet, say from rain or sweat, it might stop sensing your heart rate. Other machines might also interfere with the signals. "These are electronic devices," says Gulati, "and they're not perfect." Also, certain other variables that have little to do with your level of fitness are going to impact your heart rate. If you're dehydrated, if it's a superhot day, or if you're in pain, your heart rate might skyrocket, even if you're running at a slower pace, she adds. Gulati, herself a marathoner and triathlete, goes by feel. "Heart rate can be a good guide, but it shouldn't be the only guide," she says. "Your body is always giving you signals about what you should do."

• **The talk test.** This is one of the most widely used methods of determining whether you're running at the appropriate level of effort. Informal as it sounds, research has shown that it's an accurate predictor of intensity. In recent studies where subjects were asked to recite the Pledge of Allegiance[5] while running on treadmills, those who could comfortably do so also had heart and breathing rates that were within their target aerobic zones. The converse was also true: Those who were huffing and puffing their way through the recitation were generally running too hard.

Cross-train. Running is hard on your body, no doubt about it. So it's easy for the muscles, joints, and connective tissues to wear down from all this shock absorption. Cross-training is a great way to maintain your cardiovascular fitness while giving your body a break from the pounding of running. Activities like yoga, Pilates, and strength training can help build muscle and promote recovery. Swimming, cycling, elliptical training, and rowing will burn a lot of calories and improve your aerobic fitness. They also help you develop a strong upper body, which can help you run faster with less effort and maintain good form in the late stages of a race, when you're fatigued. Unfortunately, running fitness doesn't directly translate to other activities that use your muscles and joints in different ways. Runners tend to have weak upper bodies, poor flexibility, and muscle imbalances, all of which can lead to injuries while cross-training. When you're starting any new form of cross-training, take the same careful approach you do on the roads: Start slowly, build gradually, and seek advice from athletes and coaches who know the sport well. When you're in group exercise classes, let the instructor know that you're a runner and what level of experience you have. If you start a strength-training regimen, buy a few sessions with a personal trainer to get into a good routine and make sure you maintain proper form.

Watch your form. When you're just starting to run, don't worry too much about your form; your body will naturally gravitate toward its most efficient way of running. You have natural biomechanics that are determined by your strength and flexibility and the structure of your body. That said, there are a few basics to running form that will help you run more comfortably.

• **Look ahead.** Keep your gaze straight in front of you, not down at your feet. This keeps your neck and head in proper alignment.

What it takes to . . .
Lose 100 pounds and become a marathoner

Belynda Warner, 39, Dallas, TX
Business owner, mother of two
Experience: 3 marathons; 6:53 PR; 14 Half-marathons; 2:07 half-marathon PR
Runner's World Challenge Race: 2010 San Francisco Half-Marathon

I vividly remember the turning point that turned me into a runner. We were on a family road trip, and I was chasing a fast-food meal with a king-size bag of M&M's and a giant Diet Coke, fretting about health problems related to my weight. I had been a standout sprinter in high school and still walked regularly, but two pregnancies and a sedentary lifestyle had left me 100 pounds overweight. I was desperately tired of feeling sick and tired. I realized that if I created the problem, I could also solve it. I joined Weight Watchers, started adding bouts of running to my walks, and started dropping weight. Running was the natural progression to keep the weight loss going. It was tough at first, and often painful, but the more I ran, the more I lost, and the better I felt, so I just kept going. In 2001, I walked my first marathon. I was 265 pounds. During my third marathon, I broke my ankle, but finished anyway. My running partner is my 17-year-old daughter, Tory. We finished eight half-marathons using a run/walk method, and I have dropped 100 pounds. I have learned a lot by running with her—patience, tolerance, when to slow down, when to press on, and when to shut up. It's fun to celebrate milestones with her and share the excitement of new bling each time we earn a medal.

• **Drop your shoulders.** Keep your shoulders low and loose, and don't let them creep up to your ears, especially when you start to feel fatigued. Tense shoulders steal energy you need to run. If you find yourself tensing up, shake out your hands and arms to release the tension.

• **Run tall.** Keep your back straight, at a 90-degree angle to the ground. Don't lean forward, except when you're running uphill, as this can lead to lower-back pain and can make you fatigue faster.

• **Swing your arms.** Hold your lower arms at about a 90-degree angle to your body, about level with your belly. Let your arms swing in rhythm with your legs. Make sure to swing them forward and back, not across your body.

• **Loosen your grip.** Keep your hands in unclenched fists, with your fingers lightly touching your palms. Imagine yourself trying to carry a piece of paper in each hand without crushing it. This will release the tension in your upper body.

• **Plant your feet.** Your foot should hit the ground lightly with each step—landing between your heel and midfoot—and then quickly roll forward. Keep your ankle flexed as your foot rolls forward to create more force for push-off. As you roll onto your toes, try to spring off the ground.

• **Maintain a short stride.** Your feet should land directly underneath your body. If your lower leg (below the knee) extends out in front of your body, you're overstriding, which can lead to injuries and slow you down. With a shorter stride, you'll land softer and with less impact. To shorten your stride, work on increasing your stride rate (how frequently you take each step). Check your watch for a minute, and count each time your foot strikes the ground. If the count is below 80 for each foot, practice shortening your stride. With practice, this will feel more natural.

Warm up and cool down. It's hard enough to get in your prescribed miles for the day, so it's tempting to skip the warmup and cooldown. But taking the time to ease in and out of a run can make the running feel easier and can help you avoid injury. A 5- to 10-minute warmup will gradually raise your heart and breathing rates, get blood flowing to your muscles, and get them prepared for the work ahead. Inserting strides at the end of the warmup wakes up your nervous system and gets the fast-twitch muscle fibers firing. Ending a run with a 10-minute cooldown of easy running allows your heart rate to fall gradually. Stop abruptly after a hard run and the blood can pool in your legs, making you feel faint.

The kind of warmup you do depends largely on what kind of workout you're doing that day. In general, the faster or farther you intend to go, the longer and more thoroughly you should warm up. For an easy run of, say, 4 miles, you might just walk for a few minutes to loosen up your muscles and joints, then start slowly jogging before gradually ramping up to your target pace. If you're sore or tired, it may take longer to get the kinks out.

If you're hitting the track, a longer warmup of 1 to 2 miles will make it easier to hit your target paces and avoid injury. You might also include some dynamic stretching in the form of drills, such as skipping and high knees, or by doing strides.

Enduring Questions

If I want to get faster, why do I have to run so slow in training?

Doesn't it make sense that in order to race fast, you have to train fast? Yes. But you need to build a solid aerobic base first. Run-

How the Yasso 800s Were Born

by Bart Yasso

It all began in 1981, when I was 25 and eying a 2:50 to qualify for Boston. Once a week, I'd hit the track and do this workout: I'd run 800 meters and jog 400 to recover, and I'd repeat the cycle 10 times. The plan worked, and I ran a 2:50 and qualified for Boston. So this became my standard speed workout for marathon training.

A few years later, I was reviewing some old logs and I noticed that the average time it took me to run 800 meters 10 times was equal to my marathon finishing time. If I ran each 800 meters in 2 minutes and 40 seconds, I'd run a 2:40 marathon. If I ran the 800s in 2:50, I'd run a 2:50 marathon. In 1993, while training for the Marine Corps Marathon, Amby asked me about my goals. I told him I was going to run a 2:47. "You're certain?" he asked. "Absolutely," I said, and explained my system. Amby looked over my running logs and eventually wrote about my system in the October 1994 issue of *Runner's World,* christening the workout the Yasso 800s. I have to say that I was terrified at first. I was afraid that it wouldn't work for anyone else and that people would blame me for ruining their marathon dreams. But the Yasso 800s became popular, and soon I couldn't go to any race without someone coming up to me and either thanking me for helping them reach their goals or letting me know that they were cursing my name during their track workouts. People write to me all the time and thank me for helping them, but I don't take the credit—they did all the work. I hear from people like Chris McKee, who used Yasso 800s to run a 3:20 to qualify for Boston. "Everyone has a milestone workout, and that was mine," McKee says. "Once I did

ning seems simple, but it is a learned activity and it takes practice. The more you practice running, the more proficient you become. You become more comfortable on the road and more efficient, so you can run faster with less effort. Running at an easy aerobic pace—say 70 percent of your max heart rate—allows you to get the most practice possible, without getting hurt.

"The primary reason for the easy run is to stay injury free," says exercise physiologist Stephen McGregor, PhD, of Eastern Michigan University. "It allows the body to recover from the harder, faster runs, and it keeps the body fresh for the next workout."

If you take your easy days too fast, you risk feeling too zapped to give your all to the quality workouts, where you're pushing your body to run faster and longer than you ever have before. Run too hard on the easy days, and you'll be tired for your speed sessions and long runs, and you'll miss the opportunity to take your fitness up a notch. And if you're running hard all the time, without giving your body an opportunity to recover, you run the risk of injury and burnout.

my 10 Yasso 800s, it was the moment when I believed that I might be able to pull this off. And indeed, I ran a 3:20 on the dot."

What's the magic behind the workout? Amby reasons that Yasso 800s offer a nice "meaty" workout. It feels challenging, but not like you're going to blow your lungs out. You're just sustaining this comfortably hard effort for a short distance. And since it's 50 seconds faster than marathon goal pace, by comparison, race pace should feel easy. It's also a really simple workout to do. There are no complex algorithms you have to compute or scary numbers to crunch, and that makes it easy for runners who haven't done speedwork before.

Now I'll be the first to admit that Yasso 800s aren't a guarantee. You have to start with sessions of 5 or 6 × 800 and build up to 10 over a training season. You can't just go out once, do a set of 6, and expect that you have the key to the city. You still have to build up your weekly mileage, run long each week, and run on hills when you're training for a marathon. And even if you do, the Yasso 800s can't help you if you end up injured or it's 90 degrees on race day.

But I think Yasso 800s do more than train your body—I think they give you the belief that you can do it. I strongly feel that when you set your heart on a race goal, you have to get in the mind-set that it's doable. You've got to trust that your body can handle it, and then you can train for it. That way, you come to race day confident that even if it's hot or something goes wrong, you did the work necessary to reach your goal. And finishing the Yasso 800s in your goal time gives you the evidence you need to really believe that *yes you can.*

But even beyond that, important physiological changes occur when you're running easy.

"By running at very easy aerobic paces, you're building the foundation that's going to support your faster running on race day," says Janet Hamilton, an exercise physiologist and coach of Running Strong (runningstrong .com). "You're improving the aerobic infrastructure that's going to determine how well and how long you can keep energy supplied to those exercising muscles."

For example, you're building more capillaries, so you can deliver more oxygen in the blood. You're increasing the stroke volume, or the amount of blood you can pump with each heartbeat. You're stimulating your body to create more and larger mitochondria—the power plants of cells that make the energy you need to run. You're also recruiting more muscle fibers. Muscle fibers are often classified as slow-twitch, fast-twitch, or "convertible" fast-twitch fibers (which can be trained to work as fast- or slow-twitch). When you run at an easy, aerobic pace, you're recruiting your slow-twitch muscle fibers and training them to be more resistant to fatigue. At the same time, you're training the fast-twitch muscle fibers to work as slow-twitch and also stimulating the fast-twitch "convertible" fibers to be more efficient at working aerobically, like the slow-twitch fibers do.

So in the end, you'll have more muscle fibers working for you, and they'll be more resistant to fatigue.

Is it okay to run or cross-train on a rest day?

Most runners don't have a problem pushing themselves. But when you're focused on your race goal, it's easy to forget how important rest is. If you don't get enough rest, you'll start to break down rather than build up. Recovery is the key ingredient, whether you're shooting for a PR or just trying to get to the starting line. Ideally, you'll have at least 1 or possibly 2 days each week of complete rest, so that you give your body a chance to recover.

If you get antsy when you don't exercise, it's fine to cross-train, or even to run an easy 2 miles. The key is to keep the effort easy.

Nonimpact forms of cardio training, such as cycling, pool running, or working out on the elliptical machine, can help facilitate recovery while improving your aerobic fitness. Just don't go extra hard on the elliptical to compensate for the fact that you're not running. It is okay to run on a rest day to loosen up your muscles, fend off sluggishness, and get enough fresh air to improve your mood. Maintain an easy pace at less than 65 to 70 percent of max heart rate. As long as you keep the volume and intensity very light, you can still get the recovery benefits.

And try to take one day completely off each week. One day off won't set you back; it will help you restock your glycogen stores, reduce fatigue, and build your strength. And since most injuries come from overuse, a day of cross-training, rest, or easy miles can prevent 3- or 4-week forced breaks caused by, say, IT band syndrome.

How can I go 26.2 or 13.1 miles if I don't run the full distance during training?

How long should your long run be? There are a variety of opinions out there. The Hansons-Brooks Distance Project has plans for beginners and advanced runners that peak at 16 miles; some coaches have runners do all 26.2 miles in training. That would certainly be a confidence-booster, but here at *Runner's World,* we're not in that camp. Most marathon plans top out at 20 to 23 miles. We feel you should have run at least two 20-milers before race day to prepare you. In a pinch, you can get away with a little less.

Here's why you don't need to go the whole distance: "Race day magic" is a very real phenomenon, and a very powerful one. On race day, you'll be strong and tapered. With luck, the weather will be better than that nasty summer heat or frigid winter in which you trained. The course will be lined with cheering spectators, and the race organizers will provide plenty of aid stations en route. The races are a lot easier than the marathon and half-marathon rehearsals—your long training runs.

The goal of long runs should be to build your endurance without pushing you over the brink and into injury. That's why it's okay to go a little bit shorter and stay a little bit healthier. Run 1 to 2 minutes slower than goal race pace, at a pace that feels comfortable and makes you think you could go forever. You won't be able to, because glycogen depletion and muscle soreness will eventually get you. But the pace should be smooth and comfortable. If you run with a friend or two, you should be able to hold a normal conversation with them as you run.

How do I know if my form needs fixing?

Between the minimalist running craze and the popularity of techniques like ChiRunning and Pose Method, more people than ever are trying to fix their running form in the hopes of eliminating injuries and improving performance.

Each school of running form has its converts who swear it's the miracle cure. But experts say there's not enough research to definitively say that any of these methods prevents—or causes—injuries. "None of these methods are the be-all and end-all or total evil," says biomechanist Reed Ferber, PhD, an associate professor at the University of Calgary and director of the Running Injury Clinic. The biggest problem is that runners, desperate for a quick fix, make radical changes to their form and end up injuring themselves.

"There is no silver bullet," says Ferber. Your running mechanics are determined by the strength and flexibility of certain muscles and how your body is built. Try to manipulate one of those variables without considering the others, he warns, "and you're setting yourself up for injuries."

So how do you determine whether your form needs fixing? As long as you're running comfortably and injury free, there's no reason to believe it does, says Ferber. "If it isn't broken, don't try to fix it."

No single method will make you faster, he says. That's where the principles of smart training come in: Gradually increase your miles and your speed, and give yourself plenty of recovery time to adapt to the training stresses.

If you do try to change your form, slash your mileage in half and reduce your speed as you experiment with this new way of running. So if you usually run 5 miles a day at a 10-minute pace, drop to 2.5 miles a day at a 12-minute pace. Then, if you feel good, gradually add back mileage and speed by about 10 percent each week. Start on a treadmill, where you don't have to negotiate obstacles like curbs and potholes. Once you transition to running outside, cut your mileage in half again and reduce your speed again, and gradually build back up.

If you are injured, your best bet is to go to a running clinic or sports medicine doctor who can evaluate your gait, strength, and flexibility. He or she can suggest footwear that offers the support you need, plus exercises to help offset any muscle imbalances.

I've never done speedwork and I don't have access to a track. How do I get faster?

For most folks, the term "speedwork" evokes haunting memories from gym class; they associate fast running with physical pain and fear. But it doesn't have to be such a big deal. First of all, you don't absolutely need a track. It's okay to do your speedwork on a flat stretch of road. Your first speed session can be fun, simple, and informal, and you can do it anywhere. Start with the fartlek. From the Swedish word for "speed play," on these runs you choose how far and how fast you want to run. Many great athletes, including the Finnish Olympic medalist Lasse Virén, have done speed training this way. Don't worry about total distance or pace at first; just focus on getting more comfortable running faster than you usually do. Before you begin your fartleks, make sure to do 10 to 15 minutes of easy running to warm up. Then pick a telephone pole, mailbox, stop sign, or any other landmark up ahead and run to it.

Or pick a length of time, like 30 to 60 seconds, and run faster for that long. As you're holding the faster pace, focus on relaxing your body; don't scrunch your shoulders up to your ears. Do two or three fartlek segments on your first workout, and over the course of a few weeks build up to six, running easy between each bout of fast running.

I'm so beat at the end of a long run. Does that mean I'm not ready for the race?

Not necessarily. Long runs are one part of a mileage buildup that pushes your body more and more each week. Cumulative fatigue is normal, says Ali Molnar, who is a running and triathlon coach from Ludington, Michigan (smithsports.us). "But if you're so spent that you can barely jog at the end, adjust your pacing and start your long runs slower," she says. Remember that your taper—and your big day—will rejuvenate you. "You'll tap into the extra energy plus the adrenaline rush and psychological boost of racing," says Molnar.[6]

How do I maintain my form when I get tired?

"The three biggest form errors that occur when you're fatigued are sloppy arms, a loose core, and shuffling," says Meghan Kennihan, a 2:55 marathoner and running coach in the Chicago area (trainwithmeghan .com). Sound familiar? Correct those mistakes by doing the following drill after long runs and speed workouts to train your body to maintain form when it's sapped of energy: Hold a 2- to 5-pound dumbbell in each hand, and march slowly for 10 steps, using a short, high-knees stride and an exaggerated arm swing. Then, while still holding the dumbbells, run 10 steps fast with high knees and a normal arm swing. Repeat 10 times. The exaggerated movement reinforces correct arm swing, strengthens the abs for better stabilization of the upper torso, and eliminates the shuffle by increasing lower body strength and flexibility, Kennihan says.[7]

I have to do most of my marathon training on a treadmill. How will that affect my race?

Treadmill training is a great way to get in shape, though it's not optimal for marathon preparation because you're doing most of your running on a softer surface than you'll encounter on race day. Translation: Your legs might suffer and ultimately rebel. Whenever you can, get outside and run at your planned marathon pace. Meanwhile, set your treadmill to a negative incline and do several tempo runs or marathon-pace runs at minus 2 percent. This will increase the pounding you experience, which will strengthen your legs and prepare you for the stress of your race effort.[8]

CHAPTER 3

INTEGRATING TRAINING INTO YOUR EVERYDAY LIFE

One of the most common questions we get from *Runner's World* Challengers has to do with sticking with the training plan. Is it okay to swap my long runs around? I ran 4 miles instead of 5. Will I still be ready?

In most cases, the answer is yes.

The fact is that marathon and half-marathon plans are designed to prepare a person's body for the challenge of covering the race distance, but they don't deal with the reality that is your life during any 2- or 4-month period of time. You're going to have to work late, care for sick kids, get snowed in, and take vacations. That's life, but you won't find it on any training schedule.

That's where *you* come in. The key to reaching the starting line healthy and accomplishing your goals at the finish line is to work the plan around your everyday life. We're all real people with messy, chaotic lives that don't neatly fit on a 10- or 16-week training grid. Workouts will need to be rearranged; some will be missed altogether.

Amby's Advice

It's okay to swap your workouts around. There's no cardinal rule that says you have to do your long runs on the weekends or your speedwork on Wednesdays. Switch around your workouts any way you need to. Just make sure not to do hard workouts back-to-back. Don't put a speed session the day before a long run, and follow any hard runs with easy days or rest days so you won't get injured.

There will be days when you'll have to go to great lengths just to get in an easy 4-miler. Other times, you'll have to take shortcuts. Having a training buddy or a running group will help you stick to the plan, but meeting up with them will require an entirely new set of logistical gymnastics.

"Training should be integrated into our daily lives," says Susan Paul, coach of the Orlando Track Shack Foundation training program and author of the *For Beginners Only* blog on runnersworld.com. "Even when you have to break up workouts or move them around, it's better than not running at all. We need to get away from the all-or-nothing kind of thinking."

We were constantly amazed at the great lengths that Challengers would go to in order to get their training in. Ryan Lawrence, an engineer with the Canadian Air Force, was deployed shortly after he started training for the Flying Pig Marathon, and he did most of his runs circling the flight deck of his ship. He ran as far as 12 miles on the ship, which meant completing 290 laps. In order to escape the scorching temperatures of Guam, Challenger Tessa Robinson had to wait until midnight to get her long runs done while training for the 2009 Marine Corps Marathon. Nils Dahlin (page 62), a nuclear power instructor from Delaware, has run at least 10 runs of 15 miles or longer completely on a treadmill.

In this chapter, you'll get the practical guidance you need to put all of those training principles you learned about in Chapter 2 to work for you in the real world. You'll find out how to make your run work at any time of day, and you'll get tips on how to do the superhuman juggling that it sometimes takes to manage marathon and half-marathon training with work and family lives—and you'll learn it from Challengers who have already done it and reached their goals on race day.

All in the Timing

What's the best time of day to run? The time that you can most consistently get your run done.

Running the Numbers

How often do you run *exactly* what your training plan tells you to?

- **Always: 19 percent.** If it says to run 9.25 miles, I'll run 9.25 miles . . . on the nose.

- **Usually: 49 percent.** As long as I'm close, I'm happy.

- **Sometimes: 16 percent.** Hey, stuff happens.

- **Rarely: 7 percent.** I'm a human being with free will—not a machine!

- **Never: 10 percent.** My "plan" is to run as much or as little as I feel like.

Source: runnersworld.com

For Todd Pollock (below), 4:30 a.m. is the only time he can run if he's going to make the 7:30 a.m. daycare drop-off, get to work, and be at home at night with the kids. Scott Farley (page 49), an attorney for the National Oceanic and Atmospheric Administration (NOAA), has run at lunch for more than 20 years, which lets him feel energized for the afternoon and make it to his kids' games and practices after work. Colleen Fitzpatrick (page 51) savors the relaxation she feels during her evening runs. "I finish the day burning off calories and feeling good," says Fitzpatrick. "I don't feel like I'm rushing to get my run done, and after work, I have a chance to decompress after a long day."

From a physiological standpoint, your performance is going to be best in the afternoon and early evening. Why? Speed, strength, and motor performance have all been linked to a higher body temperature, and your temp tends to peak between 4:00 p.m. and 8:00 p.m., or about 10 hours after you wake up.

That said, whatever benefits you'll get from a higher body temperature are going to be largely overridden by how much you've had to eat or drink, how tired you are when you start the workout, how long that afternoon meeting drags on, and whether you're on duty for car pool. Stress can play a huge role in how you feel heading into a workout. If you've been under the gun all day, your body has been pumping out stress hormones like cortisol and epinephrine to cope with the day's pressures, says Julia Moffitt, PhD, an exercise physiologist at Des Moines University.

When those stress hormones are released, the body breaks down stored glycogen, fat, and protein to provide energy to cope with the stress. That means you're likely going to have less energy for your run. "Even though you haven't exercised, a stressful day is just going to drain your battery," Moffitt says.

— [WHAT WORKS] ————————————

Early morning runs

Todd Pollock, 42, Sellersville, PA; IT business analyst, father of two; 9 marathons; 3:19 PR; *Runner's World* Challenge Race: 2009 Philadelphia Marathon

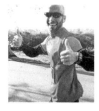

If the early morning is your only time to run, start slowly. Get up 5 to 10 minutes earlier every other day. Set the coffeemaker to go off at 4:00 a.m., so the smell of freshly ground coffee finds its way to you every morning. And whatever you do, don't turn on the computer. It's easy to get sucked into e-mail or Facebook, and you'll end up having to cut your run short!

Below we list the benefits and obstacles of running at any time of day and tips on how to get over them. If you're a morning runner and have to switch to the afternoon, or vice versa, give yourself 3 to 4 weeks to make the transition.

Morning

The payoff: Aside from sleep, chances are, you don't have anything else scheduled at 5:00 a.m. With no meetings, meals to make, or errands to run, early morning is a great time to ensure that you get your run done no matter how crazy the day gets.

The obstacles: Fatigue, a big night out, and the irresistible urge to hit the snooze button can all put your morning run in jeopardy. And once you do get up, it may take some extra effort to get loose and warmed up: Because your body has been in energy-conservation mode overnight, your blood pressure, heart rate, and body temperature are all at their lowest in the morning.

Make it happen: The night before, set the automatic coffeemaker to brew before you wake. Lay out your clothes by the door, so you're not rifling through your closets in the dark and waking up everyone in the house. Arrange an early morning running date; it's much harder to blow off a run when you know that someone is waiting for you. Turn off the computer and TV 30 minutes before bed. In the morning, get dressed in a brightly lit room; when the light hits your eyes, it signals your pineal gland to stop producing melatonin, a hormone that makes you feel sleepy.

─ [WHAT WORKS] ───────────

Run at lunch

Scott Farley, 43, Bel Air, MD; attorney for NOAA, father of two; 2 marathons; 3:37 PR; *Runner's World* Challenge Race: 2010 Marine Corps Marathon

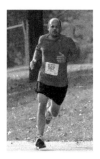

I get to work around 6:30 a.m. so that I can take 1½ hours at lunch and still leave around 4:00 p.m. to be at my kids' games and practices. Other folks are either eating or working out between 11:00 and 1:00, and few people schedule meetings during that time. That said, many things can get in the way—meetings, conference calls, and lunches with co-workers. While you need to be flexible, it's so critical to maintain the discipline to push your chair back, get up, and go. If you don't make it an absolute priority—almost equal to your work—you'll only hit half of your workouts. Make all of the important people in your workplace aware of your schedule, so there's no conflict. Make sure you've eaten and hydrated during the morning so you're energized when you go out.

What it takes to . . .
Lose 100 pounds and become symptom-free from chronic disease

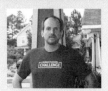

Christopher Sanford, 33, Newport News, VA
Systems database engineer
Experience: 14 marathons; 4:08 PR
Runner's World **Challenge Race: 2009 Richmond Marathon**

Marathon training helped liberate me from the debilitating effects of Tourette's syndrome and the side effects of the medication, which I have struggled with since I was young. Tourette's causes involuntary verbal tics, head jerks, grunts, coughs, shouts, and twitches. I spent so much of my childhood feeling isolated because of it. The side effects of the medication were even worse: It gave me migraines, sapped my energy, slowed my metabolism, and put my head in a permanent fog. In 2006, at 300 pounds, I started running. In 2007, I finished my first marathon in 5:26, and I have since run 13 more marathons with a PR of 4:08. I have lost 100 pounds through training. But more important, I've been released from the disease and the medication that kept me down for so long. When I first stopped taking the medication, it was like seeing a whole new world. Everything became more vivid and alive. But I wouldn't have been able to do it without running. Running has given me a sense of control and freedom. When I was overweight, I didn't realize how much pain I was in. When you're dealing with it all the time, you start to think of it as normal. Running and being fit has given me the biggest confidence boost, and overcoming the weight issues and running the marathon proved to me that you really can do anything if you set your mind to it.

Fuel up for peak performance: Eat a meal of slow-digesting carbs the night before, or have a 100- to 200-calorie snack 30 minutes before you go. Yogurt with fruit, applesauce, and oatmeal are all good choices.

Midday

The payoff: A midday break will make you more productive in the afternoon and will help you avoid hitting the wall at 3:00 p.m. at your desk. That's the time of day when melatonin (the sleep hormone) is at its lowest, and it's the time when you're most alert. A 2005 study in *Medicine and Science in Sport and Exercise* showed that workers' moods, productivity, work quality, and ability to meet deadlines improved dramatically on days when they exercised at midday.[1]

The obstacles: Unexpected meetings and emergencies can get in the way. And even if they don't, there's a strong temptation to keep plugging away and miss your run.

Make it happen: Schedule your run on your calendar just as you do other important meetings, and set a reminder for 15 minutes before you go. Put your gym bag in plain sight as a reminder. Make a running date with someone in the office. Put race numbers and inspirational quotes or photos near your desk to inspire you to get out the door.

Fuel up for peak performance: Be sure to have a carb-rich breakfast, like oatmeal or a whole wheat bagel. About 2 hours before your run, have a 200-calorie snack, like an energy bar or a yogurt. Have some protein afterwards, to help your body recover.

Afternoon/Early Evening

The payoff: Late in the day, your body temperature, blood pressure, and heart rate are at

BART SAYS ...
Don't get down and out

It's easy to get discouraged when you see the pack disappearing in the distance. This is hard, no bones about it. Just remember that everybody who is ahead of you has been the beginner at some point—and probably finished near the back of the pack when they were—so everybody knows what it's like to be in your shoes. No one starts running leading the pack, but you have to start somewhere. If you stick with it, you will improve. Most groups are really supportive and encouraging to newer runners. If the vibe is too intense, try another group. If you find a crowd you feel comfortable running with, you'll be motivated to keep joining them to run. And if you keep getting out there to run, before you know it, you won't be finishing last anymore. Then you'll be able to mentor other beginners who have found the courage to join the pack.

— [WHAT WORKS] —

Run after work

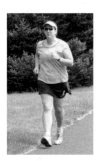

Colleen Fitzpatrick, 38, Boyertown, PA; project manager; 9 marathons; 4:54 PR; *Runner's World* Challenge Race: 2009 New York City Marathon

Eat a bigger meal for lunch so you have the energy to run later. Make sure to have a snack an hour before, so it has time to settle in your stomach and you have the energy to finish the run strong. Lay out your running gear before you leave for work in the morning, and when you get home from work, put your running gear on as soon as possible.

their peak, which is when your muscles can perform their best.

The obstacles: If you have a stressful day, you may feel drained and tired and more tempted to hit the couch than the road. If you haven't eaten, your blood sugar may plummet and you'll have a hard time getting energized for your run.

Make it happen: Change at work and go directly to the gym or trail before you get home. Join a gym so you can have access to a treadmill when snow and ice make it unsafe to run outside.

Fuel up for peak performance: Have a 100- to 200-calorie snack 1 hour before you run. Make sure it includes protein to keep you feeling full, as well as healthy, complex carbs. After your run, you may not be hungry, but you'll need to refuel. Try some hearty soup with beans, or have a glass of chocolate milk.

Running with Others

Finding a group or a buddy to run with can give a lift to your running life. A date with a group or a partner can get you out the door when you'd otherwise stay in; in a social setting, you may be able to go faster or farther than you would on your own. It's a safe way to explore new routes that you might not discover by yourself, and the acquaintances you make as the miles roll by can grow into friends for life. But going to meet another

INSIDE RUNNER'S WORLD®

JENNIFER VAN ALLEN, 37, SPECIAL PROJECTS EDITOR, PHILADELPHIA, PA

LESSON LEARNED: FIND OUT WHERE YOU'RE GOING BEFORE YOU GO

The first time I went on a group run, I went to a nearby running shop for what was advertised as an "easy 5 miles." Six men showed up, all of whom were twice my age and had run together for at least as long as I've been alive. When they asked me if an 8:30 pace was okay, I sheepishly lied "sure," even though that was a full 2 minutes per mile faster than I'd ever run in my life. For the first mile, I huffed and puffed to stay with them. During the second mile, I let myself fall behind the pack. By mile 3, I let them disappear into the distance. I was new to town and didn't know the roads, so I wandered the streets hopelessly. I finally found my way home 3 hours later, exhausted, parched, and completely humiliated. "Where were you?" my husband asked. I just shook my head, sobbed, and said, "I have no clue." Since then, I have always driven the route or mapped it out before I attempted to run it.

runner—or a group—can be daunting. Before you go, keep these things in mind.

Shop around. Some groups are competitive and serious about speed, but many others are more social and include runners with a wide range of abilities. Some days you may want to run easy, and other days you may want others to push you beyond your comfort zone. Local running shops usually have running workouts and marathon and half-marathon training programs. Before you go out for a run with a group, contact someone in the group to find out about the typical pace and distance for each group run. Try to find people who run at your pace or slower. Amy Katz (page 56), 40, a real estate accoun-tant from Irvine, California, belongs to two different clubs so that she has the option to run with people 6 days a week if she wants to. One group has runners with a wide range of abilities; the other has more advanced and competitive runners. "If I don't want to run that night," she says, "knowing that I'm meeting people will get me out the door."

Be outgoing. The opportunity to relax and socialize is often what draws people to group runs. So go ahead and introduce yourself and ask questions, just as you would at any other gathering where you are new. Chances are, when regulars spot an unfamiliar face they'll reach out to welcome you. Everyone has been the "new guy" at some point.

▬ [WHAT WORKS] ▬▬▬▬▬▬▬▬▬▬▬

Find a training partner

Denise Langhoff, 44, Marion, IA; credit research analyst, mother of three; 5 marathons; 3:45 PR; *Runner's World* Challenge Race: 2009 Richmond Marathon

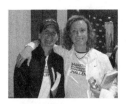

Finding a running buddy is definitely more difficult than finding a spouse. Hook up with a local running club in your area; call a local running store to find one near you. The whole group shows up and takes off running together, but soon people sort of fall into smaller packs. Listen to conversations. See who talks if you are a listener, who listens if you are a talker, and who internalizes if you would rather not be bothered with conversation. You're going to spend a lot of time with this person, so you need to be able to relate to each other, have compatible personality types, and find some common ground when it comes to humor. On top of all that, you have to run close to the same pace, have similar running goals, and have schedules that allow you to actually find time to run together. Also, you have to be very flexible when it comes to running with a partner. And it's only going to work if you're both willing to change it up, when one of you needs to.

Inventing the Hills

Hilly runs help you build the muscular and cardiovascular fitness that preps you for the more formal speed sessions down the road. So what do you do when you live in an area that's pancake flat?

You can simulate hill work on gym machines by manipulating the inclines. Most treadmills and elliptical trainers have predesigned hill programs that throw a variety of ascents and descents into your workout.

If you're suffering from cabin fever, you can also find some man-made inclines outside. Challenger Peter Kaus, of Tallahassee, Florida, runs the ramps inside the Florida State University Stadium. "The ramps to get to the upper section of the stadium are long and steep enough to run and get a good hill workout," says Kaus, who finished the Toronto Half-Marathon in 1:25.

Ben Pineau, of St. Augustine, Florida, runs the 1-mile-long Vilano Bridge for hill repeats once a week. He runs at about 90 percent of max speed to the top of the bridge (which is about 70 feet up), then recovers by jogging back down the other side. He repeats this cycle 6 to 10 times. "It's like running a sustained hill at a fairly constant incline," says Pineau, a doctor and father of two.

And the fast work seems to be paying off.

Since he started running the bridge 2 years ago, he's nabbed a 1:36 PR in the half-marathon, a 19:35 PR in the 5-K, and a 3:15 finish at the Boston Marathon.

— [WHAT WORKS]

Create your own hillwork, when the area you live in is completely flat

Andrea Myloyde, 45, Detroit, MI; supervisor, mother of one; 3 marathons; 4:30 PR; *Runner's World* Challenge Race: 2009 New York City Marathon

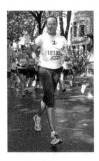

I will do anything to avoid the treadmill, and in the area where I live, there are no hills. During my lunch break, I run to a seldom-used parking garage a few miles from my office. It's 0.7 miles from the bottom to the top. I run it four grueling times, and boy, do my glutes burn by the time I reach the top! Sometimes I'll run the stairs. I'll do 7 to 12 floors; each floor has about 16 steps. When running stairs I don't really pay attention to pace. I go more by heart rate to make sure that I'm staying near or at my aerobic threshold. My theory is that if I'm working that hard, running over hills later will seem easy.

INSIDE RUNNER'S WORLD®

MARK REMY, *42, EXECUTIVE EDITOR OF RUNNERSWORLD.COM, AUTHOR OF* THE RUNNER'S RULE BOOK *AND* THE RUNNER'S FIELD MANUAL, *ALLENTOWN, PA*

LESSON LEARNED: GIVE IN TO PEER PRESSURE

I've trained myself to "just say yes" to co-workers who cajole me into ducking out for a lunchtime run. I know from experience that I almost never regret the runs that I do, but I almost always regret the ones that I skip. And when my co-workers are weak or over-whelmed, I do the same for them. It's an informal deal we've worked out. Sort of a get-off-your-butt support group. Go find enablers. It's harder to skip a run if you know others are heading out and expecting you to join them. Of course, the holy grail is to get your boss on board. If your boss is lacing up the running shoes, you can bet it's okay for you to follow suit.

The only downsides I can think of are that other co-workers might think you're crazy (or worse, a diva) for asking to reschedule lunchtime meetings so that you can run. Oh, and returning to your desk still sweating after your shower, if you're the sort of person who has that "residual sweating" problem. Which I do.

"I truly believe that combining speedwork with the bridge work has helped me reach significantly faster times," he says.

Here are more tips on improvising for your hillwork.

Stairs. Do "repeats" by running up and down stadium stairs. Just watch your step and make sure to pick up your knees—you don't want to trip!

Bridges. You can get some challenging climbs on roads leading up to a bridge and by continuing to the midpoint of the bridge. And as you're traveling across the span you'll have to contend with wind resistance, which will help you prepare in case race day is windblown.

Ramps. Ramps in parking garages can offer some quality hillwork. Just be careful of oncoming traffic. You may want to wear a headlamp and reflective gear so that cars can see you.

Treadmills. Adjust the incline of the tread-mill to simulate the feeling of uphill training. Look at the elevation chart for your race, and use the incline button on your machine to try to mimic the changes in terrain that you'll face during the race. Or try the workout in "Hills on the Treadmill," page 56.

Shortcuts for Long Runs

While training for the 2010 Toronto Marathon, Bob Gottlieb found himself in the situation that a lot of runners do. That is, he had

Hills on the Treadmill

This workout was created by Olympian Jeff Galloway, *Runner's World*'s "Starting Line" columnist.

● Start with a 3-minute warmup (or longer, if you have time).

● Raise the incline to 2 percent. Run for 1 minute.

● Raise the incline to 4 percent. Run for 1 minute.

● Recover for 1 minute at 0 percent incline.

● Raise the incline to 4 percent. Run for 2 minutes.

● Recover for 1 minute at 0 percent incline.

● Repeat as many times as you can. Once you finish, recover for 3 minutes at a comfortable pace.

Source: "Condensed Hill Run Workout," http://tinyurl.com/3w9sn9h

18 miles to run and no time to do it. With his wife out of town and his kids' busy sports schedules, it just wasn't happening. So instead of one monster-long run, he ran a 12-miler near marathon pace and followed it up with a slightly faster 10-miler the next day.

"I don't think that hurt me at all," says Gottlieb, who ran a 3:07 personal best on race day. "I needed to get the long runs in for confidence, but a one-time substitute was fine."

Indeed, the long runs are critical to building endurance, efficiency, and confidence for race day, but realistically it's not always easy to clear a 3- to 4-hour stretch of time to run, plus time afterwards to eat, ice sore spots, and shower. And all too often, the weather, your social life, or a business trip gets in the way.

The good news is, it is okay to improvise when you have to. You can replace some of

INSIDE RUNNER'S WORLD ®

TISH HAMILTON, *50, EXECUTIVE EDITOR, BERNARDSVILLE, NJ*

LESSON LEARNED: PLAN CAREFULLY FOR YOUR LONG RUN

When you're training for a marathon and you also have a small child and a husband who is training for a triathlon, you have to schedule in advance not just the time for your long run but also whatever time you need for your postrun cooldown, shower, and meal. Otherwise, you'll be tackled the second you walk in the door, commanded to fold your tired legs into a princess-castle tent, joined in the shower by a squealing 5-year-old, asked to share your fried-egg sandwich, and generally not be allowed to rest until long after the sun has set. Bonus points to anyone who manages to negotiate a nap. While your child is still in the napping age, do not use the time for a long run. It is very important for working marathoner parents to nap when small children nap because as soon as they stop napping, you will never get to put your feet up in the middle of the day again.

your longest runs with more frequent and challenging runs of 10 to 14 miles and still get the same benefit, with less risk of injury than from one exhausting effort.[2]

Stephen McGregor, PhD, an exercise physiologist at Eastern Michigan University, says runners can get similar fuel-efficiency benefits from completing two faster mid-distance runs of about 10 miles, back to back, as they would from running farther, more slowly, for 2 to 3 hours.

"If you do harder runs for a shorter distance, you should get the same underlying adaptation from a metabolic standpoint," says McGregor. On the second run, you'll be fatigued, just as you would be on the second half of the long run. Not as fatigued as you would be from a single long run, "but it's not like you'll be running on fresh legs."

The key, he adds, is to run conservatively enough in the first run so that you have the stamina for the second run.

That said, it's best not to take shortcuts all of the time. There are certain benefits and race preparation that you can only get by doing one continuous long run. The confidence you get from completing those runs, and the experience you get of hitting low points and running past them, will help you immensely in the final miles of your race.

"If you don't run long on a regular basis, you may not know what the wall is," says McGregor. "If you haven't run past your limits once from a 20-miler, a lot of times you're limited in your experience, and in turn, it limits what you do."

Doing Doubles

For many runners, finding even an hour of time for a midweek run is tricky. Between work, commutes, and car pool, plus trying to get sleep and stay fueled, it's just hard to make it all happen. For lots of folks, running twice a day gives them the latitude they need to get their miles in. Research has shown that you reap the same fitness benefits you get when you boost the duration and intensity of any one run: reduced body fat, increased VO_2 max, and improved muscle tone.

Ed Eyestone, an exercise physiologist, coach of the Brigham Young University Cross-Country team, and "Fast Lane" columnist for *Runner's World*, ran twice a day throughout his career. "You get used to training through fatigue," he says, but if you refuel and rest sufficiently, "you'll be able to hit a quality pace."

But two-a-days do take a little planning. You have to make your morning run easy enough that you're not exhausted in the afternoon. It's critical to rehydrate, rest, and refuel before the afternoon run so that you can hit your target pace. Here are some of Eyestone's tips for making the double run work.[3]

Build slowly. Start by doing doubles twice a week. Initially, the extra workout can be 20 minutes. When you first add it on, drop the length of your main workout by 10 to 15 minutes. As you get more comfortable, bring the main workout back to its original level and extend the second run to 40 minutes. Once you've done that, you can double up on as many days as you want. Just spend at least 2 weeks at each stage before adding more miles.

Recover right. Allow at least 4 hours between your workouts so you can rest and restock your glycogen stores. After the first run, be sure to rehydrate, and consume at least 500 calories within 30 minutes of finishing to help speed recovery.

Listen to your body. Stay alert for aches and pains, and fiddle with the formula until you find what works best for you. Many runners prefer to add an easy run in the morning when they know they have a hard workout in the afternoon. The easy run gets them loosened up for the hard work later. Others prefer to add extra workouts on their easy days.

What it takes to . . .
Quit Smoking and Become a Marathoner

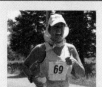

Jessica Willis, 43, Pittsfield, MA
High school English teacher
Experience: 10 marathons; 5:04 PR
Runner's World **Challenge Race: 2009 Hartford Marathon**

In 1984, when I was 16, I watched the Women's Olympic Marathon. I remember watching Joan Benoit Samuelson come into the stadium and seeing the Swiss runner Gaby Andersen-Scheiss stumble in last. She was severely dehydrated and could barely walk. She had just come 26 miles and 385 yards and had no hope of winning, but it didn't matter. The only thing that mattered was that she finished. I just couldn't fathom the idea of running that far, and I thought her struggle was so elegant. That really stuck with me. By 2004, I'd been smoking two packs a day for 20 years. I was vaguely overweight and I couldn't laugh without coughing. I got viral pneumonia and could barely breathe. I had used every excuse not to exercise—that I was too fat or too old, or it just seemed impossible. But getting sick scared me. I was tired of killing myself with cigarettes. When I crushed out that last butt, I made a commitment to myself to not smoke for the rest of the day. That day turned into a night, and into another day. I knew I had to do something to take

Missing Workouts

A few months is a long time to train, and there are bound to be times during training when life, the car pool schedule, your boss, your kids, or the weather just don't cooperate with your training plan. We get a lot of frantic e-mails from runners who missed a workout, or two, or five—or more. "Is all lost?" they wonder. "Will I still be able to finish the race?" "Can I still meet my goals?"

In most cases, the answer is yes. More often than not, life's interruptions are blessings in disguise because they give you extra time off to recover and stay fresh for the next workout. "It can be just what the doctor ordered," says Cedric Bryant, PhD, chief science officer for the American Council on Exercise. "So often runners are right on the precipice of overtraining, and that week off when they're called out of town on business allows them to get that recovery time and

my mind off smoking. So 2 weeks after I quit, I ran to the corner and back. It was about 800 yards. The next morning I had shin splints so bad that I had to walk down the stairs backward. But I kept at it. I ran 800 yards the next day and for the rest of the week. The next week, I ran to the next corner and back. A year to the day after quitting smoking, I ran 26.2 miles for the first time at the Disney World Marathon. Fear got me out the door then, and it still gets me out the door. I don't know if the runner's high is real or not, but I don't think it's a coincidence that my self-

esteem and my health improved when I put down the cancer sticks and picked up the sneakers. On days when it's tough to get out the door, I remember what it felt like to stamp out my last cigarette. I think about how good it feels when I have a rhythm going and have "disappeared" inside the run. Or how good it feels to slow to a walk after finishing the goal run for the day and having that sense of accomplishment. I think of the last 800 meters of the marathon—it's a holy time, in my opinion—and knowing that all those runs I said yes to, and didn't avoid, got me there.

come back and perform better than before."

The bigger risk is trying to cram in miles you missed, out of guilt or fear that you'll lose your fitness. Try to "make up" your miles by, say, doubling the distance of a short run or ratcheting up the intensity, and you're setting yourself up for injury.

So what should you do when you miss a run? And how do you determine when your goal is a lost cause?

It really depends on how many runs you miss, which runs you miss, when you miss them, and what kind of exercise you've been able to do while you haven't been running. If you've been off the road because you're injured, your body and your doctor will have to dictate your comeback.

As a general rule, says Bryant, for every week of complete inactivity, allow 2 to 3 weeks to get back to your previous level of fitness. Research has shown that during a 2- to 4-week break, VO_2 max decreases by about 10 percent and flexibility starts to diminish. Also, there's a decrease in your lactate threshold pace (the pace at which lactic acid starts to accumulate in your blood).

Here are some questions to consider in order to determine whether you've missed too much training time and need to reset your race goal.

How much time did you miss? One

— [WHAT WORKS] ————————————

Reset your race goals

Amy Katz, 40, Irvine, CA; real estate accountant; 32 marathons; 3:37 PR; *Runner's World* Challenge Race: 2009 Chicago Marathon

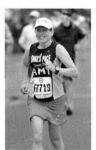

I started training for Richmond with the hopes of breaking 3:30. My PR is 3:37, and there was a part of me that wanted to finish in 3:29, because I ran my first marathon 12 years ago in 5:29. Unfortunately I developed back pain and sciatica during training and went through weeks of not being able to run, and then only being able to run in the pool. I was really looking forward to seeing friends at the race, so I had to shift my thinking from my finish line goal to just making it to the starting line. Even though I was suffering from back pain and sciatica on race day, I had a fantastic race. I really enjoyed running with my fellow Challengers, and the spectators helped me through the rough patches. I knew I didn't have a chance of breaking 3:30, but I finished about an hour faster than I expected, in 4:33. And I was thrilled to cross the finish line. I felt a huge sense of accomplishment and was proud of myself for being mentally strong. Sometimes it's important to run a race for time, but on this day it was all about finishing with a smile on my face.

week off from running usually isn't a problem, but once runners miss more than 2 weeks, it gets increasingly difficult to get back on track. That's because it can take 4 to 6 weeks to regain any fitness that was lost, says Patti Finke, an exercise physiologist and coach of Team Oregon. Beyond 2 weeks, she starts advising runners to readjust their race goals, either by scaling back any time expectations for the race or by signing up for a later race. "There are lots of races," says Finke. "You're better off changing the goal race rather than trying to run something underprepared." For a half-marathon, you should have run at least three times per week for 10 weeks before entering the race, says Tom McGlynn, an Olympic marathon trials qualifier and coach of Focus-N-Fly, an online-training service based in San Mateo, California.

How many long runs have you done? The long run is the key opportunity to get your mind and body strong enough for race day. Missing one or two long runs is no big deal. Just gradually increase the distance and work back up to the long run mileage that's designated on the training plan. Ideally, you want to have one 20-miler for a marathon, plus at least four runs that are longer than 2 hours, says McGlynn. "If you don't have that, then you have no business running a marathon," he says. For a half-marathon, you should be able to complete a 7-mile run

with only short walk breaks (less than 30 seconds), McGlynn says. "Ideally, you want to have one 9-miler and at least four runs over 75 minutes," he adds. However, if you can run 7 miles straight then you can probably gut out the race. The half-marathon distance is drastically more forgiving than the marathon distance, he points out. There's less time and strain for muscle degradation and glycogen depletion, not to mention psychological discomfort.

When did you miss your runs? If there's any "best" time to miss your runs, it's in the first 2 to 3 weeks of the training cycle, during the base-building phase. During that time you're developing a foundation of cardiovascular fitness, where you're getting into a regular running routine and gradually ramping up your mileage. You're not missing any of the critical long runs or speed workouts. As long as you had a good base of fitness going into training, you should be able to pick up the training plan in week 3 or 4 of the program without a problem. The second "best" time to miss runs is during the taper. During the taper, you're recovering from the most intense workouts, the longest runs, and the highest weekly mileage, and you're getting fresh for the race. Many runners—out of antsiness or sheer panic that they'll lose fitness—run more than they should during the taper and show up to the starting line feeling burnt out and out of energy. If an unexpected lay-off forces you to actually observe the taper, you'll be more likely to run your best on race day, as long as you've been able to get some high-intensity workouts in.

Did you do any other exercise while you weren't running? You can maintain your cardiovascular fitness with some form of high-intensity cross-training during the time that you're not running. The closer the cross-training simulates running, the easier it will be to make the transition. If you take a week off and are a complete couch potato, give yourself 2 to 3 weeks of reconditioning for every 1 week off to reach your prelayoff feeling of fitness. (See "The Back-Up Plan" starting on page 180 for a 10-week plan that shows what to do when you can't run.) Even if you're able to cross-train while you can't run, you should be careful about coming

back too quickly, particularly if you're injured, says Craig Souders, DPT, Lehigh Valley Health Network in Bethlehem, Pennsylvania. The muscles, tendons, and bones adapt more slowly to new training stress than the cardiovascular system does. "You may have the stamina to go out and do 15 miles, or run for 2 hours, but your bones and joints might not be ready to handle that if you haven't been running for a while," says Souders. "People try to pick up their running where they left off and often end up injuring themselves while trying to make a comeback." (See "Return to Running" on page 191.)

Treadmills

Most runners have a love-hate relationship with treadmills. It saves you on days when there's a blizzard or a heat wave, but the

---

— [WHAT WORKS] ————————————————

Run long on the treadmill

Nils Dahlin, 49, Wilmington, DE; nuclear power industry instructor, father of two; 8 marathons; 3:59 PR; *Runner's World* Challenge Race: 2009 Richmond Marathon

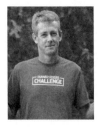

I have run two 20-milers, two 18-milers, and five runs of 15 miles on the treadmill. I survived them by breaking them into smaller segments. After each hour of running, I'd get off the machine and walk around for a few minutes, have an energy gel, refill my water bottle, and switch treadmills. That way, I could watch something different [on the gym TVs] and have slightly different scenery. Never mind the strange looks I'd get from the gym staff.

prospect of running miles and miles and miles in place on a machine is enough to make you want to quit before you even start.

We often get asked, "Is it cheating to run on a treadmill?" The answer: definitely not.

Running on the treadmill isn't exactly like running over level ground outside, but it's a lot more similar than sitting on the couch.

Conventional wisdom has always been to adjust the incline by 1 to 2 percent or to adjust

— [WHAT WORKS] ————————————————

Make the time

Mary-Pat Cormier, 40, Boston; attorney, mother of four; 2 marathons; 3:59 PR;
***Runner's World* Challenge Race: 2010 Toronto Marathon**

Mary-Pat Cormier got into running when she was 25, after being accepted into law school. "I figured it would build a mental callus that would get me through exams, papers, and court." She has run ever since, through all her pregnancies and a brutal travel schedule. Her kids are now 14, 10, and 4 years old—and the youngest are twins. She recently set a 3:59 personal best at the 2010 Toronto Marathon, and she has her eyes on a 3:50 to qualify for Boston. Here are her tips for other marathon moms.

• **Find a powerful motivator and stick with it.** It may be about weight loss, health issues, "me" time, fitting into those holy grail jeans, a sense of power and control, or meditation. At different times in life, it's going to be more one factor than another. If your motivator loses its power, find another.

• **Eschew guilt.** Sure, you are not at home doing whatever it is that you should be doing. But you give your family and boss hours of undivided attention and loyalty on a daily basis. If others try to make you feel guilty or bad about working out, that's their problem, not yours.

• **Work out when you could probably get away with not doing it.** I have run immediately after having a stomach virus, with an abscessed tooth, in the bitter cold, and through rain and snowstorms. This will remind you that if you can work out in these conditions, you can work out anytime. It also adds a bit of adventure to your running life. And hey, if you have four kids and work 70 to 80 hours a week, you've got to take your adventures where you can. This may be it.

• **If you need to miss a workout, don't stress.** But plan to be a little extra active on that day. If I'm in a big airport and have a layover, I will walk from one terminal to the farthest one and back again.

the speed by 10 to 15 seconds to make up for the lack of wind resistance that you'd get outside. But that recommendation is based on a small study with inconclusive results, says Reed Ferber, an associate professor and director of the Running Injury Clinic at the University of Calgary.

"The only way to get the feeling of really running on the ground outside," he says, "is by running on the ground outside."

While you're racking up the miles, here are some tips to keep you safe and healthy.

Don't get hurt. While the cushioned surface of the treadmill helps prevent injuries, a lot of runners report aches and pains after putting in extra time on the mill— especially those runners who are prone to conditions like plantar fasciitis. Be sure to run at a pace that you can comfortably sustain. This may take some extra effort.

When you're on the road and you start to tire, you naturally slow down, but on a treadmill, the belt is moving you so you may overstride to keep up with it when you're tired. That can put more stress on your joints. Be sure to adjust your speed or incline as you become fatigued.

Don't hold on. If you can't keep up with the treadmill without grabbing the handrails, it's a sign that you're going too fast for your abilities. It's best to back off the pace and let go. Holding on to the handrails while you run can throw off your stride and create a lot of twisting motion in your torso, and that can lead to injuries, says Ferber.

Catch up with your friends. Convince a friend to hit the gym when you're going long so that you can run side-by-side and chat while the miles roll by. You can each run at your own pace, and the miles go by faster

---

— [WHAT WORKS] ————————————

Plug in with the running world

**Tammie Kruszczak, 44, Omaha, NE; hair stylist, mother of four; 15 marathons; 4:01 PR;
Runner's World Challenge Race: 2009 Sioux City Marathon**

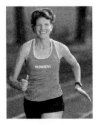

When most people hear that I'm a runner, they think I'm a nutcase. I don't know a lot of other moms who run, and I can't really plug into the local community because I have work or family obligations when they have group runs on weekends. So it can be pretty isolating. Meeting other runners at races and through the Challenge has unlocked this whole new world of incredible people who are just as passionate about running as I am. They make me feel normal.

than they would if either of you had gone solo. Rodale's senior director of employee fitness and health Budd Coates, a four-time Olympic Marathon Trials qualifier, has gutted out some 30-mile treadmill runs by scheduling friends to run shorter runs on the treadmill next to him, like a relay.

Step outside . . . slowly. If you've spent the whole winter on the treadmill, don't jump into outdoor training on the first day of spring. That could lead to injury. Gradually integrate outside running into your routine. When you're outside, your calf muscles produce 90 percent of the power needed to propel you forward on the ground, Ferber says. On the treadmill, that force is cut in half, and the smaller stabilizer muscles in the lower limbs don't have to work as hard, says Ferber. So if you're training on a treadmill and you suddenly start running outside, your calves won't be accustomed to generating that much force, and you can be vulnerable to injuries like plantar fasciitis and inflammation in the Achilles tendon.

Enduring Questions

Is it okay to do all my speedwork on a treadmill?

It's not ideal. Running outside gets you physically and mentally prepared for running hard on the surface and in the weather conditions that you'll encounter on race day,

says Dustin Jenkins, a running coach and personal trainer in Lapeer, Michigan (http://www.elitefeetrunning.com). That said, speedwork isn't a large part of marathon training. As long as you're doing the bulk of your other runs (especially your long runs) outdoors, don't worry about it. Just realize that, generally, the climate-controlled conditions of the gym or your home will allow you to hit faster paces on the treadmill than you will on the road or track.[4]

I'd like to incorporate strength training into my marathon preparation. What's the best day to do it?

It's best to do it on the same day as a hard workout, says Souders. If you're strength training on an easy day, you're not giving your body enough of a chance to recover. After you finish your run, refuel and rehydrate, then hit the weights. But the reality is, a lot of runners find that it's tough to find time to do this because track workouts and long runs already take up so much time. "If that's the case, it's okay to do it on an easy day," says coach McGlynn. "The biggest thing is to not do it the day before the hard workout," he says. "It's going to leave you sore and taxed."

Do I earn "extra mileage" on runs when I push a running stroller?

No, but there are other bonuses, says Laura Polikowsky, a personal trainer and Moms on the Run coach in Minneapolis (http://www.momsontherun.com). "If you can hit the same pace you normally run, you'll burn significantly more calories because you're pushing extra weight," she says. Even if you can't go that fast, the heavier your kid, the bigger the burn. The effort of pushing a stroller can also strengthen your deltoids, pectorals, and biceps.[5]

I'm in the base-building phase for a race. Does time on the elliptical and bike count?

Yes, it does—but not as much as time on the roads, says Amby Burfoot. Here's why: Training for running is most effective when it's most specific—that is, when you're actually running. That said, it makes sense to avoid injury and build your base with cross-training, as you are doing. At some point, however, you should try to wean yourself off the machines and put in more time on the road or track. This becomes particularly important as you get closer to your race date—specifically the last 3 to 6 weeks. You don't have to completely give up the elliptical and bike, but the more running training you do, the better you'll perform during your race.[6]

I've had to shorten a couple of my long runs. Should I make up the mileage elsewhere during the week?

Don't try to make up for "lost" mileage, advises San Diego–based running coach Carrie Grote. Your long runs train your muscles to utilize fuel more efficiently, improve your body's ability to use oxygen, and strengthen your heart and running muscles. Mentally, they give you confidence because you know that you can handle long distances. You won't get these benefits by simply tacking on more miles to shorter weekly runs. Plus, if you overload

your week, you could set yourself up for injury. It's better to look forward, with no regrets, and continue with your planned schedule.[7]

When a workout calls for strides, at what point should I do them?

If the workout is a standard distance run, meaning not a speed, tempo, long run, or hill workout (for more on the meanings of these terms, see Appendix A: A Guide to Common Running Terms on page 233), then do strides at the end, says Ryan Wolf, corporate fitness and running coach for Gallup in Omaha, Nebraska. Your body will be warmed up but not fatigued from the effort, so you'll have ample energy to focus on leg turnover and running tall. (Just remember to cool down with a 5-minute jog.) If strides are required as part of a speed workout, do them between your warmup and the first repeat so that you have sufficient energy to complete your intervals. Run two laps: Stride the straights and float the curves.[8]

Is it better to take the day off before or after a long run or speed workout?

It's best to rest or do light cross-training the day after a long run, says Scott McCoubrey, head coach of the Seattle Running Club and owner of the Seattle Running Company. Your body is fatigued and depleted of its energy supply and needs to heal and refuel (so eat plenty of protein and drink lots of water). However, it's best to skip running the day *before* a speed workout. Your body needs to be fresh, with no tightness, in order to run a maximal effort from the first repeat to the last. For long runs or speed sessions that are more exhausting than usual, consider taking a zero the day before *and* the day after.[9]

If you have to split up your long run into three parts, with short breaks between them, do you get the same benefit as from a single continuous 22-miler?

Let's say you run 6 miles, drive 20 minutes to meet up with friends, and then run another 16 miles. Does it count as 22 miles? Sometimes there is no other way to get in your long run and meet your family and social obligations. The point of LSDs (long, slow distance runs) is to train your mind and your muscles to spend hours running, just as you'll have to do on race day.

Long runs help you develop aerobic and muscular fitness, burn fat, build capillaries, and get your slow-twitch fibers up and operating so they'll be ready to fire when you need them, hours into the race. You learn to run strong through fatigue, and you'll get to rehearse your fuel, gear, and pacing strategies for the race. Certainly, a fractured LSD isn't ideal for accomplishing those goals, but it is passable, experts assure. A 20-minute break isn't enough time for your body to make any significant recovery, says Mike Broderick, head of the Boston Bound Training Program. Your metabolism is still elevated, your energy stores are still depleted from the first 6 miles, and you start the second part of the run in a fatigued state, so the cumulative effect isn't significantly different than running an easy 22-miler continuously.

→*RW* CHALLENGER PROFILE:
The Marathon Moms

Throughout the *Runner's World* Challenge, we were amazed at how much people juggled during training. We joked that we seemed to attract the superwoman demographic—people like Mary-Pat Cormier (page 63), an attorney and mother of four from Boston, Massachusetts; Tammie Kruszczak (page 64), a hair stylist and mother of four from Omaha, Nebraska; and Jenna Drury, a mother of three from Charlotte, North Carolina.

Some had run marathons before they became moms; others had only discovered marathons afterward. For them, the structure and consistency that training requires enabled them to juggle everything else in their over-stuffed lives.

"Running makes me better at everything else I do," says Kruszczak, 44, who has run 13 marathons with a PR of 4:01. She started running when the kids were 4 years old, 2 years old, and 11 months old. "Running fills up my tank, and it gives me the energy to give to everyone else."

Kathy Derrick, an emergency room nurse and mother of four, started running after her kids were born. "It just relieves a lot of anxiety and stress," she says.

Catherine Saint Louis (page 81), a newspaper reporter, decided to train for her first marathon 9 months after having her first son. She wanted to lose 25 pounds of baby weight, but the 4 months of training had bigger implications.

"It was about getting *me* back," says Saint Louis, 37, of Brooklyn, New York. "As a new mother you just become this major giver. And it was important to define for myself and my husband that I had taken one for the team. During the 4 months of training, that was his time to shoulder the burden and a way to level the playing field. I wanted something that I could be proud of—that's what kept me super-motivated. When you're giving of yourself every single hour, it's pretty important to have something like that."

Though Constance Wannamaker (shown below) had run 15 marathons before she had a baby, her running life didn't really take off until *after* she had her son Benjamin. Before him, she had a personal best time of 4:27. But months after he was born, despite working full time and the exhausting nights she spent changing diapers and attending to midnight feedings, she qualified for Boston with a 3:43 finish.

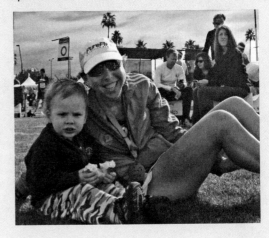

"After he was born, running became my only time for myself," says Wannamaker, 38, an attorney from El Paso, Texas. "I'd really cherish it. It gave me the energy to manage a busy job and take care of him. I was more motivated to get out there. I got more serious about my training, and I started running longer and maintaining higher weekly mileage."

But *how* do they do it?

The key is being flexible, they say. That means doing long runs during the week or in the middle of the day. Kruszczak squeezes in her run after she gets the kids off to school and before she starts work. But sometimes, she has to reschedule her run for 4:00 a.m., or as late as 9:00 p.m.

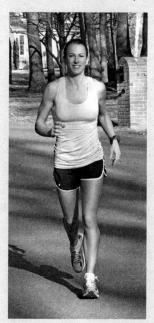

"I know people who freak out if they miss a run or don't follow a plan to a T," says Wannamaker. "But when you have a baby, you just can't do that."

For others, routine is critical. Drury (shown at left), a photographer and mother of three, has to be out the door for her run by 5:00 a.m. so she can be back in time to make breakfast, pack lunches, and get to work.

"It lets me be mentally prepared and lets my family know what to expect," says Drury, whose kids are 4, 8, and 10 years old. She finished the 2010 Richmond Marathon—her first—in 3:43.

That is not to say that there aren't exhausting days when the kids or the boss wants more than these women have to give. And there is guilt, too, and the feeling of being pulled in a million directions at once.

"When I'm getting ready for a run, my son will say, 'Mommy, don't run,'" says Wannamaker. "And I hate it, but I just have to tell him, 'Mommy will be a much better mommy when she gets back.'"

All of them say that training for marathons sets a powerful example for their kids.

"It's allowed my children to see me as more than their mother, but also as an individual that they can be proud of," says Drury. "I want my kids to see that no matter what age you are, if you set a goal and work toward it, you can achieve it. And I want them to know that when you feed your heart and soul with aspiration, what you get from it is so much more than what you give."

PART II

NUTRITION

I have never heard anyone say that they started training for a marathon so that they could eat more fruits and vegetables. In fact, most people joke that the sole reason to run long distances is to burn off a double-cheese pizza or earn the right to spend quality time with Ben & Jerry.

But every runner learns it one way or another: When you're prepping for a marathon or half-marathon, you can't run to eat, you gotta eat to run.

When you're in training, food becomes fuel. It will energize your run and help repair muscle tissue after a hard workout so that you can bounce back quickly for your next run.

Try to fuel up on Krispy Kreme or down a five-course meal before you go out and you could hit the wall halfway through or end up spending most of your run crouching in the bushes. Have a big meal the night before a long run and you could wake up with a food hangover: You still feel full and have the aftertaste of last night's meal, yet you're slightly hungry at the same time.

You can do all the training you want, but if you don't eat and drink the right things and get to know your own gut, it doesn't matter if you've got the leg and lung power of an Olympian: Your stomach will take you down every time.

In the next section, you'll find out everything you need to know about eating like an athlete. In Chapter 4, you'll learn about the best foods to include in your diet during training, how much of each nutrient to consume (as well as the best sources of those nutrients), plus how to manage special diets—like vegetarian and gluten-free—while in training. In Chapter 5, you'll learn how to eat and hydrate before, during, and after runs and how to avoid digestion problems. And in Chapter 6, you'll learn how to avoid weight gain during training, which is a surprisingly easy thing to do.

CHAPTER 4

EVERYDAY EATING

Even if you're not looking to lose weight, as you start marathon or half-marathon training, you need the right mix of foods and nutrients to feel good on your runs and to stay injury free. About 55 percent of your daily calories should come from carbs, 25 percent should come from protein, and another 15 to 20 percent should come from unsaturated fats. But there's no need to start carrying around a calculator. Don't obsess. At each meal, just devote half of your plate to carbs, one-quarter of your plate to protein, and another quarter to healthy fats.

Throughout training, your nutrition needs are going to change. During the first few weeks, when you're building your base and your weekly mileage and intensity remain low, you're not going to need as much fuel as you will later in training, when you're doing speedwork and long runs. If you'd like to know exactly how much carbs, protein, and fat to consume during each stage of training, see "The Right Fuel at the Right Time" on page 82.

Carbs. The popularity of low-carb diets over the past 20 years has given carbohydrates a bad rap. Diets like Atkins and South Beach urge people to curb carbs to help control spikes in blood sugar and insulin surges,

both of which can lead to weight gain.

That approach might work fine for dieters, but it won't work for runners. Carbs are the main source of glucose, which your muscles use for fuel. Slash your carbs too much, and you risk running out of gas on your runs. Keep carbs in your diet, and you'll be able to run faster, longer—which means you'll burn more calories. Studies have shown that athletes who consumed the most carbs had faster times.[1] But that's not license to belly up to the all-you-can-eat pasta bar. The key is to get the right types of carbs at the right time.

Some carbs are "fast," meaning that your body can digest them quickly and use them for energy in a hurry. Foods like candy, gels, plain bagels, and white bread provide a quick energy boost right before a workout or help keep you from hitting the wall during a long run. After a run, fast carbs can help restock spent glycogen stores in a jiffy.

Beyond the quick energy boost, fast carbs don't offer much benefit, and often have calories and additives that you don't need. Plenty of runners start pounding the baked goods as soon as they start training—all in the name of carb loading—but the truth is, you really need fast carbs only right before and during exercise.

Most of the foods in your everyday diet should be "slow" carbs. These foods are high in fiber, are digested slowly, and help you maintain a steady level of energy throughout a run. Fruits, whole grains, vegetables, oatmeal, and beans are all good examples of slow carbs that also provide vitamins, minerals, and antioxidants to help you stay healthy and recover quickly.

Amby's Advice

It makes sense to increase your mileage and improve your diet at the same time. You can eat more, but make it fruits and veggies and high-fiber, whole grain products. Skip sugary drinks, like sodas and juices. They only add calories to your diet and won't benefit your training in any way. Stick to water and nonfat or low-fat dairy products.

Here's more about the foods you should be loading up on.

• **Whole grains.** Whole grain foods include the bran, germ, and endosperm—the parts of the grain that contain the nutritious B vitamins, iron, magnesium, selenium, and fiber that you need to run strong. When whole grains are refined into foods like white bread, the nutrients are lost, and so is the fiber. A diet rich in fiber helps lower cholesterol, reduce blood pressure, and decrease the risk of diabetes and heart disease. Fiber also helps keep your digestive system functioning regularly, slows the absorption of sugar, and keeps you feeling fuller for longer. Good sources include bulgur, whole oats, cornmeal, popcorn, brown rice, barley, wild rice, quinoa, whole grain pasta, and buckwheat. Remember: Just because bread is brown doesn't mean that it's whole grain. Look for labels that say 100 percent whole grain, or look for these terms on the list of ingredients: whole grain, whole wheat, stoneground whole oats, and oatmeal.[2] If you see terms like enriched flour, bran, or wheat germ, chances are the bread isn't whole grain.

• **Fruits and vegetables.** When you think of carbs, you might think only of bread and grains, but fresh produce can also provide the carbs you need to run strong. In addition to providing the fuel you need to run long, they offer plenty of vitamins, minerals, and antioxidants to keep your body in peak condition. To get the widest variety of nutrients, eat as many different kinds of vegetables as possible: carrots, tomatoes, leafy greens, and more. Among fruits, choose berries, melons, grapes, apples, and oranges. And eat the skin when possible; it provides even more fiber and nutrients.

Protein. Runners need protein to help recover from the hard work of training. Protein is comprised of amino acids, compounds that help repair muscles and strengthen immunity. And since protein takes longer to digest, it makes you feel fuller for longer, which can aid with weight loss. Choose products that are lower in saturated fat, such as skinless chicken, pork, and lean cuts of beef; fish (such as salmon and tuna); soy; low-fat dairy (like yogurt and cottage cheese); and beans and lentils.

With the popularity of high-protein diets in recent years, there has been an explosion of supplements, bars, shakes, and drinks on the market, many of them containing protein from egg, soy, hemp, or whey. So, do you need them? As long as you're getting plenty of protein in your diet, probably not. It's best to get protein from whole foods, which have nutrients like fiber and iron—nutrients these engineered foods may lack. But if you can't tolerate solids after a hard workout or if you're not getting enough protein, they can be good alternatives. (For a list of good protein sources for runners, see pages 88 to 89.)

Fats. Like carbs, fat has gotten a bad rap in

the last 20 years. As a result, runners avoided oils, butter, nuts, and other fatty foods. But fat plays a key role in keeping runners healthy. Research has shown that those who consume a very low-fat diet have less endurance and fatigue sooner than runners who consume a healthy amount of fat. A 2008 study[3] found that runners who were getting a lower-than-recommended amount of fats were more likely to have running-related injuries than those who didn't.

There are a few potential reasons for that, says Kristen Gerlach, PT, PhD, assistant professor in the physical therapy program at St. Catherine University and coauthor of the study. Polyunsaturated fats (PUFAs) have anti-inflammatory properties, so they may help repair the microscopic muscle tears and bone breakdown that happen after a hard workout.

Dietary fat also helps the body absorb fat-soluble nutrients, including vitamins D and K,

BART SAYS...

Running is a lifestyle. You have to think about it 24 hours a day, 7 days a week—not just the 60 to 90 minutes a day that you spend running. With decisions you make throughout the day—when you're ordering at a restaurant or deciding to have that second beer—you've got to ask, "Is this good for my training?" You don't have to be a hermit or a purist, just be sensible and have balance.

both of which are vital for bone health, and vitamin E, which acts as an antioxidant and helps keep the body from breaking down. Omega-3 fatty acids—the polyunsaturated fats found in salmon, walnuts, and ground flaxseed—help fight inflammation and soothe aches and pains. And because fats promote the feeling of being full, they're good for runners who want to shed pounds. They also prevent blood sugar spikes and crashes, as well as the cycle of craving and overeating that can trip up your training. Some research has shown that monounsaturated fats (MUFAs) help reduce belly fat.[4]

But not so fast with that Snickers bar! The key is to eat moderate amounts of the right kinds of fats at the right time. Focus on healthy unsaturated fats from avocados, nuts, seeds, and olive oil; these fats lower bad cholesterol and help reduce your risk of heart disease. Stay away from saturated and trans fats because they raise your levels of bad cholesterol (LDL). Trans fats also lower good cholesterol levels

Fat Facts

TYPE OF FAT (OR FATTY ACIDS)	HOW IT AFFECTS HEALTH	FOOD SOURCES
MONOUNSATURATED FAT (MUFA)	Lowers total cholesterol and LDL (bad) cholesterol levels.	Vegetable and nut oils including almond, avocado, canola, olive, peanut, pecan, and pistachio.
POLYUNSATURATED FAT (PUFA) INCLUDES THE OMEGA-3 AND OMEGA-6 FATTY ACIDS ALPHALINOLENIC ACID (ALA), EICOSAPENTAENOIC ACID (EPA), DOCOSAHEXAENOIC ACID (DHA)	Promotes heart health by decreasing LDL (bad) cholesterol levels. Also linked to lower rates of heart attack and heart-related deaths.	Vegetable oils (including corn, safflower, soy, and sunflower) and nuts. EPA and DHA are found in fatty fish (such as cod, halibut, mackerel, and salmon) and enriched eggs. ALA comes from plants and can be found in flaxseed, walnuts, vegetable-oil-based soft spreads, and canola, soybean, and flaxseed oils.
SATURATED FAT	Can lead to high cholesterol.[5]	Animal-based fats including full-fat dairy, butter, lard, and marbled meats (including bacon), and tropical oils such as coconut and palm.
TRANS FATS	Raises total cholesterol levels and risk for cardio-vascular disease. Also raises LDL (bad) cholesterol while decreasing HDL (good) cholesterol levels.	Fried and baked foods (such as crackers and cookies), stick margarines, and foods that contain partially hydrogenated oils.

(HDL) and increase your risk of heart disease. It can be confusing to keep it all straight, so let the chart opposite be your guide.

Vegetarian Diets and Runners

Despite having finished six marathons by the time he was 57 years old, renowned foodie Mark Bittman was overweight and had high blood sugar and cholesterol, sleep apnea, and a bad knee. His doctor told him to become a vegan. Impossible in his line of work—Bittman writes a cooking column for the *New York Times* and has authored three books about food and cooking—yet he recognized that he did need to make a change.

"I realized I had to significantly increase the proportion of plant foods compared to everything else in my diet—both for my health and the planet," he says.

He started incorporating more plant-based foods into his diet, and soon his apnea, blood sugar, and cholesterol were under control.

"I didn't notice much difference in my running," says Bittman, who has now finished eight marathons with a 4:01 PR.

Indeed, Bittman discovered what scientists have now proven: Switching to a plant-based diet can improve your health and won't take anything away from your running.[6] In fact, because vegetarians are in many cases replacing meat—which can be high in saturated fat

and cholesterol—with fruits, vegetables, and plant-based proteins, their diets tend to be higher in fiber and essential nutrients. Vegetarians tend to have lower risks of heart disease, blood pressure, and type 2 diabetes, as well as lower cancer rates.

Researchers have found that vegetarians following a well-balanced diet get the protein, carbs, and fats they need, simply because so many plant-based foods are rich in those nutrients, as well as other vitamins and minerals. Many people just report feeling better once they make the switch. *Runner's World* Challenger Josephine DeCicco, 55, a two-time marathoner from New York, says she just feels "lighter" since she stopped eating meat 4 years ago. "I just feel better when I'm running," she says, "and I don't have that heavy feeling that I used to get after eating meat."

Not only that, but her appetite completely changed. Once she started replacing meat and processed animal products with wholesome grains, proteins, fruits, and vegetables, she found herself craving more whole foods. "I can't stand processed foods," she says. "I feel like I can almost taste the chemicals in them. And I think that's just a by-product of eating better all around."

All of those good feelings aside, it is tougher to get some nutrients if you don't eat meat—including omega-3 fatty acids, vitamin B_{12}, zinc, and iron. By consuming a diet rich in whole grains, fortified foods,

What it takes to . . .
Manage marathon training and diabetes

Ramgopal Venkataraman, 47, Dallas, TX
Assistant professor of accounting at Southern Methodist University, father of two
Experience: 9 marathons; 4:25 PR
Runner's World **Challenge Race: 2011 Big Sur International Marathon**

I was diagnosed with type 2 diabetes 15 years ago. At first I was really hesitant about exercise and would only go to the gym. But about 7 years ago, when I turned 40, a marathon became a life goal to check off my bucket list. So I started running.

Aside from taking my diabetes medication and checking my blood sugar, in a lot of ways, the way I manage my food and training isn't that different from what other runners do.

But I do have to take some precautions. During a run, I have to make sure that my blood sugar doesn't go too low, so I always carry energy gel with me. I always have my blood sugar monitor and glucose tablets in the car. I bring my cell phone, and I always make sure that someone in the group knows that I'm a diabetic.

You always have to be aware of your own body, but fear isn't necessary. The mileage ramps up gradually during marathon training, so you don't get overwhelmed and you're able to gradually get acclimated to it. And during races, if I feel like I just don't have it, I have no problem slowing down. You hear about so many people who have all different health issues because they have a fatal illness or have lost a limb, and you see that it's really not a big deal to run with diabetes. With medication and diet planning, it's nothing to be afraid of. And I just love the marathon training process. You get to be outside with friends, and what could be more fun than that?

and complete proteins, you won't have to worry about falling short. That's why, says D. Enette Larson-Meyer, author of *Vegetarian Sports Nutrition,* variety is the most important ingredient for any runner becoming a vegetarian.

"Sometimes when people make the switch they aren't familiar enough with a wide array of foods," says Larson-Meyer, an assistant professor and director of the Nutrition and Exercise Lab at the University of Wyoming. "If you're eating that same bean burrito or spaghetti every day, you're not going to get the calories you need for the hard training, or the key nutrients you need."

If you're thinking of becoming a vegetarian or just considering reducing your meat intake, don't make any sudden moves. Start with one vegetarian meal a day, and slowly start eating more plant-based foods. A gradual switch will help keep your energy level high—and your running pace intact. If you are a vegetarian, we've outlined some simple guidelines for you to get the nutrition you need so that you feel good throughout your training.

Protein. Vegetarians don't necessarily need more protein than meat eaters do; they just need to make sure they're getting enough—especially during training (see the "The Right Fuel at the Right Time" table on page 82). You can get the protein you need from a variety of soy products, beans, legumes, nuts, and whole grains, and it's best to get a little at each meal. Add peanut butter to your bagel, toss some lentils into your pasta sauce, or add chickpeas to a salad. Meat substitutes like soy burgers or crumbled soy (for use in traditional meat-based dishes such as lasagna) can provide even more. If you still choose to eat dairy products and eggs, protein won't be a problem.

Because most vegetable sources of protein don't have all of the essential amino acids your body needs, vegetarians were long advised to combine certain foods— like beans and rice—at each and every meal to ensure that protein could be absorbed properly by the body. But now experts recognize that this is really not an issue. If you eat an assortment of proteins and whole grains, seeds, nuts, and vegetables throughout the day, your protein needs will be met. If one food is low in an essential amino acid, another will make up for the deficit. "As long as you get a variety of plant proteins throughout the day," says Dawn Blatner, RD, CSSD, a spokesperson for the American Dietetic Association, "your body pools the amino acids, and you get the nutrients you need." Good grains that complement vegetable-based proteins include quinoa, which has up to 50 percent more protein than other grains, as well as calcium and B vitamins. Amaranth has protein, fiber, calcium, iron, and a balance of amino acids.

Iron. Iron is critical to running because it's involved in transporting oxygen to your muscles, and therefore aids in digestion, metabolism, and circulation. You can get your iron from beans, soy, legumes, seeds, nuts, lentils, tofu, whole grains, kale, and spinach. The body doesn't absorb iron as well from plant-based foods, but vitamin C can help with that. Pair your iron with foods like oranges, strawberries, lemons, and red peppers to help you better absorb the iron you need.

Vitamin B$_{12}$. This nutrient, widely available in animal-based foods, is essential to tissue repair, plays a role in making red blood cells, and helps your body convert food to energy. You can get B$_{12}$ from eggs, fish, and cheese, but if you don't consume any fish or dairy products, it's important to consume a supplemental source such as nutritional yeast and fortified foods (like cereals, soy milk, or meat substitutes). You don't need a lot of B_{12}—experts recommend just 2.4 micrograms daily—but go without it and you could end up with anemia and irreversible nerve damage. "B_{12} is a really important component for building tissue," says Larson-Meyer. "If you're a vegan, taking a B_{12} supplement is really key."

Zinc. Zinc boosts immune function and protein synthesis and is involved in the growth and repair of muscle tissues. Because a lot of zinc can be lost in urine after a hard workout, it's important to make an effort to replenish your body's supply. Good sources of zinc include legumes, hard cheeses (like Parmesan), whole grains, nuts, seeds, and soy.

Sodium. Healthy as many vegetarian items are, if they're processed, they can be high in sodium. When considering items like veggie burgers, look for products with less than 400 milligrams of sodium per serving, and serve them with natural whole foods, like salads and fruits, instead of chips or fries.

Gluten-Free Eating

Carbs play a leading role in any runner's diet. They break down into glucose and serve as the body's main fuel source during a run, then provide more energy afterward. Cut the carbs and you'll hit the wall, hard.

But many of runners' favorite carbs—like bread, bagels, and pasta—are also full of gluten, a protein found in wheat, spelt, kamut, barley, and rye. For runners with celiac disease (CD) or gluten intolerance (GI), consuming gluten can lead to severe digestion problems, including stomach cramping, diarrhea, constipation, and bloating. But in recent years, the explosion of gluten-free items, along with a wave of books and Web sites professing the benefits of going without gluten (saying that it eases inflammation and speeds performance), has many runners wondering whether they should give up gluten.

If you haven't been diagnosed with celiac disease or gluten intolerance, going gluten-free isn't likely to be a miracle performance enhancer for you. But if avoiding gluten means that you're staying away from cookies, crackers, and highly processed foods that have extra calories and few nutritional benefits, and you're eating more whole foods that are packed with nutrients and minerals, it's likely you'll feel better when you're on the road.

And while you won't be eating pasta or bread, other carbs will do and will provide even more nutrients. Carbs like fruits, vegetables, nuts, and beans are all naturally gluten-free, as are whole grains like quinoa, brown rice, oats, buckwheat, and amaranth.

If you miss pasta, bread, cakes, and cookies, there are a variety of gluten-free versions made with flour from rice, chickpeas, and other substances; rely on these to ease your cravings. Just beware: Some foods are full of added fats, which can lead to weight gain.

Hydration

Hydration is important, and not just when you're on the road. Fluids regulate body temperature, move waste from your body, ensure that your joints are adequately lubricated, and help flush out the damaged cells that can lead to inflammation. And proper hydration can help control cravings, which is important because it's often easy to mistake thirst for hunger.

While there's no set recommendation for daily fluid intake, a good rule of thumb is to aim to drink about half of your body weight in ounces each day. (So if you weigh 150 pounds, drink 75 ounces of water.) And you don't have to just guzzle water. Fruits and vegetables, which are about 80 percent water, can also help you stay hydrated. Plus they're packed with antioxidants, which boost muscle recovery and immunity.

— [WHAT WORKS]

Eat before you get hungry

Catherine Saint Louis, 37, Brooklyn, NY; reporter, mother of one; 1 marathon; 4:07;
***Runner's World* Challenge race: 2009 Richmond Marathon**

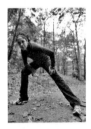

When I started preparing for a marathon, I wanted to lose 25 pounds after giving birth to my son. When you're in training you can get pretty crazy hungry. But I never let myself get to a starving place because it's just so easy to eat whatever when you're that hungry. I always kept my tank full. I was pretty calculating about snacks. I never thought, "Oh, if I get hungry, I'll just get whatever they have." I had to start asking, "What will really satisfy me?" I always packed my meals and snacks for the day. I snacked on things like dried fruit, KIND bars, and dried oatmeal biscuits with almond butter. I didn't skimp on carbs, but I ate mostly whole wheat pasta, brown rice, and sweet potatoes. If you're truly hungry, you'll be satisfied with something healthy. And by the time I got to the 2009 Richmond Marathon, those 25 pounds were gone!

The Right Fuel at the Right Time

Most nutritionists say that runners should split their calories into 55 percent carbs, 25 percent protein, and 15 to 20 percent healthy fats. But your needs will vary depending on how much you weigh and where you are in your training season. Here is a guide to designing your diet to suit your needs throughout the stages of training.

Weeks 1–6 (marathon) and Weeks 1–4 (half-marathon)

During the first few weeks of training, you're building your base and gradually increasing your mileage. If you want to lose weight, focus on doing it during this phase. You don't want to be slashing calories during the heaviest speed sessions and long runs later.

	Type of Activity	Amount Needed Daily*
Carbs	Moderate-duration and low-intensity training (30 minutes/day at a conversational pace)	2.5 g/lb of body weight/day
	Moderate to heavy training (1 hour/day)	3–4 g/lb of body weight/day
	Extreme training (>4–6 hours/day)	5 g/lb of body weight/day
Protein		0.7 g/lb of body weight/day
Fats		0.4 g/lb of body weight/day

Weeks 7–13 (marathon) and Weeks 5–8 (half-marathon)

As you start to hit the track for speedwork and your long runs stretch to 15 to 20 miles, you're going to need to rely on all the nutrients to fuel your workouts and aid recovery. If you were trying to shed pounds, it's best not to do it now.

Carbs	3 g/lb of body weight/day
Protein	0.75 g/lb of body weight/day
Fats	0.4 g/lb of body weight/day

Weeks 14–16 (marathon) and Weeks 9–10 (half-marathon)

As you taper for the race, running fewer miles but keeping up the intensity, you're going to need more carbs to restock those glycogen stores so your muscles are primed and ready to run fast.

Carbs	3.5 g/lb of body weight/day; increase to 5 g/lb during race week
Protein	0.7 g/lb of body weight/day
Fats	0.4 g/lb of body weight/day

Race Day and Recovery

Whether you cover 26.2 or 13.1 miles, it's best to take a few weeks to recover by cross-training and running fewer miles. It's common to gain weight during this time. Avoid that by decreasing your consumption of calories and nutrients.

Carbs	2.5 g/lb of body weight/day
Protein	0.6 g/lb of body weight/day
Fats	0.4 g/lb of body weight/day

*Amount needed daily is an average and is based on recent clinical research and findings, as well as anecdotal evidence provided by runners.

Putting Numbers into Practice

Now that you have a better understanding of how much fuel you need during various stages of training, you may be wondering how to design a diet around these recommendations. To help you fuel properly, the tables to follow offer sample meal plans for a 130-pound runner and a 165-pound runner.

Weeks 1–6 (marathon) and Weeks 1–4 (half-marathon)

130-pound runner:* 325 g carbs (moderate training), 90 g protein, 52 g fat

165-pound runner:* 410 g carbs (moderate training), 115 g protein, 66 g fat

Meal	130-Pound Runner	165-Pound Runner
Breakfast	2 slices whole wheat toast 1 Tbsp jam 1/2 cup low-fat cottage cheese 1/2 cup fresh berries	2 slices whole wheat toast 2 Tbsp jam 3/4 cup low-fat cottage cheese 1 cup fresh berries
Lunch	1 veggie burger patty 1 whole wheat bun 1 Tbsp shredded cheese 1 cup diced pineapple	1 veggie burger patty 1 whole wheat bun 1 Tbsp shredded cheese 1 cup diced pineapple
Dinner	4 oz grilled pork tenderloin 1 cup wild rice topped with 1 Tbsp olive oil 1 cup steamed vegetables 1 cup berry cobbler	6 oz grilled pork tenderloin 1 cup wild rice topped with 1 Tbsp olive oil 1 cup steamed vegetables 1 cup berry cobbler
Snack #1	1 cup bran flakes 1 cup skim milk 1 cup strawberry halves 1/4 cup ground nuts	2 cups bran flakes 1 cup skim milk 1 cup strawberry halves 1/4 cup ground nuts
Snack #2	1 large apple 1 cup skim milk	1 large apple 1 Tbsp caramel dip 1 cup skim milk

*Your nutrition goals may be higher or lower depending on your intensity of training, weekly mileage, and other physiological factors.

Weeks 7–13 (marathon) and Weeks 5–8 (half-marathon)

130-pound runner:* 390 g carbs, 95 g protein, 52 g fat

165-pound runner:* 495 g carb, 120 g protein, 66 g fat

Meal	130-Pound Runner	165-Pound Runner
Breakfast	3 mini whole grain bagels 1 Tbsp low-fat cream cheese 1 cup fresh berries	4 mini whole grain bagels 2 Tbsp low-fat cream cheese 1 cup fresh berries
Lunch	Wrap made with: 1 whole wheat tortilla, 3 oz lean deli meat, 1 cup chopped vegetables 1 medium peach	Wrap made with: 1 whole wheat tortilla, 3 oz lean deli meat, 1 cup chopped vegetables 1 medium peach
Dinner	3 oz grilled chicken breast 2 cups cooked pasta (choose whole wheat or whole grain) ½ cup pasta sauce 1 cup cooked spinach 1 Tbsp shredded mozzarella cheese, part-skim, low-moisture	3 oz grilled chicken breast 3 cups cooked pasta (choose whole wheat or whole grain) 1 cup pasta sauce 1 cup cooked spinach 2 Tbsp shredded mozzarella cheese, part-skim, low-moisture
Snack #1	1 whole grain English muffin 1 Tbsp margarine 1 Tbsp jam 1 cup low-fat yogurt 1 fresh orange	1 whole grain English muffin 1 Tbsp margarine 1 Tbsp jam 1 cup low-fat yogurt 1 fresh orange
Snack #2	1 medium banana 1 whole grain English muffin 1 Tbsp natural peanut butter	1 medium banana 1 cup melon 1 whole grain English muffin 1 poached egg 2 tsp margarine

*Your nutrition goals may be higher or lower depending on your intensity of training, weekly mileage, and other physiological factors.

Weeks 14–16 (marathon) and Weeks 9–10 (half-marathon)

130-pound runner:* 455 g carbs, 90 g protein, 52 g fat

165-pound runner:* 575 g carbs, 115 g protein, 66 g fat

Meal	130-Pound Runner	165-Pound Runner
Breakfast	2 low-fat waffles 2 Tbsp maple syrup 1 medium banana 12 oz green tea with 1 Tbsp honey	3 low-fat waffles 3 Tbsp maple syrup 1 medium banana 12 oz green tea with 1 Tbsp honey
Lunch	Wrap made with: 1 whole wheat tortilla, 4 oz lean deli meat, 1 cup chopped vegetables 1 medium peach 1 oz pretzels	Wrap made with: 1 whole wheat tortilla, 4 oz lean deli meat, 1 cup chopped vegetables 1 medium peach 2 oz pretzels
Dinner	1 cup cooked whole wheat or whole grain pasta topped with 1/2 cup marinara sauce 1 cup steamed vegetables, and 1 tsp Parmesan cheese 6 oz Greek yogurt	2 cups cooked whole wheat or whole grain pasta topped with 1 cup marinara sauce 1 cup steamed vegetables, and 1 tsp Parmesan cheese 6 oz Greek yogurt
Snack #1	2 packets plain oatmeal made with 1 cup skim milk 1/4 cup chopped dates	2 packets plain oatmeal made with 1 cup skim milk 1/4 cup chopped dates
Snack #2	1 large apple 1 cup skim milk	1 medium banana

*Your nutrition goals may be higher or lower depending on your intensity of training, weekly mileage, and other physiological factors.

Race Day and Recovery

130-pound runner:* 260 g carbs, 80 g protein, 52 g fat

165-pound runner:* 330 g carbs, 100 g protein, 66 g fat

Meal	130-Pound Runner	165-Pound Runner
Breakfast	2 slices whole wheat bread topped with: 1 poached egg Baby spinach leaves Sliced tomato 8 oz skim milk 1 cup pink grapefruit	2 slices 100% whole wheat bread topped with: 2 tsp margarine 1 poached egg Baby spinach leaves Sliced tomato 8 oz skim milk 1 cup pink grapefruit
Lunch	3 oz grilled salmon atop 2 cups chopped lettuce and 1 cup chopped vegetables 2 Tbsp vinaigrette dressing 6 whole wheat crackers 1 cup mixed fruit	3 oz grilled salmon atop 2 cups chopped lettuce and 1 cup chopped vegetables 3 Tbsp vinaigrette dressing 6 whole wheat crackers 1 cup mixed fruit
Dinner	1 cup vegetarian chili topped with 2 Tbsp shredded cheese 1 oz baked tortilla chips 1 cup chopped tomatoes topped with cilantro vinaigrette 8 oz skim milk	1 cup vegetarian chili topped with 2 Tbsp shredded cheese 1 oz baked tortilla chips 1 cup chopped tomatoes topped with cilantro vinaigrette 8 oz skim milk
Snack #1	1 cup raisin bran 1 medium banana 1 Tbsp roasted pecans 1 cup skim milk	2 cups raisin bran 1 medium banana 1 Tbsp roasted pecans 1 cup skim milk
Snack #2		PB & J: 2 slices whole wheat bread, 2 Tbsp jam, 2 Tbsp peanut butter

*Your nutrition goals may be higher or lower depending on your intensity of training, weekly mileage, and other physiological factors.

Put This in Your Cart

In order to fuel your marathon and half-marathon training, focus on eating foods that pack the most nutrients.

Carbs

Food	Carbs (grams)	Extra Benefits for Runners
Whole-grain pasta (1/3–1/2 cup cooked)	about 15	It contains more fiber, vitamins, minerals, and protein than white pasta. All of those nutrients help with muscle repair, recovery, and heart health.
Whole-grain bread (1 slice)	15–20	Provides fiber plus essential B vitamins.
Oranges (1 small)	15	Provides 100 percent of daily recommended intake of vitamin C, which helps lower cholesterol and prevent muscle soreness.
Sweet potatoes (1 small, about 3 1/2 oz)	28	Good source of vitamin A, vitamin C, potassium, iron, and manganese, which helps optimize muscle function.
Berries (1 cup)	20	Blueberries, blackberries, and raspberries all have antioxidants, which help ward off disease and muscle soreness.
Steel cut oats (1/2 cup)	27	With more fiber than other types of oatmeal, these oats take longer to digest, so you'll stay fuller longer. They also contain beta-glucan, which may improve immunity, along with protein, iron, fiber, calcium, folate, and vitamin A.
Raisins (2 Tbsp)	30	High in potassium and iron, which helps carry oxygen throughout the body.
Apples	19	Quercetin, a flavonoid that is also in grapes, onions, and tea, may reduce your risk of upper-respiratory infections. Be sure to eat the peel; all of the quercetin, as well as a healthy dose of fiber, is in the skin.
Kamut, black rice, amaranth, and quinoa (1/4 cup raw)	29	These ancient grains or grain-like products provide carbs and whole grains along with protein, vitamins, and minerals.
Tomatoes (1/2 cup canned)	8	Tomatoes are rich in vitamin C and lycopene, a phytonutrient that protects against various types of cancer.

Protein

Food	Protein (grams)	Extra Benefits for Runners
Chicken (4 oz of skinless, white meat)	28	Contains selenium, which helps protect muscles from free-radical damage that can occur during running, and niacin, which helps regulate how much fat is burned during a run.
Lean beef (3½ oz; cuts with *loin* or *round* or *90% lean* are going to be the best)	26	Boosts iron and zinc to keep your immune system healthy.
Pork (3 oz)	22	Pork has iron levels similar to beef, but with one-third less fat. It contains thiamin, riboflavin, and B vitamins that are involved in energy production from food.
Salmon (3 oz)	22	Choose canned for additional calcium. Choose any variety for a healthy dose of vitamin B_{12}.
Egg (1 whole)	6	Eggs are rich in protein and choline—a nutrient not found in many foods, but one that is vital for healthy brain cells and memory. Choose omega-3–enhanced eggs to increase your intake of healthy fats.
Black beans (1 cup, canned)	15	In addition to protein, black beans provide fiber and folate, a B vitamin that plays a key role in heart health and circulation.
Lentils (1 cup, canned)	18	High in iron, which helps transport oxygen. Also contains fiber.
Low-fat yogurt, plain (8 oz)	12	Provides calcium and vitamin D. Yogurts labeled "live active cultures" or "probiotics" can keep your digestive system working optimally and give your immune system a boost.
Greek yogurt (6 oz)	10–15	Greek yogurt packs more protein, calcium, and vitamin D into every spoonful. Aim for a variety that is low-fat or fat-free.
Milk (1 cup)	8	Milk contains bone-building calcium and vitamin D, so drink up for bone health (but choose a low-fat variety for heart health!).
Kidney beans (1 cup, canned)	13	Besides being rich in iron, kidney beans are also rich in fiber, providing 11 g per serving.
Chickpeas (1 cup, canned)	12–15	Provides manganese, which helps build healthy bones, and also aids with regulating blood sugar, absorption of calcium, and metabolism.
Tofu (4 ounces, firm)	20	Made from soy, it's packed with calcium and can help lower cholesterol and the risk of heart disease.

Protein (cont.)

Food	Protein (grams)	Extra Benefits for Runners
Quinoa (1 cup, cooked)	9	Grain-like and contains fiber, complex carbs, and all the essential amino acids, the building blocks for your body to make more proteins and build muscle.
Peanut butter (2 Tbsp)	8	Peanuts provide more protein per ounce than other nuts, saving you calories while helping you rebuild muscles.
Almonds (¼ cup)	8	Provide vitamin E, which helps build a strong circulatory system and acts as an antioxidant, which helps prevent cell damage. Almonds also have heart-healthy monounsaturated fats and help lower cholesterol.
Sunflower seeds (¼ cup)	6	Contains fiber, vitamin E, and B vitamins.

Fats

Food	Fats (grams)	Extra Benefits for Runners
Avocado (½ cup or ⅓ medium avocado)	11	Rich in vitamin B_6, which gives the immune system a boost; lutein, which helps with eye health; and vitamin E, an antioxidant that protects cells from damage.
Dry roasted nuts (1 oz)	12–15	Rich in magnesium, a critical component for muscle and nerve function. Also contains 5 g of protein.
Canola and vegetable oils (1 Tbsp)	14	Prized for a mild taste and ease of cooking, canola is comprised of 62 percent MUFAs and 13 percent PUFAs, leaving little room for artery-clogging saturated fat.
Salmon (3 oz, cooked)	4–7	Any variety of this fatty fish is rich in inflammation-fighting omega-3 fatty acids, which also boost heart health, reduce high blood pressure, and help control blood glucose levels.
Olive oil (1 Tbsp)	14	Rich in monounsaturated fat, which can lower your risk of heart disease. Choose extra-virgin or virgin olive oils, which are the least processed and contain the highest levels of polyphenols, which promote heart health.

→RW CHALLENGER PROFILE:
Christine and James Orr

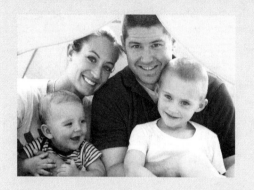

In 2010, Christine and James Orr were reeling.

Their infant son, John, had just been diagnosed with severe type A hemophilia, a rare condition that causes spontaneous internal bleeding and requires daily transfusions. Minor scrapes and cuts that a Band-Aid would fix for other kids required trips to the ER for John. He would get deep bruises just sitting in the bathtub. With health care bills piling up at a rate of $12,000 a week, they were facing losing their insurance. Having recently moved hundreds of miles away from their family and friends, and also caring for their 4-year-old son, Jimmy, they felt vulnerable and alone.

"Hearing the diagnosis, and finding out what it meant for him and for us, was a huge blow to our family," says Christine, 35, who lives in Menlo Park, California. "I felt like I had the floor pulled out from under me."

James and Christine had run casually in the past—just 3 to 4 miles for fitness—but after John's diagnosis, those runs became their daily medicine: time to wrap their heads around their new reality, brief respites from their hypervigilance concerning every move or sound John made, a temporary escape from fear's iron grip. Running helped them reach deep below the well of helplessness and vulnerability that consumed them, to tap into the physical and mental strength they so desperately needed to cope with their day-to-day reality.

"Maybe it was the sweat or the fresh air or the sense of accomplishment," says Christine, "but it always brought me a sense of peace. And it just made me feel fixed."

Soon, 3 to 4 miles wasn't enough; they needed more time and more miles and more healing. So they signed up for a marathon: the 2010 San Francisco Marathon with the *Runner's World* Challenge.

Christine hadn't run a marathon since high school and James, a former lacrosse player, had never run one at all. Though marathon training required sweat and blisters and sore muscles, the discipline and routine kept them accountable to the running that had such a healing power.

"It forced us to take care of ourselves," says Christine. "If it hadn't been for the program, we would have probably ended up on antidepressants."

And the rhythm of training gave them some quality of normality that the rest of their lives so sorely lacked. James would wake at 3:45 a.m. to get his run in before getting to the

Runner's World Challenge Race: 2010 San Francisco Marathon

office at 6:00 a.m.; Christine would run while pushing both kids in a double jogging stroller 8 to 10 miles each day through the hills of San Francisco. She would park the stroller at the track while she did her Yasso 800s.

On days when she couldn't get out, she'd do a workout DVD at home. They'd trade off watching the kids for long runs; she'd finish a 15-miler and return home so exhilarated that she wanted to do it again.

"Long runs were my solace—and my paycheck," she says. "They made me feel fresh and fixed. I would come home from a run in the rain and the fog, just grinning from ear to ear. People would look at me like I was high. I just wanted to tell them, 'You have no idea how good this feels.'"

They ran the marathon side by side for the first 17 miles. Christine finished in 4:11, and James finished in 4:45. Seven months later, Christine finished the P.F. Chang's Rock 'n' Roll Marathon in 3:31. James finished the half-marathon in 2:01. They went on to train for the 2011 Big Sur International Marathon with the Challenge; Christine met her goal and finished in 3:38; James finished in 4:33, beating his time from the San Francisco race by 12 minutes. Christine went on to run a 3:29 at the 2011 California International Marathon.

"Life had handed us a huge lemon," says Christine, "and training for a marathon was how we could make it lemonade. It was just the only way we could get through this."

CHAPTER 5

EATING BEFORE YOU RUN, ON THE ROAD, AND AFTER YOU'RE DONE

When it comes to fueling your runs, timing is everything. Go out on an empty stomach, and you could end up crashing and burning. Eat the wrong food before you go, and you might end up running for the bathroom. Neglect to refuel after a 20-miler, and you risk ruining your next run.

It's important to strike the delicate balance between getting enough fuel to stay energized and not eating so much that you end up nauseous and cramped—or worse. Get the balance wrong, and all the hard work you did developing your legs and lungs could be for naught.

"Ninety-nine percent of how well you do on race day will have to do with what you ate or drank or didn't leading up to the race," says Lisa Dorfman, MS, RD, CSSD, LMHC, director of sports medicine nutrition and performance at the University of Miami. "Even the best runners in the world have cramped up because of doing the wrong thing the day before."

Like so many other aspects of training, there are general guidelines to follow but no one-size-fits-all formula. Runners are unique in terms of how much and what kinds of foods and drinks they need, and what they can or can't tolerate. The only way to find your own foolproof solution is to use the weeks of training to experiment with different forms of fuel and find out which ones give you the most energy without leaving you with an upset stomach.

In this chapter, you'll learn everything you need to know about fueling before you go, on the road, and after you're done. We'll offer you the tools to figure out what, how much, and when to eat. Then it's up to you to figure out your own personal prescription.

Eating Before the Run

What you eat before you hit the road all depends on when you're running and what kind of workout you're planning. Many people don't have the time—or the stomach—to eat and digest food before a run, especially in the early morning. For an easy-paced run of 60 minutes or less, going without food or drink probably won't do you any harm. (Just make sure you're staying hydrated; see the tips on page 96.) But for any run that's longer or more intense—say, a session of mile repeats or a 10-mile run—prerun fuel is critical. Go out on empty and you'll fatigue sooner, plus you'll have a much tougher time hitting your pace targets.

For high-intensity workouts, like speedwork or tempo runs, prerun fuel is especially important. That's because you're burning through carbs faster than when you're ambling along at an easy pace. You may have enough stored glycogen to see you through the workout, but you'll perform better if you top off your tank before you go. Have a high-carb meal 2 to 3 hours before you run, or have a small high-carb snack or drink about 30 minutes beforehand. (An energy gel or chew will do in a pinch.)

Runner's World Challenger Adam Wall, a 3:06 marathoner from New York City, learned about the perils of running on empty during a track workout. He forgot to snack before his mile repeats, and "I just bonked horribly," says Wall, a father of two and COO of the electronic trading business of a bank. "It was the most bizarre sensation. There was absolutely nothing in the tank—no energy. In the end, I realized that I ultimately wasted the workout."

If you're running long, say 12 to 23 miles, you want to start fueling and hydrating the day before. You don't necessarily need to increase your calories—just make sure that carbs make up the bulk of lunch and dinner. Your body will absorb and store

BART SAYS...

Don't do long runs on an empty stomach. Experiment to find out what types of foods work for you. You want to find your "comfy food": That's the food that you enjoy, that goes down well, and that makes you feel comfortable while you're on the road.

Amby's Advice

There are only three times to consume simple and processed carbs, including sugar: Immediately before your run, while you're on the road, and immediately after you're done running. Don't overeat or overdrink during your long runs; there's too much risk of getting an upset stomach. Practice to find out what you can have and how much you can take without running into stomach trouble.

the nutrients, and you'll be able to rely on those fuel stores during the next day's run. Have your main meal at midday and a smaller meal for dinner so that you have plenty of time to digest before you go to sleep.

The morning of your long run, start fueling 2 to 3 hours before you go. Aim for 300 calories for each hour before your run. (So if you're going for a run in one hour, have 300 calories. If you're going for a run in 2 hours, have 600 calories.) And whatever you eat, make sure it's high in carbohydrates.

When should you fill your tank? Each runner is different, but in general, the bigger the prerun meal, the more time you'll need to digest it. After a 200- to 300-calorie meal, you could be ready to hit the road in 30 to 60 minutes. Any more calories, and you'll want to wait 60 to 90 minutes before you start your run. See "Prerun Fueling" below for easy reference.

So what's the perfect prerun meal? Familiar foods that are easy on your system, low in fat and fiber, and high in carbs will boost your energy without upsetting your stomach. Check out Appendix B on pages 242 to 250 for some ideas.

Eating on the Run

When you're on the road for less than 75 minutes, you can rely on water, sports drinks, and your body's own glycogen stores. Any longer, and you begin to deplete those stores. Your muscles run out of fuel, and your body—not to mention your attitude—starts to drag. Consuming carbs midrun can keep

Prerun Fueling

TYPE OF RUN	HOW MUCH TO EAT	WHEN TO EAT IT
Up to 75 minutes	100–200 calories of high-carb, low-fat, low-fiber food	30–60 minutes before your run
75 minutes or longer	300 calories for each hour before the run	60–120 minutes before your run
Speed session (mile repeats, tempo runs, Yasso 800s)	High-carb meal or 100- to 200-calorie high-carb snack	2–3 hours before your run for a regular meal; 30 minutes before your run for a snack

your blood sugar steady so you don't crash and burn.

The key is to fuel at regular intervals, and before you need to. Wait until you're out of gas, and you won't be able to recover from feeling hungry or weak. Your muscles will be forced to play catch-up, and you won't be able to bounce back and finish the run feeling strong.

Runner's World Challenger Kelly Schwarting (below), an 11-time marathoner from Edmonds, Washington, learned that lesson the hard way. While training for her first marathon, she figured she'd wing it with water and energy gels.

"I knew I needed to eat something, I just didn't know how much or when," says Schwarting. "It was completely hit or miss, as was the success of my runs."

Experiment with different brands and fla-vors of energy gels and sports drinks, and find out what sits well in your stomach. Each brand has its own proprietary blend of sugars and other ingredients. You may respond better to one than another, and you may prefer certain flavors or textures.

As you're road-testing your fuel sources, be sure to try the brand that will be provided at the race. If it doesn't sit well with you, plan to bring your own on race day.

Eating for Recovery

Come in from a gut-busting session at the track or a long run and all you want to do is shower and collapse, right? Not so fast.

What you do in the half hour following a long run or a hard workout can determine the quality of your next run and whether or not

(continued on page 98)

--- **[WHAT WORKS]** ----------------------------

Have a fueling strategy from the start

Kelly Schwarting, 45, Edmonds, WA; account manager, mother of three; 11 marathons; 3:32 PR; *Runner's World* Challenge Race: 2010 Toronto Marathon

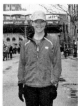

Don't wait until you're feeling weak or hungry to take in carbs. Have an energy chew or gel and water every 40 to 45 minutes to avoid hitting the wall. Don't try to gut out anything more than 10 miles without food or water in an effort to toughen yourself up. You'll destroy the quality of your run and plant the seeds of doubt that you'll bonk during the race. I made that mistake and was very nervous going into my first marathon.

Hydration: Take It Personally

"How much should I drink?" is a simple enough question. But the answer is not always so easy or so clear.

For years, runners were warned to hydrate, hydrate, hydrate—regardless of thirst—or risk dehydration. More recently, runners have been warned not to overdo the drinking, as it can lead to hyponatremia, a potentially fatal condition that comes from excessive fluid intake leading to low blood sodium levels.

So what's the deal?

Yes, you need to stay hydrated. Water affects every body function—it helps transport nutrients throughout your body, flushes waste products from your muscles, regulates your body temperature, and much more. When you're significantly dehydrated (generally that's when you lose 2 to 3 percent or more of your body weight in fluids), your body has to work harder to perform all those functions. Your blood volume drops, which forces your heart to beat faster, and it becomes more difficult to keep up with the cardiovascular demands of running. It becomes harder to concentrate, and your level of effort spikes. It's risky to your health, and needless to say, it makes your performance suffer.

Overhydrating, on the other hand, has its own dangers. Hyponatremia, or "water intoxication," happens when you take in more water (or other fluids that contain minimal or no electrolytes) than you lose through sweat. In rare, extreme cases, hyponatremia can trigger seizures, coma, and even death. Women seem to be more at risk for this condition, as are novice marathoners. "Inexperienced and slower runners have a greater risk of overconsuming because they're out on the course for longer and tend to drink at every water station," says Michael F. Bergeron, PhD, director for the National Institute for Athletic Health and Performance at Sanford Health in Sioux Falls, South Dakota.

"The faster you are, the better hydrated you are at the start, and the less you sweat during a run, the less you need to be overly concerned with getting dehydrated, losing too many electrolytes, or drinking too much," Bergeron says.

So what's a runner to do? While there's been much debate on the subject, there are a few guidelines on which the experts agree.

Customize your plan. Though many runners can stay sufficiently hydrated with 15 to 20 ounces of fluid per hour on the road, sweating—and thus fluid and electrolyte needs—vary widely from person to person based on size, speed, weather conditions, heat acclimatization, genetics, and fitness level. While one runner might be fine on 16 ounces of water per hour, another might need 32 ounces. If you're a salty sweater (your skin is covered with salt and your clothes are smeared white after a run), you may need more fluids or electrolytes than others.[1]

Use your thirst as a guide. Timothy Noakes, MD, author of *Lore of Running* and a professor of exercise and sports science at the University of Cape Town in South Africa, says that drinking to quench thirst is the best strategy. Drinking more or less than that can hurt your performance and lead to health problems.[2] But, Bergeron cautions, that may not work in all conditions. If you're running in a very dry climate, for instance, your mouth might get very dry, very fast, and so you might overdo the fluids. In other cases, just a bit of cold water in your mouth may readily quench your thirst even though you need more fluid.

Take the sweat test. If you want to get an estimate of how much fluid you lose when you run, and therefore how much you need to replace, weigh yourself naked before and after an hour-long run. (See "The Sweat Test" on page 99.) Keep in mind, though, that in order to get the best estimate of how much to drink for your marathon, you'd have to take the sweat test in the exact same conditions as the ones you'll face on race day. See what the average conditions are on race day and make sure to do the test in those conditions and run at your planned race pace. Your best bet is to take the sweat test in a variety of conditions, record your findings in your training log, and refer to it on race day.[3]

Do the bathroom test. When you're well hydrated, your urine should be pale yellow—the color of lemonade or light straw. So hit the bathroom before you head off to a run. If your urine looks dark—like apple juice—you're clearly not drinking enough.

Sip, don't swig. Set your watch to beep every 15 minutes on the road as a reminder to consider your thirst, and have a drink if you need one. You'll be a lot more comfortable taking in a little bit at a time. If you wait until you're parched and gulp 20 ounces of sports drink all at once, you could end up feeling nauseated and experience a sloshing feeling in your stomach.

Don't just use water. On any run longer than 45 minutes, choose a drink that contains a combination of carbohydrates and electrolytes, which can help sustain electrolyte-fluid balance and exercise performance.[4] There are plenty of sports drinks on the market that fit the bill. Read the labels. The carbs will help keep your energy levels stable, and the electrolytes will help prevent hyponatremia (depletion of sodium) and maintain better body water distribution.

Respect the conditions. When the temperature spikes, you're going to sweat more and fatigue faster. So when it's super hot and humid, you're going to need to drink more than you usually do. If you're really worried about dehydration, it's best to run slower so you'll sweat at a lower rate and stay in balance.

Road Rules

In order to avoid common pitfalls associated with fueling on the go, follow these rules of the road.

Practice, practice, practice. Train your gut during long runs so that it's accustomed to receiving foods and fluids while on the go.

Watch what you eat. Look at the nutrition content of each gel, chew, or other fuel source you're using. Follow the instructions to determine how much water to consume with each source.

Chase it with water. Always chase gels, chews, or blocks with water. Try to wash them down with a sports drink and you'll end up taking unwanted bathroom stops or feeling nauseated.

Carry it on. Find a lightweight, comfortable waist pack or fuel belt to easily carry your sport beans, gels, or chews. Some running shorts also include pockets designed to carry gels and chews. If you don't have gear, try fastening the packages to your shorts with safety pins.

Pack your own. When your hands are slippery, packages of gels or chews can be tricky to open on the go. Try taking your gels or chews out of their original packages and putting them in a snack-size zipper-lock bag for your long run or race.

Take it slow. Eat your gels, beans, or chews slowly. Trying to gulp down all of the fuel in one quick bite could cause you to choke or to feel stick to your stomach.

you can stay injury free throughout training, says Suzanne Girard Eberle, MS, RD, CSSD, a board-certified sports dietitian and author of *Endurance Sports Nutrition.*

The 30 to 60 minutes after your run is prime time for recovery. That's when your body is ready to restock glycogen stores and start repairing muscle tissue so you can bounce back for your next run, Eberle says.

After exercising, and particularly after a hard workout like a tempo session or a long run, blood flow to your muscles increases. At that time, your body is more sensitive to insu-

lin, which shuttles glucose into your muscles, where it's converted into glycogen and stored until your body needs it for fuel. Along with glucose, insulin also cues your muscles to pick up protein to jump-start muscle repair. Wait any longer, and your body won't absorb glucose and other nutrients as readily, and you'll end up feeling more tired. You might not feel it right away, but the cumulative effect of weeks and months of hard and long running—without proper refueling—will wear you down before you get to the starting line.

"A lot of runners miss this whole window,

and that's where they get into trouble," says Eberle. "It will start taking longer to recover, increase the risk of injury, and it can make training seem harder than it needs to be."

Refueling is most important if you're out for an intense effort—such as an interval session, a tempo run, or a long run of 1 hour or more—that taxes your muscles and drains your muscle glycogen stores. For a 30-minute easy run at less than 60 percent of maximum heart rate, refueling isn't going to be as critical. Even so, Eberle recommends eating right away, just to get into the habit of tying your meals to your workouts.

How many carbs do you need for recovery? Divide your weight in half and eat that many grams of carbs. (A 120-pound runner would aim for 60 grams.) Make sure your meal has a carbs-to-protein ratio of 4:1. (Meaning that same 120-pound runner would aim for about 15 grams of protein.) Don't stress about hitting the exact ratio; just make sure you're getting both carbs and protein. Then try to eat that same balance of carbs and protein 2 hours later. For postrun meal ideas, check out Appendix B on pages 242 to 250.

How much should you drink? That will vary widely depending on your fitness level, the weather, and how much you sweat. Your best bet is to do the sweat test (below). When you're rehydrated, your urine will be the color of lemonade. If it's darker—say, the color of apple juice—or you haven't gone for a few hours, drink more.

Rehydrating is probably the most critical step of the recovery process. Water supports

The Sweat Test

Your size, the length of your run, the weather conditions, and your pace affect what you should drink during your run. This "sweat test" is a good way to estimate how much fluid you need. Redo the test during different seasons, with different workouts, in different weather conditions, and as your fitness changes.

1. Weigh yourself without clothes right before a run.

2. Run at race pace for 1 hour, keeping track of how much you drink during the run.

3. After the run, strip down, towel off any sweat, and weigh yourself nude again.

4. Subtract your postrun weight from your prerun weight and convert it to ounces (1 pound = 16 ounces).

5. Add to that number however many ounces of liquid you consumed on your run. (For example, if you lost 1 pound and drank 16 ounces during your run, your total fluid loss is 32 ounces and you'll need to drink 32 ounces of water and electrolytes to remain hydrated on similar runs.)

so many of your body's critical functions, including bringing nutrients and oxygen to your cells via your blood and flushing waste products out of your muscles. If you're dehydrated, "the body has to work that much harder to perform all those functions," says Eberle. As a result, you're going to feel fatigued, and it's going to take longer to recover.

Running into Trouble

Dale Hammond went into his first 10-miler fully prepared to refuel on the road. One hour into the run, he had a gel and washed it down with a sports drink.

"Within 5 minutes, I was doubled over with stomach cramps," says Hammond, 36, a father of three from Spokane, Washington. "I tried to keep going, but whenever I turned up the intensity, the cramps came back. After about 30 minutes of walking, I was finally able to run again."

Hammond is hardly alone. It has been reported that more than one-third of all runners complain of stomach distress during a race.[5] Gastrointestinal issues can lead to cramps, nausea, bloating, and diarrhea. These symptoms can make finishing a workout painful, or even impossible.

To some extent, stomach trouble is unavoidable. When you run, blood is diverted to your leg muscles and away from your gastrointestinal (GI) tract, which disrupts the normal digestion process. Even more blood is diverted during intense runs like races and speedwork, which is why so many folks only get sick on those occasions. But you can take steps to reduce the chances that you'll run into trouble.

• **Watch the timing.** The more you eat before a run, the more time you'll need to digest. Allow 3 hours between a big meal and your run. And, of course, try to empty your system before a run. Coffee, tea, or any warm beverage can get your intestines moving, but watch the caffeine, as it can cause problems of its own. (For more on caffeine, see page 102.)

• **Make lunch your main meal.** What you eat in the 24 hours before a long run can have an impact on how your gut feels while you're on the road. Make lunch your main meal the day before your race or long run, so you have plenty of time to digest it, and then have a smaller meal for dinner.

• **Go low-fiber, low-fat, and low-protein.** All of these nutrients are good for your everyday diet, but they can wreak havoc on your stomach during a run. Stay away from certain vegetables, like broccoli, cauliflower, and cabbage, which can lead to bloating and gassiness. And keep fat and protein to a minimum.

• **Eat white.** Processed carbs that you keep out of your everyday diet make for ideal prerun meals. Foods like plain bagels, regular pasta, and white rice are easy to digest and provide fast energy.

• **Don't overdo the dairy.** The lactose in milk, cheese, and other dairy products can be hard for some people to digest. Try substituting your daily dairy with soy, rice, or almond milks, which don't contain lactose. Or look for milk and yogurt that contain live and active cultures. These products have added good bacteria that can help break down lactose.

• **Don't overload your system with carbs.** Your stomach can process only so many carbs at once, so if you take an energy gel, chase it with water, not a sports drink. If you're having a sports drink, don't take a gel at the same time.

• **Watch the sweeteners.** Some forms of sugar—like sorbitol, mannitol, fructose, glucose, and high-fructose corn syrup—that are used in energy gels and drinks just don't sit well with some runners. Different brands use different sweeteners, so check the ingredients and find the blend that works for you.[6]

Caffeine

Many runners rely on a prerun cup of coffee for an energy boost and to get the GI tract moving. While it has long been thought that caffeine leads to dehydration, recent research suggests that this might not be the case.

In a 2005 study in the *International Jour-*nal of Sport Nutrition and Exercise Metabolism,[7] moderate consumption of caffeine (59 men consumed 500 milligrams per day, or the amount in 4 to 5 cups of coffee) had the same effect on hydration status as a caffeine-free diet. And a group of studies found that caffeine lowers fatigue and perceived exertion; increases speed; boosts mood, endurance, and energy; and can boost performance by 3.2 to 4.3 percent.[8]

But Dr. Lawrence Armstrong, professor of exercise and environmental physiology at the University of Connecticut, cautions that each athlete is going to feel the effects differently. Some people get revved up from caffeine, while others feel no effect or have stomach troubles after consuming it. So it's important to test out caffeine during training and figure out how it affects you.

Runner's World Challenger Steve Maki drank only a single cup of coffee on weekdays, but on the morning of the 2010 Flying Pig Marathon, he ran into trouble after having one cup coupled with energy gels containing caffeine.

"I figured it wouldn't hurt, and it would wake me up a bit," says Maki, an accountant and father of six. "Big mistake."

About 40 minutes into the race, he felt nauseous and dizzy. His heart rate soared, and he had to walk for about a mile, dashing his hope of a 3:30 finish. "It was just a lesson I had to learn the hard way," he says.

Armstrong emphasizes that moderation is

Caffeine Cheat Sheet

A guide to the caffeine content of some common go-to drinks for runners:

- Brewed coffee (8 ounces): 133 mg (Can range from 102–200 mg)[9]
- Starbucks Café Latte (16 ounces): 150 mg[10]
- Decaf coffee (8 ounces): 5 mg (Can range from 3–12 mg)[11]
- Pepsi (20 ounces): 63 mg[12]
- Red Bull (1 can): 80 mg[13]
- Coke (20 ounces): 57 mg[14]
- Hershey's Dark Chocolate Bar (1.45 ounces): 25 mg[15]
- Hershey's Milk Chocolate Bar (1.55 ounces): 11.7 mg[16]

key. Studies haven't been done on the effects—good or bad—of caffeine in the long term or in doses higher than 600 mg per day.

"I wouldn't necessarily recommend starting to drink a caffeinated beverage if you're not already doing so," says sports nutritionist Nancy Clark, RD, author of *Nancy Clark's Food Guide for Marathoners*. "But if you already enjoy a cup of coffee, there's nothing wrong with it prerun."

And coffee isn't the only option to get your intestines moving, says Clark. Any warm beverage—like hot water, tea, or even decaf coffee—will do the trick, she says.

Alcohol

It goes without saying that running 13.1 or 26.2 miles is hard enough. The idea of taking on that distance drunk—or hung over—could be dreadful, not to mention dangerous. Yet many races offer beer at aid stations and at the finish line. And many marathoners belly up to the bar the night before the race.

Yes, beer can help replenish carbs. And studies have shown that in moderation wine, beer, and spirits help increase levels of HDL (good) cholesterol, prevent LDL (bad) cholesterol from clogging arteries and causing heart attacks, and lower blood pressure. Plus, resveratrol, an ingredient in red wine, can act as an antioxidant to help reduce cell damage.

However, the American Council of Sports Medicine (ACSM) says there are distinct downsides for runners. Drinking before a run will hurt your strength, power, speed, coordination, VO_2 max, and muscular and

INSIDE RUNNER'S WORLD ®

JEFF DENGATE, 35, *SENIOR EDITOR, RUNNER'S WORLD, JERSEY CITY, NJ*

LESSON LEARNED: WATCH WHAT YOU EAT THE NIGHT BEFORE A MARATHON

The night before the 2009 Adirondack Marathon, I ate a sausage sandwich at midnight. I'm not saying there's any connection here, because the sandwich sat well. But the next day, I couldn't hold down any fluids at all. Undeterred, I pressed on, trying to finish the marathon old-school—with no gels and no fluids. I was in second place in that race through 22 miles. Somewhere after mile 20, as the day heated up and the sun beat down on me, I started to lose my head; body control soon followed. I couldn't sense when my feet were actually connecting with the pavement. I was only able to pick up my legs and drop them, my forefoot slamming into the roadway. My pace slowed dramatically and there was little I could do. I fought on for a mile or so before coming to terms with my day ending early. I only finished that race because it would be quicker for me to walk and jog the rest of the way back to the finish/start area than it would have been to hitch a ride. The funny thing is that, over those last few miles, I could stomach all the Gatorade and water I wanted—too little, too late. I finished about 30 minutes off of my goal time. In races, I'm still struggling with what to take in. I don't like gels, plus those sugar loads make my energy levels feel too uneven, rising and crashing. Mostly I don't like having to carry anything, so on longer training runs, I'll head out with just a bottle of Cytomax.

cardiovascular endurance, and can lead to dehydration. What's more, alcohol will interfere with your muscles' ability to absorb glucose, the preferred source of fuel. [17]

So what's the deal? Do drinking and running mix?

A little wine or beer probably won't harm your running, as long as you're smart about it. It's best not to have a beer before a hard race or workout, or to drink while you're on the road. A drink or two is probably fine afterwards, experts say, as long as you rehydrate and refuel with nonalcoholic substances first. [18]

Following are some general guidelines on drinking and racing.

• **Wait 48.** The ACSM advises skipping alcohol for up to 48 hours before a marathon or half-marathon. Other experts say one drink with dinner the night before a race should be fine, as long as you take in plenty of water and carbs at the same time.

• **Food first.** Before lifting a glass at a

postrace party, have your recovery meal (a snack with a 4:1 ratio of carbs to protein) and rehydrate with 16 to 24 ounces of water or sports drink. If you start "recovering" with a beer, and then another, that important recovery snack may fall by the wayside.

• **Add water.** To combat alcohol's diuretic effect, drink an 8-ounce glass of water for every alcoholic beverage you consume.

• **Know your limits.** Moderate consumption of alcohol is fine, experts say. So what's moderate? For men, two drinks a day. For women, one drink a day. What's a drink? A 5-ounce glass of red or white wine, 12 ounces of regular beer, or 1½ ounces of 80-proof distilled spirits.

• **Know your own risk.** If you have certain health conditions, such as heart problems, high blood pressure, or type 1 diabetes, you are more at risk for complications from drinking. If you have a family history of alcohol abuse, then you are at a higher risk for developing drinking problems, as well.

Enduring Questions

I do my long runs at 5:00 a.m. and I can't get up at 3:00 a.m. to eat, nor can my stomach tolerate it. How do I fuel up for my runs?

If you can't—or don't want—to eat anything before a long run, that's okay. But if that's the case, it's especially important to make sure that you have high-carb meals at lunch and dinner the day before. Try to have your main meal at lunch and a smaller meal at dinner, so that you have plenty of time to digest them before you run. On your run, start fueling earlier than you might otherwise. If you're going out for, say, a 3-hour run, start fueling 30 minutes into your run, instead of waiting longer.

I have tried every brand of energy gel and chew on the market, and I can't stomach any of them! Are there any "real" foods I could eat during my long runs?

Try honey, dried fruit, or even pretzels. If you can't stomach those, either, you can use sports drinks to provide the carbs and electrolytes you need for your long runs.

I know I need to refuel, but I feel sick to my stomach after runs. I can't eat anything. What should I do?

Feeling queasy after a hard effort is very common. Studies have shown that aerobic exercise reduces hunger and affects hormones that suppress appetite.[19] Even if you don't feel like eating, it's best to try to get something down, as it will help you feel better and speed your recovery. If you feel too sick to stomach anything, it's okay to get your sodium and fuel from a recovery drink, energy bar, or gel, and then have a full meal a few hours later. You might want to try chocolate milk; it provides that 4:1 ratio of carbs to protein but probably won't strain your stomach. Or try bland foods like Cream of Wheat, crackers and cheese, or even a banana. You might also consider a smoothie. Smoothie recipes start on page 107.

Prerun Meal Ideas

Here are some high-carb, low-fat, low-fiber prerun meals to provide the energy you need to run your best. They're packed with nutrients to keep your body in peak condition throughout marathon training. Mix and match any of these foods to suit your tastes.

MEAL	NUTRITIONAL INFO*	HEALTH BENEFITS
6 oz low-fat fruit yogurt 1 medium peach	231 calories 46 g carbs	The peach offers carbs for fuel, plus potassium and antioxidants to boost immune function. The yogurt offers calcium and vitamin D to keep bones healthy.
2 oz pretzels (40 small) 2 Tbsp hummus	263 calories 49 g carbs	The pretzels offer simple carbs, plus sodium to help you stay hydrated. The hummus adds iron and a little protein.
2 whole grain waffles (frozen) 2 Tbsp maple syrup	294 calories 56 g carbs	Whole grain waffles offer slow carbs for long-lasting energy, while maple syrup adds some fast carbs, plus B vitamins that help with cell growth and metabolism.
PB&B sandwich: 1 medium banana 2 slices whole grain bread 1 Tbsp peanut butter	337 calories 53 g carbs	The whole grain bread offers slow carbs for energy and the banana adds B vitamins and potassium to help with muscle contraction. Peanut butter adds protein and healthy fats, plus niacin, which aids in recovery.
16 oz sports drink	125 calories 28–30 g carbs	Fluids with electrolytes help you stay hydrated and provide plenty of energy if you can't stomach solid foods.
2 oz honey whole wheat pretzels dipped in 1 Tbsp natural peanut butter	320 calories 49 g carbs	The easy-to-digest pretzels provide B vitamins such as thiamin, while the peanut butter provides long-lasting energy and heart-healthy fats.
1 cup apple cinnamon O's topped with 1 cup skim milk and 1 medium banana	255 calories 55 g carbs	The cereal offers carbs, plus it's fortified with vitamins and minerals. The milk offers calcium and vitamin D, while the banana adds B vitamins and potassium.
Turkey sandwich on 100% whole grain bread 1 apple	420 calories 72 g carbs	Whole grain bread provides long-lasting energy. The apple provides more energy, plus fiber, vitamin C, and antioxidants to help reduce cell damage.

*Estimates based on USDA nutrition database; specific calorie and carb counts may vary according to brand.

Postrun Meal Ideas

After you're done running, it's important to refuel fast—within 30 minutes—to restock your glycogen stores and jump-start muscle repair. These snacks meet your needs for carb and protein replenishment, and most have the 4:1 carbs-to-protein ratio you're looking for. Plus, they're packed with vitamins and minerals to keep you healthy throughout your training.

MEAL	NUTRITIONAL INFO*	HEALTH BENEFITS
8 oz low-fat chocolate milk 1 serving fresh fruit	225 calories 40 g carbs 9 g protein	Fresh fruit and milk help you rehydrate while providing calcium, vitamin D, and other vitamins and minerals.
1 oz pretzels dipped in 6 oz low-carb (protein-rich) yogurt	275 calories 50 g carbs 12 g protein	Pretzels offer carbs, plus sodium to help replenish electrolytes. Yogurt adds calcium and vitamin D.
Turkey sandwich with 2 slices whole grain bread, 4 thin slices deli turkey, and extra veggies	310 calories 55 g carbs 17 g protein	Higher in protein, this is your best choice following a tough workout or during a high-mileage week.
1 medium banana spread with 2 Tbsp peanut butter 8 oz recovery shake	380 calories 55 g carbs 12 g protein	The sports drink replenishes electrolytes and fluids, while the banana offers potassium to help with muscle contraction. The peanut butter adds healthy fats, plus niacin, which helps recovery.
1 whole egg (cooked in a nonstick skillet) on a toasted whole wheat English muffin 1¼ cups fresh blueberries 6 oz light yogurt	400 calories 67 g carbs 20 g protein	This snack is low in saturated fat and high in fiber. Blueberries contain antioxidants that help with muscle soreness and the yogurt adds calcium and vitamin D to keep bones healthy. The egg provides protein, B vitamins, and choline, all of which keep your immune system strong and your muscles ready for action.
Smoothie made with: 6 oz low-fat vanilla yogurt 2 Tbsp peanut butter 1 medium banana 2 Tbsp fat-free chocolate syrup	415 calories 66 g carbs 13 g protein	This meal is easy on the stomach if you can't tolerate solids after a hard workout. Yogurt provides calcium and protein, while peanut butter offers healthy fats and niacin. The chocolate syrup adds carbs and a sweet taste!

MEAL	NUTRITIONAL INFO*	HEALTH BENEFITS
2 whole grain pancakes topped with ½ cup canned fruit (drained) 12 oz English tea mixed with ½ cup skim milk and 1 Tbsp honey	330 calories 65 g carbs 13 g protein	Whole grains and fruit replenish your carbs and offer antioxidants. Tea provides antioxidants and phytochemicals, which can help prevent the months of heavy training from wearing you down. Milk provides calcium, and honey offers energy and other immune-boosting phytochemicals.
3 cups air-popped popcorn 8 oz low-fat chocolate milk	280 calories 46 g carbs 11 g protein	Popcorn provides carbs, fiber, and iron, and any salt you add will help you rehydrate. Milk provides calcium and carbs. And together they can satisfy a sweet-and-salty craving.

*Estimates based on USDA nutrition database; specific calorie and carb counts may vary according to brand.

Postrun Smoothies

Easy Run Low-Calorie Cooler

Your body doesn't need a ton of nutrients to recover from an easy run. That's why this smoothie uses almond milk—it has nearly half the calories of low-fat milk. Spinach, which has just 7 calories per cup, is one of the richest plant sources of iron, a mineral that helps transport oxygen to your muscles. Kiwis are high in vitamin C, which increases iron absorption. Frozen, creamy banana chills the smoothie and offsets the slightly bitter greens. This recipe is by sports nutritionist Cassie Dimmick, RD.

½ cup unsweetened almond milk

1 cup fresh spinach

1 kiwifruit, sliced

½ banana (preferably frozen), sliced

Place the milk, spinach, kiwifruit, and banana in a blender and blend until smooth.

Makes 1 serving
Per serving: 128 calories, 28 g carbs, 6 g fiber, 2 g protein, and 2 g fat

Crunchy Coffee Fix

Caffeine and carbs at the same time help your body restock muscle glycogen stores faster than carbs alone can. Natural cocoa powder—not Dutch-processed or alkalinized—provides anti-inflammatory antioxidants and delicious flavor for just a few calories. Bananas are rich in potassium, which helps maintain fluid balance. Almonds not only add a crunchy texture, but also contain heart-healthy fats that help keep you full. This recipe is by Cassie Dimmick, RD.

> **4 oz chilled coffee**
>
> **4 oz fat-free milk**
>
> **1 banana (preferably frozen), sliced**
>
> **2 Tbsp whole almonds**
>
> **2 tsp natural cocoa powder**

Place the coffee, milk, banana, almonds, and cocoa in a blender and blend until smooth.

Makes 1 serving
Per serving: 252 calories, 35 g carbs, 6 g fiber, 10 g protein, and 11 g fat

Savory Surprise

The carrot juice in this savory smoothie is rich in vitamin A, which helps regulate the immune system. Fresh ginger adds a sweet, peppery flavor, and studies have shown that it can reduce postexercise muscle pain. Avocado adds heart-healthy monounsaturated fats, and the capsaicin in cayenne pepper can boost metabolism, helping you burn a few extra calories. This recipe is by sports nutritionist Ilana Katz, RD.

> **6 oz carrot juice**
>
> **1/4 avocado**
>
> **1 Tbsp fresh lemon juice**
>
> **2 oz water**
>
> **1 Tbsp freshly grated ginger**
>
> **Pinch cayenne pepper**

Place the carrot juice, avocado, lemon juice, water, ginger, and pepper in a blender and blend until smooth.

Makes 1 serving
Per serving: 161 calories, 23 g carbs, 5 g fiber, 3 g protein, and 8 g fat

Breakfast to Go

Greek yogurt and milk provide lots of protein to repair your muscles after long runs. Oats are fiber-rich and digest slowly, providing long-lasting energy. Blueberries have a high level of antioxidants and help neutralize free radicals caused by exercise. Ground flaxseed provides a dose of omega-3 fatty acids that can help lower cholesterol. This recipe is by Cassie Dimmick, RD.

   1 cup fat-free milk

   ½ cup frozen blueberries

   ½ cup plain, fat-free Greek yogurt

   ¼ cup uncooked old-fashioned oats

   1 Tbsp ground flaxseed

Place the milk, blueberries, yogurt, oats, and flaxseed in a blender and blend until smooth.

Makes 1 serving
Per serving: 290 calories, 41 g carbs, 6 g fiber, 22 g protein, and 5 g fat

Maple Pumpkin Pie

Pumpkin is high in fiber and beta-carotene, an antioxidant that protects eye health. Silken tofu lends a thick consistency and, along with the soy milk, provides a nondairy source of protein, making this smoothie an ideal choice for lactose-intolerant runners. Studies show that regularly eating nuts and nut butters (including peanut butter) can lower your risk of developing heart disease and type 2 diabetes. Maple syrup adds sweetness as well as compounds that have anti-cancer properties, while cinnamon helps keep blood sugar levels steady. This recipe is by Ilana Katz, RD.

   ½ cup plain soy milk

   ⅓ cup canned pumpkin

   ⅓ cup silken tofu

   1 Tbsp natural peanut butter

   1 tsp real maple syrup

   ¼ tsp cinnamon

Place the milk, pumpkin, tofu, peanut butter, maple syrup, and cinnamon in a blender and blend until smooth.

Makes 1 serving
Per serving: 212 calories, 17 g carbs, 5 g fiber, 11 g protein, and 12 g fat

CHAPTER 6

WEIGHT MANAGEMENT

Like a lot of people, when Scott Alder started training for his first marathon, he figured he could eat whatever he wanted. After all, he had started running while trying to lose weight with the Jenny Craig diet plan, and the pounds had melted off.

But once he started preparing for the 2010 Portland Marathon, he quickly broke all the eating rules he had been following so carefully.

"I started putting in more miles, and I definitely let myself go overboard," says Alder, 50, who is in sales for a software security company from Portland, Oregon. He finished the race having gained 15 pounds, and he wanted to lose them before his next race.

"I learned that I can't eat everything I want just because I'm in marathon training."

While many people do lose weight while preparing to run marathons and half-marathons, training is certainly no guarantee. Plenty of folks maintain their weight or even end up at the starting line a few pounds heavier than before they started training. In fact, a 2010 Tufts University study of 64 marathon trainees found that just as many of the runners gained weight as lost.[1]

Why is that? Running alone—even marathon and half-marathon training—won't make you lose weight. If you want to shed pounds, you have to cut calories, too.

But where and what to cut? Conventional dieting strategies, like drastically slashing calories or cutting out carbs and fat, aren't the best approach. You'll end up feeling deprived and drained on all of your runs, and you'll be at risk for injury. And if the diet isn't sustainable, chances are that you'll end up regaining the weight.

But shedding pounds during marathon or half-marathon training isn't an impossible mission. The key is to strike a balance. You have to eat the right things at the right times and cut calories in all the right places.

Losing Weight on the Run

If you are trying to shed pounds on the way to the starting line, here are some rules to keep in mind:

1. Drop pounds early. If you're going to slash calories, do it before you start training or during the first 4 weeks of training, when the mileage and intensity are low. The closer you get to race day, the more you want to focus on adequately fueling and recovering from those speed sessions and long runs.

2. Take it slow. Aim to lose ½ pound per week, which means cutting about 250 calories per day—the equivalent of an energy bar or soda. Over the course of the week, that's 1,750 calories, which is ½ pound. By slowly tweaking your diet, you'll avoid severe feelings of deprivation. You'll give your body time to adjust to the reduced calorie load, and you'll have a better chance of sustaining it for the long term.

3. Stay in balance. In order to stay energized for your runs, and therefore perform well and burn the most calories, you're going to need the same balance of calories that all runners do: Roughly 55 percent of your calories should come from carbs, 25 percent from protein, and 20 percent from fats. Take out one of those nutrients, and you'll find your workouts will feel harder, you won't recover as well, and you'll feel drained all the time. Just make sure to include high-quality foods from each group. For carbs, choose fruits, vegetables, whole grains, beans, and lentils, which are also rich in fiber (to help you feel full longer), vitamins, and minerals. Choose unsaturated fats like olive oil, flaxseed oil, nuts, seeds, and avocados. The best sources of protein are lean meats, low-fat dairy, eggs, legumes, beans, and fish.

4. Get the timing right. You're going to need food most before and right after a run. Before a run you'll need carbs to get fast energy; right after a run you'll need carbs to restock your glycogen stores and protein to help repair muscle tissue. Eat your highest-carb meal of the day a few hours before your workout (see page 82). If you need a daily indulgence, have that sweet shortly

Amby's Advice

Many runners overestimate the number of calories they burn on a run and underestimate how many calories they take in after they're done. Unfortunately, it's hard to burn a lot of calories and easy to take in too many—especially through fast, fatty, sugary processed foods. Where possible, steer clear of processed, packaged foods, and choose whole foods instead.

after a run—during that 20-minute window when your muscles can quickly soak up the sugar to replace spent energy stores.

5. Eat real food. Many diet foods are too low in carbs, fiber, or protein to give you the nutrients you need to train, feel satisfied, and keep your body in peak condition. "Often foods that are trying to compromise one thing [like sugar or fat] don't make up for the nutrients that you'd get from the whole food," says Lisa Dorfman, MS, RD, CSSD, LMHC, director of sports medicine nutrition and performance at the University of Miami.

6. Become a food-label detective. Just because a food package says "healthy" or "organic" or "natural" doesn't mean that what's in it is good for you. Inspect nutrition-

Labels Matter

Food labels can be confusing. Here's how to decode them so you can watch what you eat.

Serving Size: Read the serving size first. Even some foods that look like they contain a single serving are actually two servings.

Fats: Total fat should be no more than 30 percent of total calories.

Sodium: Aim for less than 200 milligrams (mg) per serving most of the time.

Fiber: Aim for 25 to 30 grams (g) of fiber daily, or 14 g for every 1,000 calories consumed.

Saturated Fat: Less than 10 percent of calories should come from saturated fat; ideally, make it more like less than 7 percent.

Trans Fats: Try to avoid them completely. If you must consume them, keep total consumption below 2 g per day.

Ingredients: Listed in descending order by weight. If an ingredient is toward the beginning of the list, the product contains a large amount of it. If the ingredient is toward the end, the product contains only a small amount.

What It Says	What It Means
All natural	The food is minimally processed and contains no artificial colors or ingredients. May be high in sodium, fat, and salt.
Reduced fat	Contains at least 25 percent less fat per serving than the original version. Watch for added sugar, which can boost the calories.[2]
Low saturated fat	Contains 1 g or less of saturated fat per serving.
Low cholesterol	Contains 20 mg of cholesterol or less per serving. Contains 2 g or less of saturated fat.
Low fat	Contains 3 g of fat or less per serving.

fact labels and ingredient lists to figure out how healthy an item is, and compare it with other items. Research has shown that adults who read nutrition labels are more likely to lose weight than those who don't.[3] There's also the potential to go overboard on diet foods, figuring that if the Oreos are low-fat, that's license to eat the whole package. A 2006 study[4] found that people ate 28 percent more chocolate candies if the treats were portrayed as "low-fat" rather than "regular." Researchers concluded that low-fat labels make people underestimate calories and eat more. "Calories will add up even if they're from fat-free products or low-sugar products," Dorfman says. It's important to know what the claims on the labels really mean. (See below.)

What It Says	What It Means
Light	No standard definition. Sometimes means lower in fat and calories than similar products. (In the case of olive oil, just means it's lighter in color, but same number of calories and fat.)
Cholesterol free	Contains fewer than 2 mg of cholesterol per serving. But unless it contains eggs or milk, it probably didn't have any to begin with.
Low calorie	Contains 40 calories or less per serving.
Reduced sodium	Contains at least 25 percent less sodium than the original version.
Low sodium	Contains 140 mg of sodium or less per serving.
Very low sodium	Contains 35 mg of sodium or less per serving.
Reduced sugar	Contains at least 25 percent less sugar than the original version.
Low sugar	No standard definition.
No sugar added	Contains no table sugar, but there may be other added sugars or sweeteners like corn syrup, dextrose, fructose, glucose, maltose, or sucrose. Keep in mind that the American Heart Association recommends no more than 6 teaspoons of sugar for women and no more than 9 teaspoons of sugar for men.[5]
Sugar free	Contains less than 0.5 g of sugar per serving.
Fortified	Nutrients have been added that weren't in the original ingredients.
Recommended Dietary Allowance (RDA)	This is the government-recommended daily amount of various nutrients, vitamins, and minerals for healthy adults.

7. Vary your workouts. Running most days of the week will set the stage for weight loss, but stay too long in your comfort zone and eventually you'll reach a fitness plateau. "If you run the same 5-mile route at the same pace over and over," says exercise physiologist Pete McCall, a spokesman for the American Council on Exercise, "your body will become very efficient at it. To gain speed or strength, you've got to change some aspect of the training program, such as distance, intensity (exertion level), or volume (number of miles per week)." Boost your intensity and do different types of workouts—like cross-training, hillwork, or a long run—and you'll torch more calories and speed up weight loss. Try any of the rut-busting workouts starting on page 251 before you start marathon training, or during the first few weeks. These are hard workouts, so make sure to follow each with a rest day or an easy run.

8. Lift weights. Runners often avoid the gym. But pumping iron will help you burn more calories, increase lean body mass, and shed body fat. Each pound of muscle burns an additional 5 to 7 calories each day, says McCall. So when you build muscle, you increase your body's ability to burn calories. Research has shown that runners who add 3 days of resistance training exercises to their weekly program increase their leg strength and endurance.[6] And the stronger you get, the better your muscles become at producing a consistent amount of force over a long period of time, so it will be easier to maintain good form even when you're fatigued. McCall's advice: Twice a week, do a strength-training routine for your legs, chest, back, and shoulders. Exercise your

---

— [WHAT WORKS] —————————

Use portion control

Adam Wall, 36, New York, NY; COO of an electronic trading business of a bank, father of two; 4 marathons; 3:06 PR; *Runner's World* Challenge Race: 2009 Richmond Marathon

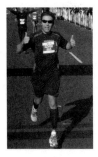

You're much better off having a small meal and then a snack, rather than just eating big meals. Before I started marathon training, I always ate healthy food—I was just eating way too much of it, like 800 to 1,000 calories for breakfast, dinner, and lunch. Eventually, I realized that I was much better off eating smaller meals and snacks. It's much more manageable that way. I ate fewer calories overall, and I didn't feel hungry. In just under 2 years, I was able to go from 230 pounds to 180 pounds and from a 3:54 marathon to a 3:06.

core, which stabilizes your body during running, three or four times a week.

9. Write it down. A 2008 study in the *American Journal of Preventive Medicine* found that among 1,700 overweight runners, those who kept a food diary more than 5 days a week lost almost twice as much weight as those who didn't, and they kept the weight off.[7] But even if you aren't looking to shed pounds, a food diary can provide valuable insight into what best fuels your running life and which unhealthy habits might be tripping up your training. Try to keep a journal for at least 3 days, and make sure one of those is a weekend day. And be honest: It can

Sample Food Diary

Monday, January 3

Today's goals:

- 2,000 calories
- Less than 15–20 g of saturated fat
- 275 g of carbs, 125 g of protein, 40 g of fat
- At least 28 g of fiber; less than 2,300 mg of sodium
- At least 30 minutes of physical activity

Meal & Time	Food	Calories	Fat	Carbs	Protein	Fiber	Sodium	Activity
Breakfast								
Morning snack								
Lunch								
Afternoon snack								
Dinner								
	Total intake							
	Goals	2,000	40 g	275 g	125 g	28 g	<2,300 mg	30 minutes of physical activity
	Differences (+/–)							

only help if you include everything! Take notes on:

- Anything that passes your lips—all meals, snacks, drinks, and condiments.

- The day, date, and time that you ate the food.

- Calories, carbs, fat, protein, fiber, saturated fat, and any other nutrients you'd like to track.

- The cooking method used (baked, fried, steamed).

- The brand name of any store-bought foods.

- The time and intensity of physical activity performed.

10. Catch some zzzs. Research has linked sleep loss to obesity and suggests that people who don't get enough sleep may weigh more. Without enough sleep, your energy levels, immune system, and mood drop—the only thing up (besides you) will be your appetite. Research has shown that

— [WHAT WORKS] —

Keep a food journal

Robert Nagle, 49, Paradise Valley, AZ; attorney, father of two; 12 marathons; 4:10 PR; *Runner's World* Challenge Race: 2011 Big Sur International Marathon

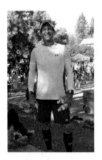

I used to train for marathons, and either my weight would remain the same or worse, it would go up slightly. I started logging what I ate and the calories I consumed. I started measuring my servings and found that smaller amounts were frequently enough to satisfy my hunger. So rather than a handful of almonds, I'd have ¼ cup (one serving size), which was sufficient. Rather than 300-plus calories, I had 160. Being able to see how much I was overeating and where there was room for improvement really helped. A food journal allows you to see how you're doing for the day and week, and where the big calories are coming from. For instance, I was having two cups of coffee with heavy cream each morning. Using the log, I realized that I was consuming hundreds of calories before I had put a single piece of food in my mouth. So I switched to 1 percent milk and one cup of coffee, for 37 calories. My acid reflux vanished. I've lost 50 pounds, and my body fat is down to 15.6 percent. Instead of extra-large shirts, I wear mediums. But most important, I never go hungry. I pretty much eat whatever I want (but with "normal" portion sizes), and I never have to pass on dessert. I had been 225 at one point, had gotten down to 180 using the Atkins diet, but then gained back to 195 pounds. Atkins was a good start, but like most diets, it ended up being a short-term solution because no one can live that way forever. You need to be able to just roll with everyone else.

people who get less sleep eat more snacks, especially high-carb ones.[8]

Avoiding Weight Gain

Rebecca Bosman always ate healthy; she wouldn't even have dressing on her salad. But once she started training for her first marathon, that all changed. "I felt like, 'Well, I ran 15 miles, I can have a cheeseburger with fries,'" she recalls.

Bosman ended up at the starting line 7 pounds heavier than before she started training.

"You spend all your time working out, trying to make your weight go one way, and it goes the other," says Bosman, 30, a mother of two from Troy, Michigan. "It's pretty frustrating."

Bosman experienced what so many other runners do: weight gain on the way to the starting line. While you are burning more calories once you start running more, it is way too easy to eat back those calories—and then some— during your training. Overcompensation, experts say, is one of the biggest issues that lead to weight gain during marathon training. Marathon coach and wellness consultant Mary Kennedy, the lead author of the Tufts study on weight gain among marathoners, found that many people tend to feel entitled to eat more food—and less healthy foods—just because they are training for a marathon. For others, it's the calories from high-carb snacks at aid stations, at the ends of long runs, and when they're out for celebratory events that can make people pack on those extra pounds.

Whatever the case, being mindful of what you put in your mouth is the key to training for a race without gaining any weight. "It's so important to pay attention to what you're eating and why you're eating it," says Kennedy. "Just because you're training doesn't give you license to eat whatever you want."

There are times during marathon training when you're going to be hungrier, she concedes, and you should eat more. But it's important to stick to the fundamentals of healthy eating.

Following are some tips on how to avoid tipping the scale on the way to the starting line.

Celebrate your successes with non-food rewards. Reward yourself for finishing your first long runs, setting PRs for distance,

BART SAYS...

I think 80 percent of runners would love to be 5 pounds lighter. But if this is your sport and your passion—not your livelihood—you've got to be smart about it. Don't think that you should deprive yourself of happiness. Those extra 5 pounds are not the end of the world. Try to get to your racing weight, but don't go overboard. There's a fine line between feeling good and feeling too light and weak.

Mars and Venus Get on the Scale

When it comes to losing weight, are there differences between men and women? Yes, and in this particular battle of the sexes, women aren't on the winning side. Studies have shown that men are more likely to lose body fat during an exercise program than women are. And a recent study showed that in women, exercise accelerates certain shifts in appetite-regulating hormones (resulting in higher levels of acylated ghrelin and lower levels of insulin), which leads women to be hungrier postexercise. As a result, they eat more and gain weight.[9] Researchers speculated that this is the female body's way of fighting energy deficits in order to preserve reproductive capability. (When women aren't getting enough calories, ovulation and hormones that make reproduction possible get suppressed.) Men are not as susceptible to these hormonal fluctuations, which makes them less likely to put on extra pounds.

and other achievements—just make sure those rewards aren't food. Get a new pair of running shoes, buy some cool new gear, go for a manicure, or treat yourself to a night out with friends.

Ask the experts. Lots of runners find that they get good guidance when they see a sports dietitian. Be sure to look for the credentials RD (which stands for registered dietitian) and CSSD (which stands for certified specialist in sports dietetics). Both credentials require testing and many hours of practice, so you can be assured that whomever you are working with will know what he or she is talking about. "Figuring out your [calorie] targets should be one of the first things you do during training," says Kennedy. "Just like you go and get fit for the right sneakers and figure out what clothing and running gear works best for you, you should take an hour to meet with a dietitian at the beginning of your train-

ing so you can understand what your calorie needs really are."

Cut the junk. If you radically reduce your calorie intake while increasing your calorie burn, injury and fatigue are all but assured. But if you slowly increase your training while slowly cutting back on those "extras" that aren't doing you any favors anyway, you can easily shed a few unwanted pounds without suffering fatigue and muscle breakdown. Replace your soda with water; swap whole grain bread for white; have dried fruit and nuts instead of M&M's; and trade your ice cream for nonfat Greek yogurt. You'll be surprised at how far a few small changes can go.

Watch the "sports" foods. There is a dizzying array of drinks, gels, and bars that advertise their benefits for recovery and energy, but many of those products are laden with calories and fats that most runners don't need for most of their runs. You'll want to have sports drinks and energy gels with you during long runs and on hot days, but beyond that, it's best to stick to whole foods. "People feel like they need to have all of these products because they're in training," says Kennedy. "And it takes a while to figure out that they don't need them."

Enduring Questions

Do gym machines accurately calculate calorie burn?

If you run on a treadmill, train on an elliptical, or pedal a stationary bike, the number of calories you actually burn can be 10 to 15 percent lower than what's displayed on the screen. That's because most machines don't take into account your percentage of body fat, height, sex, age, or resting heart rate, or if you're holding on to the handles, which reduces workload, says McCall. Also, the mechanical assistance of machines allows your body to do less work. That doesn't mean you should totally ignore an exercise machine's stats; use the calorie readout as a barometer of your progress. If the number goes up from one session to the next for the same workout, you know you're working harder toward your weight-loss goals.[10]

If I lose weight, will I get faster?

Healthy runners will race about 2 seconds per mile faster for every pound they lose. That is, as long as they stay in a healthy weight range (between 18.5 and 24.9 body mass index). Weight loss boosts maximal aerobic capacity (VO_2 max), because the less weight you carry around, the more miles per gallon you get from oxygen. And because losing a few pounds makes running easier, you should be able to increase your workout distance and speed. So losing weight helps you train harder. University of Dayton physiologist and runner Paul Vanderburgh, EdD, devised a calculator that he calls the "Flyer Handicap Calculator" to "equalize" performances among runners of different weights and ages."[11] (You can find it at snipurl.com/agesexweightcalc). Since the calculator factors in age, weight, and gender, it can be used to compare, say, a 25-year-old woman who weighs 120 pounds with her 55-year-old mother who weighs 165.

Do walking and running burn the same amount of calories?

Nope. In a 2004 study, researchers found that running a mile burned about 50 percent more calories than walking the same distance.[12] Why is that? When you walk, you keep your legs mostly straight, and your center of gravity moves along in a smooth, level way. When you're running, you actually jump from one foot to the other. This continual rise and fall of weight requires a tremendous amount of force (to fight gravity) and requires a lot more energy. That's why running burns more calories than walking. And since you can run 2 miles in the time it takes to walk 1, you can burn more calories in less time by running. That's not to say that walking is a waste; it's an excellent form of exercise that builds aerobic fitness, strengthens bones, and burns calories.[13]

Is it true that you always burn about 100 calories per mile when you're running, no matter how fast you're running?

Not exactly; 100 calories is just an estimate. A number of factors play into your running calorie burn, including your weight (the more you weigh, the more energy it's going to take

	TOTAL CALORIE BURN/MILE	NET CALORIE BURN/MILE
Running	0.75 × your weight (in lb)	0.63 × your weight (in lb)
Walking (3–4 mph)	0.53 × your weight (in lb)	0.30 × your weight (in lb)

to make your body run, so the more calories you'll burn), and your gender (men tend to have more muscle mass than women, so they burn more calories). The best way to determine the calorie cost of any activity is to determine the "net calorie burn," the amount of calories you burned during the workout minus your "sitting metabolic rate" (what you would have burned if you were sitting on the sofa doing nothing).[14] For more information, see chart above.

And keep in mind that how much you burn is going to change over time, depending on the following factors:

Weight loss. If you lose weight, and particularly if you lose body fat, you're going to start burning fewer calories per mile. You'll be carrying a lighter load, so it will take less energy (and fewer calories) to cover the same mile.

Experience. The more you run, the more efficient your biomechanics become, which means it will take less effort to run a mile than it did when you were just starting out.

Intensity. Studies have shown that the more intense the exercise, the longer your metabolism will stay elevated after the workout. In a study published in *Medicine and Science in Sports and Exercise,* athletes who cycled at 75 percent of VO_2 max for 20 minutes burned more calories after their workout than they did after cycling at just 50 percent of VO_2 max for 30 or 60 minutes.[15]

I've heard that running at a lower intensity burns more fat. Is that true? If so, isn't running slower the most efficient way to lose weight?

Not exactly. Higher-intensity workouts are actually going to be your biggest calorie burners and lead to weight loss. For most of your easy runs and long runs, when you're running between 50 and 70 percent of your max heart rate, your body is going to be burning equal amounts of fats and carbs. These lower-intensity runs make your legs and lungs stronger, and they increase your metabolism. But once you start running at a higher intensity, once you're working at 80 to 90 percent of max heart rate (say, during a tempo run or at the track), you'll start burning a higher proportion of carbs, and more calories overall. And since weight loss is the result of calories in being less than calories out, total calorie burn is the key. Plus, since higher-intensity exercise keeps your heart rate and metabolism high after you're done with your workout, you'll burn more calories even after you're done.[16]

I crave junk food during marathon training and have candy and chocolate far more often than I normally do. Why am I craving this stuff when I don't usually eat it?

One school of thought says cravings are your body's way of telling you it's in need of a certain nutrient. That may be the case if you're craving salty snacks (which have sodium) or even lots of red meat (which has iron). But when you're jonesin' for ice cream, cookies, or a candy bar, it's unlikely the result of a nutrient deficiency. Instead, you're either extremely hungry, or you're in the mind-set of "I just ran 10 miles—I deserve that Snickers bar!"

When you're piling on miles, you're burning more calories than you're accustomed to, and you're going to feel hunger pains and drops in blood sugar far more often than you're accustomed to. When that happens, anything that's not tied down starts to call your name. Instead of answering the call of the vending machine, try fortifying your diet with filling, nutritious foods like nuts and beans, which have protein to help

you feel fuller for longer. Snack on raw vegetables and hummus, and be sure to stay hydrated by sipping fluids throughout the day. (It's easy to mistake thirst for hunger.) So have about half your body weight in ounces. If you weigh 170 pounds, drink 85 ounces of fluids per day. If you're craving something sweet, plan ahead and pack an afternoon snack. Try some fruit, yogurt, and granola, or a banana-and-peanut-butter sandwich. If you're craving something salty, try air-popped popcorn; it's a whole grain, it's high in fiber, and it's filling. If you're bored and get into mindless eating, try sipping on flavored water or herbal tea. Any of these snacks will fill you up without filling you out.

INSIDE RUNNER'S WORLD ®

SEAN DOWNEY, 43, *SENIOR EDITOR, DOWNINGTOWN, PA*

LESSON LEARNED: LOSING WEIGHT HELPS YOU GET FASTER AND STAY INJURY FREE

When I started working at *Runner's World,* I was a 230-pound runner with shin splints who'd never covered more than 10 miles. I felt a little out of place amid all of the incredibly fit runners. I ran my first marathon in 2006 and finished three more over the next 2 years. As I trained, the extra pounds started slowly falling off. By the time I broke 4 hours at the 2007 Philadelphia Marathon, I weighed 207 pounds. I felt strong and fit, even though I was still sporting a spare tire. I figured that I didn't need to change my diet—I'd just run more. I started a food log, which was a major pain but extremely helpful. It helped me realize that it wasn't *what* I was eating, it was *how much.* I wasn't blowing my calories on cheeseburgers and ice cream; I was loading up on second helpings of stir-fry. And it made me reconsider those mindless small bites between meals—samples at the grocery, treats in the office, leftovers on my son's plate—because I didn't want to have to log every little thing. So I started snacking; a piece of fruit was all it took to take the edge off. Then I reduced the sizes of my meals and made some substitutions. I'd have a smaller bowl of cereal, for instance, and add blueberries. I lost 17 pounds and 2 inches off my waist in the 4 months leading up to the 2009 Richmond Marathon. And after maintaining my weight loss, I ran a 3:38 at the 2010 Richmond Marathon, setting a 17-minute PR, and I dropped down another belt size.

→*RW* CHALLENGER PROFILE:
Tony Digaetano

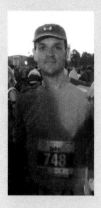

Tony Digaetano distinctly remembers his "get up or give up" moment: He was on a camping trip with friends, fell out of a raft, and endured merciless teasing as he tried to haul himself—at 275 pounds—back in.

"The teasing was good-natured," says Digaetano, a software developer from Crete, Illinois, "but it resonated pretty deeply."

But the signs that he needed to do *something* had been accumulating. Fears about diabetes, high blood pressure, and high cholesterol gnawed at him. He was tired all the time. He couldn't concentrate, and he frequently had an upset stomach.

But starting to run at age 37, after twenty years of slacking off, wasn't easy. He got on a treadmill, pressed some buttons, and hated every second—all 30 of them. Things hurt that he was sure weren't supposed to—first his shins, then his calves, and then his knees.

"I'd say I was seriously out of shape," he says, "but honestly, I was never in shape to begin with."

But every hurt eventually passed, and he got back on the treadmill and stuck with it. The running itself started to feel better, and he felt better mentally, no matter how badly his body hurt. A little less than a year after he started, he ran in a half-marathon, and 3 months later he ran in another one, finishing in 2:57.

"I fell in love with the physical and mental peace that accompanied a slow, steady rhythm," he says, "and I loved seeing such measurable improvements in pacing and speed, then taking that to a race to try to outdo myself."

His wife, Pam, began running too, and they started training and racing together. He also started eating less junk food and keeping a food journal to make sure his eating was supporting his running. He gave up caffeine, soda, and artificial sweetener. The less fat he ate, the less fatty food he could tolerate. He cut back on his meat, swapping turkey for steak, and eventually stopped eating meat altogether. Three years ago, dinner may have been two lean hamburgers, Tater Tots, and a diet soda or two. Now dinner might be whole wheat pasta with crushed tomatoes and spinach, or lentil tacos. Water is the drink of choice.

"I'm trying things that I just had no interest in tasting before—things like sweet potatoes, spinach, and chickpeas," he says. "I've discovered that these foods can actually be really tasty, which actually encourages me to eat well."

By the time Tony ran the Flying Pig Marathon in May 2010, he was 100 pounds lighter and deeply in love with running. He crossed the finish line in 4:52 feeling elated, like running a marathon again the next weekend. He ran the Air Force Marathon 4 months later in 4:43 with Pam, as she covered 26.2 miles for the first time.

Being 100 pounds thinner and becoming a runner is "like being a completely different person," he says. Each day, Tony bounds out of bed at 6:00 a.m., energized enough to go for a run or take on whatever the day may hold. He sleeps better, has an easier time focusing, and no longer has fears about cholesterol, high blood pressure, or diabetes.

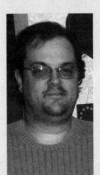

"I haven't felt this good for as long as I can remember," he says.

But the biggest changes he notices are the ways that running has changed him from the outside in. Family and friends say that he's much more friendly and open than before.

"I suspect that the huge boost marathon training has given to my self-image has actually allowed me the freedom to be less introverted," he says. Instead of being worried about what others think of him, he can think more about other people.

And life is much more directed than before, and not just when it comes to running. Projects that he tinkered with over the years now get done.

"Before I started training for a marathon, goals were hardly spoken, never quantified, rarely achievable, and never reached," he says. "They were just wishes."

But now that he's gone 26.2, he has evidence of just how strong he is, and he has the courage to go after the life that he wants. "It's one thing to know intellectually that I can do anything, but it's another to realize the truth of it," he says.

"I can see new challenges ahead, and they're not going to stay unconquered for long. Whether it's triathlons, trail races, ultras, or back-to-back races, it's all out there and I'm eager for more."

PART III

INJURY
PREVENTION

The most difficult challenge to conquer in any race, we often say, is getting to the starting line. Yet when most people sign up for marathons and half-marathons, they don't realize how formidable that challenge is.

We are constantly inundated with e-mails telling us about stress fractures, strained tendons, screaming IT bands, raging cases of plantar fasciitis, torn hamstrings, and runner's knee, not to mention sunburns and bloody blisters. In nearly every case, regardless of which body part is broken or bruised, the emotional fallout is usually worse than the physical injury.

"A few days before my marathon, I was diagnosed with a stress fracture and I was devastated," says *Runner's World* Challenger Katie Livingood, 29, of Jenks, Oklahoma. She had to take 6 weeks off. "I cried—a lot! It's a big deal to put so much effort into training for something, then have it taken away." Indeed, what runners often find once they get into training is that once you start to reap the emotional, social, and physical benefits of the sport, plus gain daily satisfaction from working toward your goal, it becomes much tougher to rest than to run.

Whenever sidelined by injury, "I feel like I'm on the fast track to getting old," says *Runner's World* Challenger Deb Dellapena, 45, of Wayne, Pennsylvania. "I feel less fit, get cranky, stress out about little things, and have trouble making decisions."

In this section, you'll hear from experts, as well as runners, on how to prevent injuries and how to deal with them when they—inevitably—occur.

CHAPTER 7

STAYING HEALTHY

In the mid-1970s, *Runner's World* medical editor George Sheehan, MD, confirmed that he was hardly the only runner beset by injuries: A poll of the magazine's readers revealed that 60 percent reported chronic problems. "One person in 100 is a motor genius" who doesn't have injuries, concluded the often-sidelined Sheehan.

With all of the amazing advances in sports medicine, you'd think our rates of shin splints and stress fractures would have dropped since Sheehan's era. But 30 years after running's first big boom, we continue to get hurt. A runnersworld.com poll revealed that 66 percent of respondents had suffered an injury in 2009.

After we interviewed the world's best injury-prevention experts on biomechanics, sports podiatry, and physical therapy, certain principles began to emerge. From them came the following laws of injury prevention. Incorporate these guidelines into your training, and you'll spend more time on the road and less time in rehab.[1]

1. Build mileage gradually.

It's easy to get injured; anyone can do it. Just run too much, too soon. "I firmly believe that every runner has an injury threshold," says physical therapist and biomechanist Irene Davis, PhD, director of the Spaulding National Running Center and a member of the department of physical medicine and rehabilitation at Harvard Medical School. "Your threshold could be at 10 miles a week, or 100, but once you exceed it, you get injured." Various studies have identified injury thresholds at 11, 25, and 40 miles per week. Your threshold is waiting for you to discover it.

Of course, your goal is to avoid injury. Runner and sports podiatrist Stephen Pribut, DPM, of Washington, DC, warns runners to beware the "terrible toos"—doing too much, too soon, too fast. Every research paper and every expert agrees that this is the number one cause of self-inflicted running injuries. The body needs time to adapt to training changes and increases in mileage or intensity. Muscles and joints need recovery time so they can handle more training demands. If you rush that process, you could break down rather than build up.

Experts have recognized this problem and long ago devised an easy-to-use 10 percent rule: Build your weekly training mileage by no more than 10 percent per week. If you run 10 miles the first week, do 11 miles the second week, about 12 miles the third week, and so on.

Yet there may be times when even a modest 10 percent increase proves too much. Biomechanist Reed Ferber, PhD, an associate professor in the faculty of kinesiology and director of the Running Injury Clinic at the University of Calgary, says he sees a lot of newly injured runners during the third month of marathon training, when a popular 16-week Canadian program pushes the mileage hard. Meanwhile, his clinic's 9-month marathon program for first-timers increases mileage by just 3 percent per week.

"We have a 97 percent success rate getting people through the entire program and to the marathon finish line," Ferber says.

Be the tortoise, not the hare. Increase your weekly and monthly running totals gradually. Use the 10 percent rule as a guideline, but realize that it might be too aggressive for

you—especially if you are injury-prone. A 5 or 3 percent increase might be more appropriate. In addition to following a hard-day/easy-day approach, or more likely a hard/easy/easy pattern, many top runners use a system where they scale back their weekly mileage by 20 to 40 percent on a regular basis, such as once a month. And keep in mind that mileage isn't the only issue. Experts point out that an overly aggressive approach to hill running, intervals, or trail running—indeed, any change in training—can produce problems. Keeping a detailed training log can help you gauge your personal training threshold. Record your weekly mileage and how you feel after your runs. Look for patterns. For instance, you may notice that your knees ache only when you're logging more than 40 miles a week.

2. Listen to your body.

This is perhaps the oldest and most widely repeated advice for avoiding injuries, and it's still the best: If you don't run through pain, you can nip injuries in the bud. Most running injuries don't erupt from nowhere and blindside you. They produce signals—aches, soreness, persistent pain—but it's up to you to address those signals. "Runners can be crazy, the way they'll run through pain," Ferber says. "They need to pay more attention to pain and get to the root of what's causing it." If you don't, you could hurt something else as you try to change your gait to accommodate the pain.

At the first sign of an atypical pain (discomfort that worsens during a run or causes you to alter your gait), take 3 days off. Substitute light walking, water training, or bicycling, if you want. On the fourth day, run half of your normal easy-day amount at a much slower pace than usual. If you typically run 4 miles at 9 minutes per mile, do just 2 miles at an 11-minute pace. Success? Excellent. Reward yourself with another day off, then run 3 miles at a 10-minute pace. If you're pain-free, continue easing back into your normal routine. If not, take another 3 days off, then repeat the process to see if it works the second time around. If not, you have two obvious options: Take more time off or schedule an appointment with a sports medicine specialist.

3. Shorten your stride.

Overstriding is a common mistake that can lead to decreased efficiency and increased injury risk. If you shorten your stride you'll land "softer" with each footfall. "A shorter stride will usually lower the impact force, which should reduce injuries," says biomechanist Alan Hreljac, PhD, a retired researcher from California State University, Sacramento.

For the last decade, Davis has been researching runners' abilities to change their stride. "We have shown that running and walking gait can be altered in such a way as to reduce pain, improve function, and reduce injury risk," she says.

If you've had frequent running injuries, you might want to experiment with making your normal stride just slightly shorter; try to reduce it by about 10 percent. "This will help reduce your stride so you have more turnover," Davis says. "The number of footstrikes or repetitions trumps having a longer stride because it reduces your impact load." Start with a short distance, like ¼ mile, when making this change. If you have an injury that's related to your gait, see a physical therapist. Adam St. Pierre, an exercise physiologist and 2:54 marathoner from the Boulder Center for Sports Medicine, notes that he often sees runners with shin splints, stress fractures, and hamstring strains who have stride rates below 160 steps per minute (80 steps on each foot). Increasing stride rate—say to 170 or so—often decreases the symptoms and prevents them from recurring. This change is often accompanied by other beneficial changes, he says, like better posture while running and better use of the arms—both of which can lead to improved performance.

4. Strength train to balance your body.

You need something to keep your body properly aligned when you're running down the road at 450 pounds of crunching, twisting-in, and torquing-out force per stride—and what better than muscle? According to Ferber, it's particularly important to strengthen your hip muscles. He claims his clinic has cured

92 percent of knee injuries with a hip regimen.

"Strengthening the hips is optimal for effective rehabilitation, as opposed to treating the area where the pain is located [for example, your knee]," he says. "When you strengthen the hips—the abductors, adductors, and glutes—you increase your leg stability all the way down to the ankle."

You don't want to train for bulging muscles. You need just enough core, hip, and lower-leg strength training to keep your pelvis and lower-extremity joints properly positioned. "Healthy running should be as symmetrical and fluid as possible," says Michael Fredericson, MD, associate professor of sports medicine at Stanford University School of Medicine. "If you don't have muscle balance, then you lose the symmetry, and that's when you start having problems." St. Pierre recommends exercises to build strength in the gluteus medius, which controls rotation of the femur and which will affect leg and pelvis biomechanics during running. "It's chronically weak in people who only run and bike, because it is not worked by those activities," he says. "The gluteus medius is worked by lateral or side-to-side motions." Often, this weakness doesn't cause any trouble when you're running shorter distances at a lower intensity. "Then, as soon as you step up the mileage or intensity, it puts you past the biomechanical threshold and you start to notice it," he says.

5. RICE works.

When you've got muscle aches or joint pains, there's nothing better than Rest, Ice, Compression, and Elevation (RICE) for immediate treatment. These measures can relieve pain, reduce swelling, and protect damaged tissues, all of which speed healing. The only

Cold Therapy

Icing an injury can reduce swelling and inflammation—if you do it right. When the ice hits your skin, it decreases blood flow to the area. Once the ice is removed, the blood flows back to the area, flushing out toxins in the process, says Joseph Dykstra, head athletic trainer at Calvin College in Grand Rapids, Michigan. Here are some key things to remember when it comes to icing.

Ice postrun. Ice the area as soon as you get home from your run—don't ice before you go. "If you numb that area up, you're not going to know how it's feeling, and you could end up pushing through an injury and setting yourself back," says Dykstra.

Keep at it for 15 to 20 minutes. Leave it on for longer, and you'll risk frostbite. Leave it on for 10 minutes or less, and you won't reduce the inflammation. Some redness is normal, but if you start to feel numbness, remove the ice. As a precaution, wrap the ice in a T-shirt or paper towel to separate it from your skin.[2]

problem with RICE is that too many runners focus on the "I" while ignoring the "RCE." Ice reduces inflammation, but to ice and run, ice and run, without giving the tissues enough time to heal, is a little like dieting until 6:00 p.m. every day, then pigging out. So Bruce Wilk, an orthopedic rehabilitation specialist in Miami, Florida, has added another letter to the acronym: PRICE. The P stands for "Protection," which means don't run until the injury is better.

RICE is most effective when done immediately following an injury. If you twist your ankle or strain your hamstring, plan to take a few days off from running (see Rule 2 on page 128). Apply ice for 10 to 15 minutes at a time, several times a day. A homemade ice pack—a plastic bag filled with ice cubes and water—is best. A bag of frozen vegetables is also effective. If you can, elevate the area (easy for foot and ankle injuries, not so much for hip or hamstring issues) to limit swelling. Compression can also further reduce inflammation and provide pain relief, especially when you first return to running. Depending on the location of the injury, an ACE bandage can be the simplest way to wrap a swollen area, but Amol Saxena, a sports podiatrist in Palo Alto, California, uses a compression dressing with Coban, a self-adherent over-the-counter product. He then uses Kinesio Tex Tape or a Darco Body Armor Walker when the swelling goes down. "The tape pulls up the skin slightly, allowing more blood to flow to the injured area," he says. He teaches runners, including 2008 Olympic bronze medalist Shalane Flanagan, how to put it on themselves.

6. Run on a level surface.

Here's another factor that could have a significant impact on running injuries but that has been rarely studied: road camber. No doubt you always run on the left side of the road facing traffic. That's good for safety reasons, but it also gives you a functional leg-length discrepancy, since your left foot hits the road lower on the slope than your right foot does. You're also placing your left foot on a slant that tends to limit healthy pronation and your right foot in a position that encourages overpronation. And you're doing this—running in an unbalanced way—160 to 180 strides a minute, mile after mile, day after day, week after week. Clint Verran, an elite marathoner and a physical therapist in Lake Orion, Michigan, sees the results of this cambered running in his clinic, where he treats a higher incidence of left-hip injuries in runners than right-hip injuries.

True, it's not easy to escape cambered asphalt. And safety concerns demand that you run on the left side of the road. So you've already got two strikes against you. To avoid strike three, remember that road camber can cause problems. If you're increasing your mileage, feel an injury coming on, or are returning from an injury, try to do some of your training runs on a level surface, like a bike path or dirt trail. The local track also provides a firm, essentially flat surface that's great for slow-paced running. (When you do faster interval training on a track, you put unequal torque on your feet and legs due to the need to keep turning left, so be careful if you are injury prone.) Also consider the treadmill. It's hard to imagine a better surface for balanced running. At the very least, a treadmill provides a great surface for beginning runners, runners who are recovering from an injury, and perhaps even marathoners aiming to increase mileage without increasing their injury risk.

7. Don't race or do speedwork too often.

Researchers have found a correlation between injuries and frequent race efforts. This connection might extend to speedwork, since intervals also require a near-maximal effort. So if you train fast once or twice a week and then race on the weekend, that's a lot of hard effort without sufficient rest, particularly if you follow this pattern week after week. Some experts are cautious about recommending regular speed training for certain runners, especially those who get hurt easily. It's fine for those chasing podium placements or age-group awards. But for mid- and back-of-the-packers? "You might get 5 percent faster, but your injury risk could climb by 25 percent,"

Verran says. "That's a bad risk-benefit ratio. I think most runners can hit their goals without going harder than tempo pace."

Recognize that races take a heavy toll, so give yourself plenty of recovery time. If you are trying to quicken your pace for a specific goal, add a weekly speedwork session to your training plan, but be judicious about it. Even Olympic gold medalists do only 5 percent to 10 percent of their training at 5-K race pace or faster. If you're coming back from an injury or have chronic issues that you're fearful of aggravating, consider Verran's advice: Do your faster workouts at tempo pace (5-K pace plus 25 to 35 seconds per mile).

8. Stretch selectively.

Few running practices are as hallowed as stretching, and none have been debated as much in recent years. Studies have failed to reliably show that the addition of stretching to a warmup before activity reduces overuse injuries. "The jury's been out on stretching for about a decade," says Michael Ryan, PhD, a postdoctoral fellow at the University of Wisconsin–Madison. "And as far as I can tell, it hasn't come in yet." Yet few experts in the field are ready to abandon stretching. The reasoning: Runners are tight in predictable areas, they get injured in and around those areas, and therefore they should increase flexibility in those areas. The muscle groups at the backs of the legs—the hamstrings and calf muscles—top most lists of "best muscles for runners to stretch." Hamstring and hip-flexor flexibility seems to improve knee function, and calf flexibility may keep the Achilles tendon and plantar fascia healthy.

Little evidence indicates that stretching prevents overuse injuries. That said, knee and Achilles problems are among runners' most frequent complaints, so experts recommend increasing the range of motion of muscles that can strain these areas if there is underlying tightness. Before a workout, stick to dynamic stretching, which uses controlled leg movements to improve range of motion and loosen up muscles, as well as increase heart rate, body temperature, and blood flow so you run more efficiently.

"It can be a fun part of mental preparation, help you loosen up, and be a good warmup," says Nikki Kimball, a champion ultrarunner and physical therapist based in Bozeman, Montana. Save static stretches (holding an elongated muscle in a fixed position for 30 seconds or longer) for after your run. "If you have an area that's tight and needs to be stretched—the calves, hamstrings, hip flexors, IT bands, or quads—stretch it after your run," says Kimball. "It won't do any harm, as long as you're smart about it."

9. Cross-training provides active rest and recovery.

Running is hard on your body, and experts acknowledge that force can reach two to three times your body weight with each stride, and even more on downhills. It's no surprise that our muscles, joints, and connective tissues get weary from all of this shock-absorbing. So

Keep It Safe

Cross-training can help you stay fit when you can't run, but choose wisely, says runner and sports podiatrist Stephen Pribut, DPM, of Washington, DC. Some activities may exacerbate an injury. Below is a chart that indicates whether a cross-training activity is safe to do depending on the type of injury you've experienced.

	STATIONARY BIKE	ELLIPTICAL	SWIMMING	ROWING MACHINE
Runner's Knee	Sometimes	Sometimes	Yes	No
IT Band Syndrome	Sometimes	Sometimes	Yes	Sometimes
Calf Strain/Achilles Pain	Yes	Yes	Yes	Yes
Plantar Fasciitis	Yes	Yes	Yes	Yes
Shin Splints	Sometimes	No	Yes	No
Stress Fractures	Sometimes	No	Yes	No

experts agree that most runners can benefit from at least one nonrunning day a week and that injury-prone runners should avoid consecutive days of running. Cross-training offers a great alternative.

Use cross-training activities to supplement your running, improve your muscle balance, and keep yourself injury free. Swimming, cycling, elliptical training, and rowing will burn a lot of calories and improve your aerobic fitness, but be careful not to aggravate injury-prone areas (see "Keep It Safe," page 133).

10. Get shoes that fit.

Running shoes have changed a lot over the years. They breathe better, are more likely to come in various widths, and are constructed from superior materials. Most important, there are far more shoes to choose from (racing, training, track, cross-country). There are even minimalist shoes designed to mimic barefoot running (although there's no scientific evidence that forgoing shoes decreases injury risk). Of course, you still have to figure out which shoe will work best for you, which is no easy task.

"There's no single best shoe for every runner," says J. D. Denton, who has owned a Fleet Feet running store in Davis, California, for 14 years. Not only that, but it's impossible to say that shoe ABC will eliminate injury XYZ. Denton and his staff are careful to draw a line between giving medical advice and suggesting a top-notch shoe. "We're careful not to say, 'This shoe will cure your plantar fasciitis,'" Denton says. "Shoes aren't designed to cure injuries. Our goal is to make sure you get the shoe that fits and functions best on your feet."

Others are less cautious than Denton. They point out that while a given shoe isn't guaranteed to heal a given injury, the right shoe on the right runner can help. Verran says he has been able to help patients overcome injuries by suggesting a better fit. "It happens all the time," Verran says. "It's a matter of finding the shoe that's right for a certain foot type."

Don't expect shoes to correct an injury resulting from training error or muscular imbalance. However, when you need new shoes, go to a specialty store to get expert advice. Studies show that shoes perform best when they fit best. Ask the sales staff, "Why is this the best shoe for me?" If you don't get a sound answer, find another store. Keep track of the mileage on your shoes so you know when to replace them. Note the date that you bought them in your training log. How often you should replace your shoes depends on a lot of factors. You should get at least 350 miles from a solid training shoe, and you can reasonably expect another 100 or 200 miles. You'll probably get fewer from a lightweight trainer and far fewer from racing shoes. Whatever the case, it's a good idea to make a note of the date of purchase in your training log so you know when it's about time to get a new pair.

11. Be flexible with your plans.

There's nothing more motivating than signing up for a race, putting it on the calendar, and working toward it. It will help you get out the door when you'd rather sleep in and keep your routine on track so you won't get injured. But build a few extra weeks of cushion into your training schedule so that you have some room to maneuver in case you get hurt. "Have a degree of flexibility in your training that allows for a day or two off in case something happens," says Verran. "You don't want to set up your training so that it's a house of cards, and it's so fragile that if you miss a few days, it's all going to be ruined."

Most training plans for marathons and half-marathons include enough of a time cushion each week and throughout the program to provide that flexibility. That's why it's better to follow a plan, rather than trying to wing it or "cram" for a race.

Ice Baths

In *The Runner's Rule Book,* author Mark Remy jokes that the idea of taking an ice bath to ease muscle soreness is an elaborate practical joke dreamed up by running bigwigs to torture gullible newbies—and he refuses to fall for it.

"All I know is, I've never sat in an ice bath," he writes, "and I don't intend to."

Joking aside, it's easy to see where he's coming from. Sitting in a tub full of ice seems like some ancient form of torture—and just about the last thing anyone would want to do after gutting out a 20-miler or a speed session. In fact, *Runner's World* Challenger Hillary Trout, from San Luis Obispo, California, used to do the opposite, hopping into the hot tub for relief postrun.

But studies show—and seasoned runners swear—that ice baths help reduce the aches and pains of tough training so that you can bounce back strong. A 2007 study found that ice baths reduced soreness and muscle damage after a 90-minute run.[3]

"All of my runners who really want to do hard workouts and not be injured do it," says Kimball. She recommends ice baths after long runs, speedwork, hill repeats, "or after any workout that's hard enough that you're going to be sore the next day."

During an ice bath, the blood vessels in your skin constrict to conserve body heat, says Joseph Dykstra, head athletic trainer at Calvin College in Grand Rapids, Michigan. When you get out of the water, the blood rushes back in to rewarm the skin. In the process, it flushes out toxins that build up after a hard workout. It's the same concept as icing a sore muscle, "but this works well to cool off a big area," Dykstra says.

And what about those long soaks in a hot tub? Not a good idea, experts say. It can actually cause further inflammation to the muscles and joints and prolong recovery, says St. Pierre. It can also worsen dehydration, he says.

For the ice bath, Kimball recommends filling the tub with cold water (50° to 59°F, or 10° to 15°C) until it's waist-high when you sit down, adding ice, and then sitting in it for 15 to 20 minutes.

"The first one is going to be awful, but by the fourth or fifth one, it's not painful anymore," says Kimball. "It's not comfortable, but your body does accommodate it."

And there are ways to make it more palatable, she says. Put on some neoprene socks or kayaking booties, make a hot drink, bundle up your torso in a jacket or fleece, put on a hat, and get some magazines to help the time pass quickly. When the weather permits, Kimball even uses Mother Nature's ice bath, wading into an ice-cold river with her buddies after a long group run. "You don't even notice it's cold," she says.

Trout tried ice baths after her first 16- and 20-milers. Though it was tough at first ("There was a sort of screeching meow that came from me," she says), she did adjust. "My legs felt better the rest of the day as they recovered," she says. "Much better than the times I would soak in the hot tub."

As for Remy, he's still not convinced. He swears he's never taken an ice bath and never will. "Closest I've come is turning the water on cold for the last minute or so of my shower," he says, "and aiming the jet at my legs."

BART SAYS...

I always felt that the biggest mistake people make is that they go by the watch when they're running in the heat. If it's warm and humid, you have to adjust. Early in the run, look at your pace, and if you can't sustain it, back off. Within a mile, you're going to know whether you can sustain that for the distance or the workout, or if you have to make an adjustment.

Staying Safe on the Road

In 2007, 1 month after his first marathon, *Runner's World* Challenger Christopher Sanford went out on a 4-mile easy run. From a safety perspective, he was doing everything right: running on a sidewalk and against the traffic flow. He came to an exit driveway of a church parking lot, where a car had stopped before making a right turn. He assumed she saw him, so he started to run across the street.

"Next thing I knew I was rolling across her hood, spinning in the air, and then on the ground," says Sanford, 34, of Newport News, Virginia.

He suffered a broken nose, displaced pelvis, abrasions on his face, elbows, and knees, and a good cut inside his upper lip. The fact that he was wearing tights and long sleeves, he figured, saved him from worse injuries. Doctors said his sunglasses probably saved his eyes. He spent 8 weeks in physical therapy and was out of running for 6 weeks.

Considering how much worse it could have been, "I came out of it pretty lucky overall," says Sanford. "And the lesson I learned was 'Don't assume that drivers see you.'"

Collisions between runners and motorists are occurring with steady frequency in the United States. While state and federal officials don't track car accidents specifically related to runners, a *Runner's World* search of newspaper and online reports found that nearly 20 runners had been killed by cars or trucks during the first 10 months of 2009, and more than 40 runners have been killed

Vision Quest

It's pitch black and you're out running. At what distance will a driver spot you? A *Runner's World* field test, conducted by *Runner's World* contributor Lisa Jhung, revealed the best-case scenarios—as well as the worst.[4]

VISIBILITY	WHAT YOU'RE WEARING/CARRYING
½ mile	**Headlamp or handheld light** The whitish beam is a color the eye sees clearly at night. And with your motion causing the light to move—the headlamp a little, the handheld a lot—a driver should recognize you as a runner.
¼ mile	**Reflective vest or blinking red light** If you don't feel comfortable wearing a headlamp or holding a flashlight, at least run with a reflective vest or a blinking red light. Drivers won't always identify you as a runner, but they'll have a hard time ignoring your motion. The light should have a bright LED, and the reflective material should cover half of the vest.
150 yards	**Brightly colored jacket or top** This will help get a driver's attention. Yellowish green and bright orange are your best bets. Reflective panels on the sleeves can help a driver to better detect your motion.
100 yards	**Reflective details** At any distance within 100 yards, you put yourself at the mercy of a driver's reaction time. Do yourself a favor and wear clothes and shoes with reflective details.
50 feet	**White T-shirt** Although a white T-shirt becomes visible before a dark one does, the difference is negligible—especially if a driver is moving at a fast clip.
30–40 feet	**Dark clothing** You're asking for trouble by running in dark pants and a dark shirt. Drivers won't notice you until they're dangerously close.

since 2004. A *Runner's World* poll of 2,400 runners revealed that 138 respondents (6 percent) had been hit while running, though most sustained minor or no injuries (and just two said they were nearly killed).[5]

To prevent a close encounter with a vehicle, it's best to stick with some basic rules of the road: Face traffic by running on the left side of the street; wear bright or reflective attire; and avoid using iPods or wearing headphones, so you can hear oncoming traffic.

But as Sanford learned, there are no guarantees you won't be hit. Drivers are increasingly distracted behind the wheel, programming GPS units, dialing cell phones, and texting. An estimated 20 percent of 1.5 million crashes resulting in injuries were reported to have involved distracted driving in 2009, according to the US Department of Transportation. And

Rules of the Road

1. Don't assume a driver sees you. In fact, imagine that a driver can't see you.

2. Run against traffic so you can react to any mistake an advancing motorist may make.

3. At stop signs or lights, wait for drivers to wave you through—then acknowledge with your own wave before crossing.

4. Allow at least 3 feet between you and passing vehicles.

5. Be prepared to jump onto the sidewalk or shoulder of the road.

6. During group runs, go single file when cars need to pass.

7. Use hand signals to show which way you plan to turn.

8. Respect drivers' right to the road.

9. Run with proper ID and carry a cell phone with emergency contacts taped to its back.

10. Check with the police for local traffic rules.

11. When cresting a hill, remember that a driver's vision can suddenly be impaired by sun glare. Dress in highly visible clothing and be prepared to go off-road until the driver is on the other side of the hill.

12. If you are going to run with headphones, run with only one earbud in; you want to make sure you can still hear outside noises, such as the sound of approaching vehicles.

13. If you run before dawn or in the evening, watch out for impaired drivers on the road. People may be tired from just waking up or heading home after a long day. In the early morning, look out for motorists who have not cleared frost from their windshields; they may not be able to see you clearly.[6]

16 percent of crash fatalities were related to distracted driving.[7]

As a runner, it's important to protect yourself. The following guidelines can help you stay safe.

Beating the Heat

Living in Fort Lauderdale, Florida, Chris Cano has gotten to know the signs that he's been hurt by the heat.

"I start to get angry at the smallest things—a car coming too close, trash that someone hasn't picked up—no matter how trivial it is, it will set me off," says Cano, 32, who has finished five marathons and 13 triathlons. "I'll start chafing, get cotton mouth, and just feel hotter than usual. When I first started, I would convince myself that I just wasn't physically ready for the miles I was doing," adds Cano. "After a while, I wised up."

Now that Cano recognizes the signs, he's able to cool his jets quick. He walks, has some water, consumes about 100 to 200 calories, finds some shade, or even goes into a restaurant to cool off.

"The first thing that I have to come to terms with is that my workout is over," he says. "Then the goal becomes getting home safely and making sure that I can go again tomorrow or the next day."

Indeed, what Cano has learned is one of the hardest things for most runners to grasp. "People can never match their same intensity

Race Day Forecast: How Heat Affects Your Marathon Pace

A number of studies have investigated how weather up to 77°F affects marathon performances. One published in 2007[8] looked at temperatures and results from 140 marathons, and found 50°F to be close to ideal for marathoners. The data suggest that slower runners are affected more by rising temperatures than faster runners are. A 2:25 marathoner would slow 1.1 percent for about every 10°F increase in temperature, while a 3-hour marathoner would slow by 3.2 percent. As a rough guide, you could expand these findings to 4- and 5-hour marathon runners. But the decrease in performance would likely be much greater, as the progressive slowing would be partially attributed to how long each runner is exposed to the environmental conditions.

50°F	60°F	70°F	80°F	90°F
3:00	3:05:24	3:10:48	3:16:12	3:21:36
4:00	4:07:12	4:14:28	4:21:36	4:28:48
5:00	5:09:00	5:18:00	5:27:00	5:36:00

in the heat that they can in a cooler climate," says Douglas Casa, PhD, ATC, chief operating officer for the Korey Stringer Institute at the University of Connecticut. "That's hard for people to get."

Even if you don't push the pace, running in hot weather forces your body into overdrive. During a hot run your heart rate soars, your body temperature rises, and the decreased blood flow to your muscles gets in the way of your leg muscles functioning efficiently. Blood volume contracts and you get dehydrated, which forces your heart to work harder to push blood to your legs and to your skin to cool it.

More important, heat illnesses, such as cramps and heat exhaustion, can begin when core temperature rises only a few degrees above normal, which is often related to dehydration from sweat losses. Losing just 2 percent of your body weight through sweating and dehydration can diminish your running performance by up to 20 percent in normal conditions and as much as 60 percent in a hot environment. Casa has done studies on trail runners that show that for about every 1 percent that you're dehydrated, your heart rate goes up about five beats per minute. That's why it's so important to know your sweat rate. (See "Hydration: Take It Personally" on page 96.)

"Runners rarely get heat illness during training, it's races when they tend to get into trouble because they're trying to hit a specific

Turning Up the Heat

In 2008, Amby Burfoot went to work with Douglas Casa, PhD, ATC, chief operating officer for the Korey Stringer Institute, at the University of Connecticut environmental chamber to find out just what happens to the body when running in the heat. He ran identical workouts—1 hour at an 8:30-per-mile pace—on consecutive days. The first run was in 53°F conditions, the second at 90°F. On the hot run, his heart rate, temperature, and sweat loss spiked to levels that diminish performance while increasing health risks, which the doctors said was normal. [9]

BODY MEASUREMENTS	53°F	90°F
Heart rate	158	175
Rectal temperature	101.98°F	103.45°F
Lactate	0.978 mmol/liter	4.04 mmol/liter
Sweat loss	27.05 ounces	54.10 ounces
Percent dehydrated	1.3	2.6
Plasma volume	-0.2%	-10.9%

time," says Casa. "They override their internal cues that something's wrong."

The problem also comes when runners train in the cold and get an unusually hot race day, or when there's a sudden heat wave. That's what happened at the 2007 Chicago Marathon, when temperatures that normally range between 42° and 63°F hit 88°F less than 4 hours from the start. Organizers ended up halting the race, but 185 runners went to the ER, and one runner died.

Yet it can be difficult to distinguish the normal feelings of discomfort that go along with a hot day from a real heat illness that requires medical attention. When there's a

heat issue, fatigue often sets in earlier or after less effort than normal. In a session of mile repeats, for instance, you might be spent after the second mile, while you'd usually make it through the whole workout. "Back off your pace and save that workout for another day," says Casa. "Often runners will get weird sensations in the top of the head or neck, light-headedness or dizziness, headache, nausea, vomiting, loss of appetite, and thirst."

When you recognize these symptoms, "in almost all of the conditions the most important thing to do is back off the intensity," says Casa. "If you're running hard, back off. If

(continued on page 144)

INSIDE RUNNER'S WORLD ®

DAVID WILLEY, 44, *RUNNER'S WORLD* EDITOR-IN-CHIEF, BETHLEHEM, PA

LESSON LEARNED: MAKE TIME TO HYDRATE

I learned about heat illness the hard way. It was 1989, and I had arrived home from my college graduation in time to run a local 10-K with my dad. I was sleep-deprived and undertrained, but I decided I was going to break 40 minutes for the first time. It was an unusually hot June afternoon, and I started fast, and skipped all but one of the water stops. (No time!) By the time I crossed the finish line, I saw Rorschach tests in my peripheral vision. I wobbled into the medical tent, where I was given Gatorade and told I was probably suffering from heat exhaustion. Then I threw up. If I'd known then what I know now, I probably would've broken 40 minutes (missed it by 7 seconds, natch) and not ruined my first 2 days of summer vacation. But at least I am reformed. I never blow by a water stop in a race these days. Before long runs, I stash water bottles and sports drinks in bushes and mailboxes along my route. That sub-40 10-K is still out there. But I no longer have poor hydration as an excuse.

What it takes to . . .
Lose 100 pounds and walk/run a 2:49 marathon

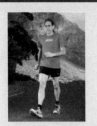

Ian Kitley, 29, Cambridge, United Kingdom
Software engineer
Experience: 3 marathons; 2:49 PR
Runner's World **Challenge Race: 2011 Prague Marathon**

When I was young I ran cross-country, but I was always at the back of the pack, and as I got older, my interest waned and I stopped. Then, about 3 years ago, a friend of mine was complaining about his weight and had found a run program he wanted to try, so I offered to help. Eventually around 10 of us started meeting up to run a few times a week and the bug firmly bit. Over the next year, as my running developed, I would always run by time—not miles—and one day I realized that I was covering the same sorts of distances I would need in order to train for a marathon. I would go for a 2½-hour run and end up covering 20 miles. And so the idea of doing a marathon began to gnaw at me.

Around this time I was finding that when I did my long runs, I'd end up getting tired and feeling beat up before the end. About 3 miles into a 15-K run my internal voice would be crying, "I want to walk, but I can't walk because I have to run the whole way!" Over time, as I got more into my program, I pieced together a run/walk schedule that I was comfortable with. Right from the start, I would run for 10 minutes and walk for 45 seconds any time I ran more than 15-K.

Whenever I would start running again after one of these walk breaks I'd find that I had so much more energy, and the aches and pains I had been experiencing before would fade away. And the following week, I was able to return to my training far quicker. Walk breaks allowed me to increase my distance much faster, while at the same time reducing my risk of injury.

I entered the Dublin marathon with the "if at all possible, crazy idea goal" to break 3 hours. And I did it, finishing in 2:56 and enjoying it so much that I went on to enter marathons in Rome and Prague. In both I used run/walk schedules, amazing myself by finishing Rome in 2:53 while walking 40 to 45 seconds every 5-K and Prague in 2:49 by walking for 30 seconds every 10 minutes. I found myself feeling so refreshed after each walk.

When I began this journey, I was 264 pounds. Today, I weigh 167. It was only when I began to get serious about what I was eating that I really began to drop the weight. My diet wasn't great, but it wasn't awful, either. Mostly it was just inconsistent. When I

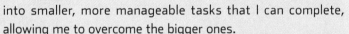

started getting serious about dieting, around October 2009, the first thing I did was ensure that I had breakfast and split up my meals throughout the day, instead of gorging at various points when I would get ravenous. I also started cooking for myself more regularly, instead of relying on takeout once, twice, or even more each week. By cooking, I could limit what I was eating to what I actually felt like, portionwise, rather than feeling like I had to eat everything someone else gave me.

Finally, I came to peace with junk food. In the past, whenever I attempted to cut it out of my diet, I would just end up gorging on it later. Now I allow myself to indulge just a little each day and a little more on the weekends. This way, I don't go overboard and I don't feel bad about my indulgences. I've also found healthier alternatives to junk—such as fat-free yogurt and dried fruit—and I enjoy these just as much as the junk. It helps that I love the alternatives and (usually) they're better for me than chocolate or cookies.

This journey, this experience, has helped me in so many ways. I had never had to put in this much work to achieve something, but in doing so I've seen that I can accomplish so much if I put my mind to it. Losing the weight and being able to set and attain these goals has shown me that I can make a commitment and stick with it all the way to its successful end, making sure it gets done. It also taught me to split bigger challenges

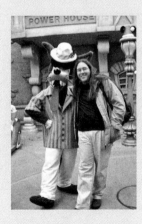

into smaller, more manageable tasks that I can complete, allowing me to overcome the bigger ones.

I've been able to translate these skills into all areas of my life. At work, I find myself more confident in both my abilities and my ideas, allowing me to communicate them more clearly. And along with this I have begun to notice that others are a lot more willing to listen to me and treat me with more respect.

Losing this weight and running this fast—I know how completely strange and weird and insane it all sounds—but I'm living it. I've succeeded in accomplishing so much more than I ever would have thought myself capable of. And now I'm just hoping that I can continue with it.

you're running at a medium effort, walk. If you're doing a walk, get the heck inside, or take a break in the shade."

Tips for Running in the Heat

- Run a shorter distance than you might normally run in cooler weather.

- Run slower than you would in cooler weather. Don't expect to match the times that you achieved in better conditions; it's not possible in the heat.

- Run with friends, or let someone know where you're running and when you'll return.

- Give yourself 8 to 14 days to acclimate to hot weather, gradually increasing the length and intensity of your training. In that time, your body will learn to decrease your heart rate, decrease your core temperature, and increase your sweat rate.

- Run at the coolest time of day, usually in the morning before or just after sunrise.

- Run in the shade—on trails or tree-lined roads—to avoid heat gain from direct sun.

- Wear light fabrics and as little clothing as possible to encourage the evaporation of sweat.

- Listen to your body, and back off when something doesn't feel right.

- Hydrate appropriately before, during, and after your run. But be careful not to overhydrate; that can lead to hyponatremia, a potentially fatal condition resulting from overly diluted blood.

How Heat Can Hurt

It's important to recognize—and deal with—harmful heat ailments before they get out of hand. Almost all of these ailments can be prevented by hydrating adequately (see "Hydration: Take It Personally" on page 96) and by acclimating to the environment.

Heat Cramps

Watch for it: Spasms in the abdomen, arms, calves, or hamstrings during or after intense exercise; dehydration; thirst; sweating

Treat it: Rest, stretch, and massage the affected muscle. Have fluids or foods that contains salt, such as a sports drink, to help retain water. After you rest and rehydrate, you can return to running.

Heat Exhaustion

Watch for it: Heavy sweating, paleness, weakness, headache, dizziness, nausea, fatigue, vomiting, decreased urine, decreased muscle coordination

Treat it: Stop running, get in the shade, remove excess clothing, lie down and elevate your legs, and cool yourself with ice bags. See a doctor if symptoms continue. Wait 24 to

48 hours before returning to running. When you do return to running, gradually increase the intensity and mileage.

Heatstroke

Watch for it: Confusion, rapid breathing, fainting, increased heart rate, disorientation, irrational behavior, vomiting, extreme hyperthermia (usually 104°F or higher)

Treat it: Stop running, call for emergency help, get in the shade, remove excess clothing, and immerse yourself in aggressively circulated cold water (35° to 39°F). Cool until your temperature is back down to 102°F.[10] If you've experienced full-blown heatstroke, see your doctor and wait until he or she has given you the go-ahead before you start running again.

Cold Weather Running

Having done 20-milers when temperatures dipped as low as 22 below zero, *Runner's World* Challenger Jill Turner has come to take pride in her cold-weather training; she even looks forward to it.

"If you are dressed warmly, it can be a very pleasant experience," says Turner, 41, a 10-time marathoner who lives in Edmonton, Alberta. "I love the quiet, the smell of the wood-burning fireplaces, the refreshing and cool air, and the way I feel toasty warm. Then I come home with icicles hanging from my hair and eyelashes, feeling like a running warrior."

Cavalier as Turner might sound, her attitude toward cold-weather training is right on, experts say. Snow can create hazards (see "Snow Tips" on page 151), but if you dress appropriately, stay dry, and keep up your intensity, there's no reason you can't run in the cold.

"As long as you have the right gear and take the right precautions, there's no reason why you can't enjoy exercising in almost any environment, no matter how cold," says John Castellani, PhD, an exercise physiologist at the US Army Research Institute of Environmental Medicine who helped write the American College of Sports Medicine's guidelines on exercising in the cold. "The biggest thing in winter is the road conditions. Other than that, there's nothing that should hold people back from running."

Studies have shown that if you're exercising at 60 percent of VO_2 max—a level of intensity you'd maintain for an easy run—you can produce enough body heat to offset the cold. The problem comes if you're exercising at a lower intensity, don't properly cover your skin, or get wet. All of these factors could leave you vulnerable to hypothermia or frostbite, says Castellani.

"Your exercise intensity will play a big role in whether your core temperature starts to fall," he says. "Typically you're generating heat through exercise that's equal to what you're losing in the cold."

Hypothermia strikes when your body loses more heat than it can produce and your core temperature falls below 95°F (35°C).[11] Symptoms of hypothermia can vary widely, but typically it starts with severe shivering and numbness and progresses to confusion, lack of coordination, and in extreme cases, even death.

You're most at risk for hypothermia when it's rainy or snowy out or your skin is damp from sweat. That's because water transfers heat away from your body much more quickly than air does. You can get hypothermia on a soggy 40-degree day twice as fast as on a much colder day that's dry, Castellani says. "The one thing we don't want people to do in the cold is to get wet."

The time to worry is when you're doing a longer run or race (out for 4 to 6 hours), you end up damp from sweat, and you're not exercising at a high enough intensity to generate more heat than you're losing. In those cases, it's important to take extra precautions. Make sure you wear clothing with zippers and vents to get sweat away from your skin, carry an extra base layer, and stay well fueled, says Castellani.

Frostbite is the other major risk. This happens when skin temperature falls below 32°F (0°C) and most commonly strikes the nose, ears, cheeks, fingers, and toes. Frostbite can start with a feeling of coolness, tingling, burning, aching, and redness, then progress to numbness, and eventually a sort of wooden sensation in the area. Windy and wet days are the riskiest times for frostbite. When the wind chill falls below –18°F (–27°C), you can develop frostbite on exposed skin in 30 minutes or less.

Dr. Bill Roberts, medical director for the Twin Cities Marathon and a professor in the department of family medicine and community health at the University of Minnesota Medical School in St. Paul, doesn't go out if it's colder than –20°F and the wind chill is –40°F. "Colder than that, you've got to be prepared. You can get frostbite really fast if you're not covered."

Your race performance shouldn't necessarily suffer if it's cold, as long as your muscles stay warm. When the temperature dips lower, a lot of factors, including the terrain and the wind speed, can impact running economy. The limiting factor, Castellani says, is that if it gets cold enough, you might have to wear more layers, to the point that it might restrict your range of motion.

Winter Warnings

Here are some tips from experts and *RW* Challengers who are cold-weather veterans to help you keep your training on track during the winter months.

Don't overthink it. The biggest hurdle to cold-weather running may be psychological. Most runners agree that the worst part of winter running is the few minutes of dread before you go. "Don't let the cold weather

Three Common Questions About the Cold

I always seem to shiver when it's cold out. Why does that happen? And should I be worried?

Shivering is a reflex; your body shivers to increase heat production and help offset heat loss. If you're shivering while you're exercising, it typically means that the intensity of your workout isn't generating enough heat to offset what you're losing, says John Castellani, PhD, an exercise physiologist at the US Army Research Institute of Environmental Medicine. It's best to run faster, put on more clothing, or fuel up as quickly as you can.

Sometimes my toes get numb while I'm running, and they don't warm up during the entire run. Why is that?

If your toes are getting numb, it means that not enough blood is getting to them and that you could possibly get frostbite. The best thing to do is to stop and find a place where you can warm them up. To prevent your toes from getting numb in the first place, make sure that your shoe has a big enough toebox, and make sure to get winter running shoes that offer more covering and less mesh, to help keep your feet warm and dry, says Dr. Bill Roberts, medical director for the Twin Cities Marathon and a professor in the department of family medicine and community health at the University of Minnesota Medical School in St. Paul.

Do mittens keep hands warmer than gloves?

Mittens keep hands warmer than gloves because there is less area for heat to be lost. On really cold days, wear a thin liner glove under your mittens and as your hands warm up from exercising, take off the mittens. If your hands get cold, just put the mittens back on.

freak you out," says *Runner's World* Challenger Alissa Messner of Edmonton, Alberta. "It's never as bad as you think it will be."

Cover your extremities. When your core body temperature falls below 95°F (35°C), your skin clamps down to limit the amount of heat that's lost from your body into the environment and to direct blood flow toward your core and your internal organs, explains Castellani. That's why your hands, feet, earlobes, and nose—which are farthest from your core—are the first places to freeze up when you get outside. So be sure to wear a hat, mittens or gloves, a neck gaiter, a balaclava, a headband, and socks that wick away moisture. If you're running in snow, get some lightweight gaiters to keep the moisture out of your shoes. Don't bother with Vaseline or other lubricants; they don't offer you any additional protection against the cold.

Cover your mouth. When the air gets

(continued on page 150)

What it takes to . . .
Run marathons with two reconstructed knees

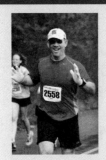

Todd Wilson, age 48, Chesterfield, VA

Program manager for Crop Production Services, an agricultural supplier

Experience: 7 marathons; 3:05 PR

Runner's World Challenge Race: 2009 Richmond Marathon

My adult quest for the marathon began in 2006 when, at the age of 46, I had the privilege of receiving ACL replacements on both of my knees.

Needing the replacements wasn't a huge surprise to me, as I had reconstruction surgery on my right knee when I was injured in high school (by a very rude fullback). I tore everything up in that one—ACL, MCL, PCL, muscle. I shattered my kneecap and even severed the nerve. After 30 years, I guess the warranty on that repair had finally run out.

I don't know why having both of my knees cut on awakened my long-latent desire to run. I had run in my youth, posting a personal best 3:05 marathon. But running had taken a backseat to the normal distractions of life—wife, children, job—and so here I was, a typical middle-aged, overweight desk jockey. And now I had bad knees to go along with it.

My physical therapist started me running while rehabbing from surgery. Somewhere in the process, as I groped along on the treadmill—rehabbing my lungs together with my knees—I found that I was actually enjoying myself. I lost weight, firmed up, and had more energy than I'd had in 15 years. I guess I kind of owe my good health to my bad knees!

I celebrated the anniversary of my surgeries by running a 10-K, and I followed that with a half-marathon and a marathon that same year.

I ran five more marathons, with my last as a *Runner's World* Challenger in Richmond in 2009. I was training for another marathon when the old right knee started flaring up again, aggravated by a misstep while officiating a flag football game. For the fourth time, I went under the knife, where they found quite a bit of torn cartilage and some arthritis. Additionally, the surgeon discovered that the replacement ACL was deteriorating and would not likely hold up much longer.

If the ACL continues to degenerate and I lose stability in the knee, they will have to replace it again. I've been fitted for a brace that is supposed to take some pressure off of the joint when I run, which should buy me some time. My doctor tells me that eventually I will require knee replacement. The more I run, the quicker I will need it.

And I will continue to run. Maybe not as far and certainly not as fast, but I will continue to run—until I can't run. And when I can't run, I will know that I ran all that I could when I could. Some may consider that a destructive attitude, but as the old saying goes, "I'd rather wear out than rust out."

I've been asked what it takes to run a marathon with two reconstructed knees. For me, it has required a love for running that overwhelms the adversity of running. For most runners, the adversity is part of what we love, so with my personal challenges, I've been blessed with a little extra of what I love when I've run them.

Although none of my injuries were the result of running, marathons are probably not the best prescriptions for them. Even so, I have no regrets. Maybe running as many miles as I have the last few years wasn't the best thing for me, but, looking back, I honestly don't know which mile I would have chosen not to run. I've loved every mile that I have run—even the miles that I hated to run.

We runners have an overwhelming wonder of what's around the next corner. I believe that this has been a necessary part of it for me. The journey that I have been on and am now continuing has had its share of disappointments. Honestly, this recovery has been slower than the others, and until recently the setbacks have outnumbered the gains. I've had to draw on the lessons of perseverance that the marathon has taught me in order to continue. I take comfort in believing that this is not the way things are, it's just the way things are right now. And there is always this next corner to turn with a new adventure just beyond it.

I will never take running for granted again. I'll be 50 years old this fall and everything below the waist hurts at some time or another, so I just take it one day at a time. I'll never see another 3:05 marathon, but that's okay, because I'm on a new adventure now.

I run now because there was a day when I couldn't and there will probably be a day when I can't. And I continue to run with considerable thanksgiving for every previous mile the Lord has allowed me to run. I have "run and not grown weary" and will do so until it is time to "walk and not grow faint."

cold it can cause a burning sensation in your throat as you run. That happens because cold air dries out your airways, causing some constriction, Roberts explains. But it won't cause any damage to your lungs. To prevent that burning sensation, cover your mouth with a scarf or a balaclava to warm the air before you breathe it in.

Wear layers. Dress in thin, light layers that you can add to or take off to suit your temperature. Layers trap air between them, providing insulation. Wear a lightweight polyester or silk layer against your skin to wick away moisture, a middle layer of fleece, and an outer layer to block the wind and wet weather. Do not wear cotton, which absorbs and holds moisture against your skin. Once you start sweating, "you're creating your own little wet environment, and that sucks the heat out of you," Castellani says.

Don't overdress. Dress as though it's 15 to 20 degrees warmer than it is. You should feel slightly chilled when you walk out the door. As you warm up and your body temperature starts to increase, you'll feel better. You want to reduce your risk of overheating and sweating excessively, which can prompt the chills and lead to hypothermia. Wear clothing with zippers and vents so the sweat can evaporate, says Roberts. "If you're not wearing clothing that wicks away sweat, you'll get colder faster."

Watch the wind chill. When you're check-ing the weather forecast, watch the wind chill, which is how cold it actually feels once the wind hits your skin. According to the National Weather Service, as the wind speed increases, it drives down body temperature. If the temperature is 0°F and the wind is blowing at 15 miles per hour, the wind chill is –19°F (–27°C), and at that temperature you can develop frostbite on exposed skin in 30 minutes or less.

Protect your private parts. Men should wear wind-blocking underwear or something to block the genitalia when it's windy out, says Roberts. When the wind blows, you're more prone to frostbite. "The wind isn't very discriminating," he says. "It will go right through your tights."

Start into the wind. Start your run going into the wind, so it's at your back on the way home. That way, when you're fatigued and sweating more, during the second half of your run, the wind will be at your back, making the effort feel easier, says Roberts.

Warm up inside. When it's below freezing, try to do part of your warmup indoors. Start your run on a treadmill, then head out once your legs feel ready but before you start sweating.

Eat and drink as you would on regular training days. "Hydrate and take in fuel the same way you would on a warmer day," Castellani says, even if you don't feel like it. You're likely to sweat less on a cold day than you would in the heat, so you may not be as likely to take a drink, plus the cold reduces your thirst drive. But it's just as easy to get dehydrated, which can lead to fatigue and hurt your performance. Make sure you're well hydrated before you go out. Likewise, be sure to fuel up. You're likely to spend more energy in the cold weather, especially if you have to negotiate snowbanks and icy patches. Shivering—your body's reflex to produce heat—also burns glucose that your muscles need for energy.

Defrost as soon as possible. Damp clothes increase heat loss. As soon as possible after your run, change into dry, warm clothing, like a fleece and sweats.

Snow Tips

Running in the snow may seem crazy to some, but for those of us who live in cold climates, it's a reality that can't be dodged. Here are some tips to help you safely keep up with your training in a winter wonderland.

Watch your step. You'll get better traction on snow that's been packed down, and fresh powder can cover up ice patches. Run on the street if it's been plowed (as long as it's safe from traffic), and watch out for black ice. Run on the sidewalk if it's clear of ice.

Don't go out when it's freezing. Snow is most slippery when it's freezing (right around 32°F), says Roberts. "That's when I don't run," he says. "There's poor traction,

and you can hit an ice patch and go down in a heartbeat." You'll get better traction when the temperature drops below zero, he adds.

Expect some soreness. Between slipping in the snow and ice and navigating nonuniform, snow-covered surfaces, you have to adjust your gait, so get ready for a little extra postrun soreness. "With all the small adjustments your feet and ankles are making," says Messner, "you wind up straining something somewhere." *Runner's World* Challenger Wayne Horseman, of Minneapolis, Minnesota, agrees. "It's easy to let your shoulders slouch inward, which can lead to neck and shoulder pain," he says. "Snowy trails and maneuvering around icy patches can take their toll on calves and ankles."

Shorten your stride. When you're running on ice or snow, shorten your stride to help prevent slipping and falling. Focus on getting in the time rather than hitting a certain pace or running a preset distance on challenging weather days. Use products like Yaktrax to reduce your risk of falling.

Take it inside. If the roads are covered with ice, take it to the treadmill. If you can't stand the 'mill, cross-train on the bike or elliptical trainer for the same amount of time you'd spend running. (See "The Backup Plan," starting on page 180.)

Be flexible. To avoid missing workouts, always have a plan B. If you're usually a morning runner, be willing to run in the afternoon.

If the street is an ice rink, head to the gym. It's better to reframe your workout than to ditch it altogether. Even if you can do only a 20-minute workout, you'll feel better.

Buddy up. Run with a partner or a group whenever you can. If you're running alone, let someone know your route and how long you plan to be gone, and carry a cell phone, says Horseman. "Cold weather isn't the time to go out and run on your own out in the country," says Roberts. "Have a few bailout loops that are safe and close to home, where you can find someplace indoors to warm up if the weather gets bad."

Skin Issues

Four weeks from the Big Sur Marathon in 2011, *Runner's World* Challenger Scott Francis was feeling pretty confident. He'd beaten some IT band issues and was ready to go, except for one thing: a blister under his big toenail that became red, swollen, and painful, and caused him to cut his long runs short. "I didn't know whether to lay off, keep running, or rip the darn thing off with a pair of pliers," says Francis. "I didn't want to mess up my training."

He saw a podiatrist, had it removed, and had to take 3 days off from running. "I definitely underestimated the toll it would take," he says.

While in training, we tend to fret most about tweaked hamstrings and stress fractures. But as Francis learned, seemingly superficial issues—like blisters, chafing, sunburn, or athlete's foot—can be just as disruptive. Even if your muscles and bones are in working order, an irritated piece of skin the size of a hole punch can put you out of commission.

"Runners have a ton of skin ailments that they either don't attribute to their run or they just ignore," says Brian Adams, director of the sports dermatology clinic at the University of Cincinnati and a five-time marathoner. "But they can really get in the way of training."

Luckily, most of these issues are easy to treat and prevent. And, if they're treated correctly, they won't derail your training.

Blisters

Caused by friction, which can happen when your shoes rub against your skin, blisters can be irritating and painful, and can stop you in your tracks. Heat and moisture set the stage for blisters, since both make the skin swell. That's why blisters tend to be more common during the hot summer months and on rainy days. Blisters are often the result of poor-fitting shoes.

Treat it. If the blister is smaller than the size of a pencil eraser, you can leave it alone to heal on its own. If you're going to keep running on it and want to keep it from getting bigger, take a piece of moleskin, cut a hole the size of the blister, and place the moleskin around the blister. Cover the whole thing with gauze. For a bigger blister, draining the fluid will help relieve the pain. Take a needle, wipe it with rubbing alcohol to sterilize it, lance the edge of the blister, and drain the fluid out. It's tempting to remove the roof of the blister, but it's best not to. "That can lead to infection, and the skin underneath is going to be really raw and painful," says Lee Firestone, a podiatrist in Chevy Chase, Maryland, and Washington, DC. Cover the lanced blister with an adhesive bandage or another covering, such as moleskin with a hole cut out of it and a layer of gauze. If you return from a run to find bloody socks and blisters that have already been popped, clean the blisters with antibacterial soap, apply an antibiotic cream (like Neosporin), and cover them. If the area around any blister is extremely warm or has red streaks on the skin or a green discharge, see a doctor. Those are all signs of an infection.

Prevent it. Making sure your shoes fit is the first line of defense against blisters. Before you run, slather Vaseline or a sports lube on any hot spots on your feet that are prone to friction, or put an adhesive bandage over areas where blisters pop up, says Adams. If you're going to be out for 2 hours or more, forgo the Vaseline, warns Adams. It can lose its effect. Firestone suggests using duct tape to cover blister-prone areas. "It's a little stickier, it contours better over the skin, and it glides a little bit easier" against your sock, he says. If you feel an area of your foot start to get hot during a run—a sign that there's friction between your foot and your shoe, and that a blister isn't far behind—loosen your laces and adjust your socks. A bunched-up toe or misaligned seam could be causing irritation. Adams suggests using the lacing technique in "Banish Blisters" (below) to prevent any friction from developing in the first place.

Banish Blisters

This lacing technique, suggested by Brian Adams, director of the sports dermatology clinic at the University of Cincinnati, will help prevent your heel from slipping out of your shoe, which can lead to blisters.

1. Lace your shoe normally, but leave the last hole on each side undone.

2. On the last hole, lace the shoestring through the hole on the same side.

3. Pull the end of each lace to the opposite side, pulling it through the loop formed in step 2.

4. Pull the laces up, out, and tight before tying them.

Chafing

As with blisters, friction is the main culprit of chafing. Anything that rubs against your skin—shorts, sports bra, or a cotton T-shirt—can chafe your skin into a red, raw state that can be painful, lead to infection, and make that postrun shower downright unbearable. Moisture and heat can make chafing worse. Among male runners, nipple chafing is common.

Treat it. Wash the area with soap and water, apply an antibacterial ointment, and cover the chafed area with an adhesive bandage. It should heal on its own.

Prevent it. Wear technical clothing that wicks moisture away from your skin. Cut the tags off your clothing. Make sure your clothing fits: too snug, and it can dig into your skin; too loose, and excess material can irritate your skin. Men should use nipple guards, which are sold in most running stores. Keep areas that are prone to chafing covered with an ointment like Vaseline, Aquaphor, or a sports lube.

Sunburn

The bright red hue you get from staying out in the sun too long is a sign that your skin is damaged. "Sunburn is your body's alarm system," says Brooke Jackson, a Chicago-based dermatologist and 10-time marathoner. "It's like putting meat on the grill." More worrisome is the risk of skin cancer. Studies have shown that marathoners and outdoor athletes have a higher risk of malignant mela-noma. (See "Skin Cancer," opposite.)

Treat it. If your skin is red and sore after a day in the sun, apply a cold compress or some lotion, take a cool shower or soak in an oatmeal bath, or take some Tylenol to relieve your discomfort. If the burn is severe enough that you develop blisters, you might be susceptible to infection and it's best to get treatment. Applying aloe can have a cooling effect, but beware of aloe gels, Jackson warns. Gels are alcohol-based, and the last thing you want to do is put alcohol on a burn. Moisturizing lotion works just as well.

Prevent it. Avoid running between 10:00 a.m. and 4:00 p.m., says Adams; that's when the most potent ultraviolet rays shine. The impact of the sun can be amplified if you're running in an area surrounded by snow. Wear a hat and sunglasses to protect your face and eyes. Guys should keep their shirts on while running, and women should avoid running in nothing but a jog bra. "Wearing some sort of sun protection from your clothes is the best way to prevent sunburn," says Jackson. Look for running clothing that offers UV protection, or wear darker colors, which block more UV rays than light colors do. Use a sunscreen with an SPF of 30 or greater. It should be labeled "broad spectrum," which will protect you from UVA and UVB rays. Make sure that you apply enough sunscreen; the amount that could fill up a shot glass should cover your entire body before you go outside. Apply it 20 minutes before you go out so that it has time to be absorbed into your skin. If you're going on a long run, reapply the sunscreen once each hour, Adams says.

Black Toenails

Seen by some runners as badges of honor and by others as unsightly war wounds, black toenails develop when the toenail, often on the second toe, gets slammed against the toebox of your shoe. When all that force is directed back to the nail bed, it causes bleeding under the nails. Downhill running, which puts even more force on the toenail, can make it worse. Black toenails are often caused by ill-fitting shoes that don't have a deep enough toebox.

Treat it. As long as the nail doesn't hurt, leave it alone, and the black part will grow out in a matter of weeks, says Adams. If the nail becomes malformed or the nail plate begins to come off, it may become vulnerable to infection, so it's best to see a doctor. Be sure not to go barefoot in showers, hotels, and locker rooms, where it is easy to pick up a fungus that could lead to infection.

(continued on page 159)

Skin Cancer

A 2006 study published in the *Archives of Dermatology*[12] showed that runners had significantly more atypical moles and liver spots, indicating a greater risk for malignant melanoma. The authors of the study suggest that, in addition to longer exposure to the sun—the more miles the runners ran, the higher their risk—runners' higher risk may have to do with suppression of the immune system during endurance sports. In addition, sweating may make your skin more sensitive to ultraviolet radiation, causing it to absorb it better.

"You're out there doing this wonderful thing for your body and getting in great shape, but you're doing this horrible thing for your skin," says Brooke Jackson, a Chicago-based dermatologist and 10-time marathoner. That said, there are plenty of measures you can take to prevent skin cancer or catch it at an early stage.

In addition to covering your skin with clothing and sunscreen before you head out (see "Sunburn" on page 154), the most important thing to do is to familiarize yourself with your skin, says Jackson. Know what your moles look like, and look for any changes in size or color. Also, note if you have new lesions. A pimple should heal up within a week or so. If it's not healing, or it's bleeding or growing, see a doctor. "Just get to know your own body and know when it's not behaving, just like when you think you have a sprain or a shin splint," says Jackson. Get an annual skin cancer screening by a dermatologist, who can look at the small nuances and pick up early warning signs. "The earlier the diagnosis," says Jackson, "the better the prognosis."

All the Right Moves

Dynamic Stretching

Maybe you've heard that stretching before a run is a big mistake. Indeed, studies show that static stretching—holding a muscle in an elongated, fixed position for 30 seconds or more—could hurt performance if done before a workout. (Save those stretches for after your run.) But dynamic stretching, which uses controlled leg movements to improve range of motion, loosens up muscles and increases heart rate, body temperature, and blood flow to help you run more efficiently. This prerun routine, developed by Nikki Kimball, a champion ultrarunner and physical therapist based in Bozeman, Montana, targets the muscles used for running. Start slowly, focusing on form. As the exercises get easier, pick up speed. Use small movements for the first few reps, and increase the range of motion as you go.[13]

Leg Lifts

While standing, swing one leg out to the side, then swing it across your body in front of your other leg. Repeat 10 times on one side, then repeat on the other side. Feel wobbly? Hold on to a stable object.

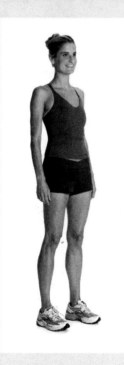
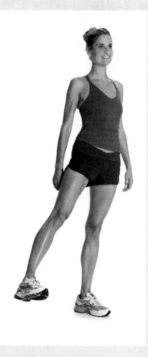
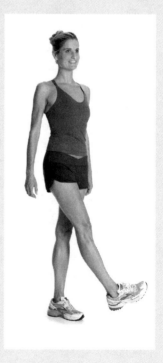

Butt Kicks

While standing tall, walk forward, kicking your heels up to your glutes. When this is easy, try it while jogging. Do 10 reps on each side, alternating sides.

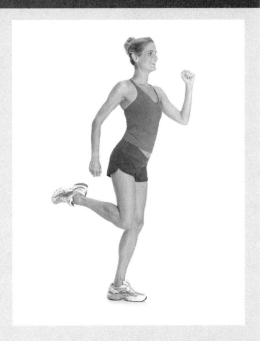

Pike Stretch

Get into a "pike" position, with your hips in the air. Put your right foot behind your left ankle. With your legs straight, press the heel of your left foot down. Release. Repeat 10 times on one side, then repeat on the other side.

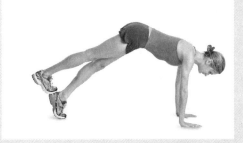

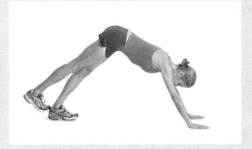

All the Right Moves (cont.)

Hacky Sack

Lift your left leg up, bending your knee so it points out. Try to tap the inside of your left foot with your right hand without bending forward. Repeat 10 times on one side, then repeat on the other side.

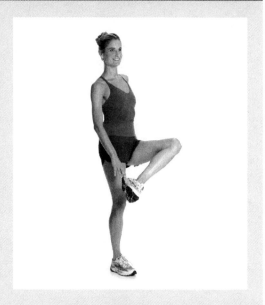

Toy Soldier

Keeping your back and knees straight, walk forward, lifting your legs straight out in front of you and flexing your toes. When you can do this comfortably, add a skipping motion to make it more challenging. Do 10 reps on each side, alternating sides.

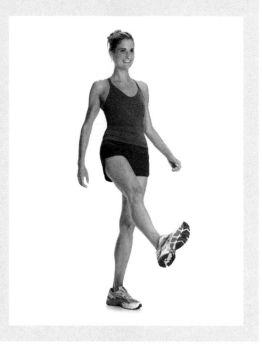

Walking Lunges

Step forward using a long stride, keeping your front knee over or just behind your toes. Lower your body by dropping your back knee toward the ground. Maintain an upright posture and keep your abdominal muscles tight. Do 10 reps on each side, alternating sides.

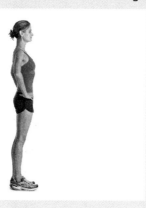 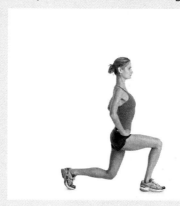

Prevent it. Buy shoes that fit, and use the lacing technique described on page 153. This will reduce how much your foot moves in your shoe and keep your toe from slamming into the toebox.

Athlete's Foot

This is one of the most common ailments among runners. "Fungus loves warm, dark, moist areas, and runners have the sweatiest, warmest feet," says Adams. Athlete's foot can cause itching, burning, and dry cracks on your heels or between your toes. But runners often don't even know they have it. "If you have dryness and itchiness of your skin that persists for more than a month and won't improve with moisturizer, see a doctor," says Firestone.

Treat it. In most cases, an over-the-counter treatment like Lamisil, twice a day, can treat the symptoms of athlete's foot.

Prevent it. Make sure that you dry your feet completely before putting on socks. Wear moisture-wicking socks, and shower right after your run. Don't go barefoot in public showers or locker rooms, or on pool decks; wear sandals or flip-flops, instead. Firestone recommends rotating your shoes every day to let each pair dry out. After a run, take off your shoes and take out the insoles to let the shoes dry out and to prevent moisture from building up.

(continued on page 163)

Six Postrun Stretches

These six poses, developed by yoga instructor and *Runner's World* contributor Sage Rountree, target runners' tightest and weakest spots, improving range of motion and strength to keep muscles and joints healthy. As a bonus, you'll also develop balance, core strength, and focus. Done together, these exercises make the perfect postrun routine.[14]

Hold each of these for 5 to 10 breaths (or more). You can run through the sequence on one side, then the other, or do both sides before moving to the next pose.

1. Triangle

The payoff: Stretches your outer and inner hips and thighs and strengthens your core and legs.

The move: Take a wide stance, right toes forward, left toes angled to the right. Lean over your left leg and reach your right arm high.

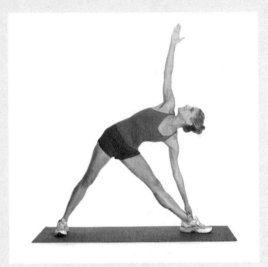

2. Pyramid

The payoff: Stretches your hips and hamstrings and strengthens your quads and core.

The move: Square your hips and fold over your left leg. Bend your knees as much as necessary to keep your hamstrings happy.

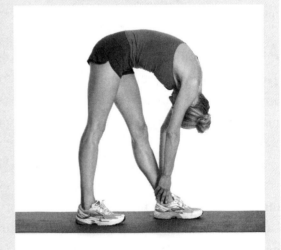

3. Quadriceps Stretch in Lunge

The payoff: Stretches your front leg's hamstring and your back leg's hip flexors and quadriceps.

The move: Drop your right knee to the ground and lower your hips toward your left heel. Reach your right hand for your right foot.

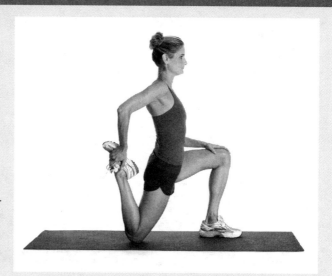

4. Pigeon Forward Fold

The payoff: Stretches your hip muscles, including the piriformis, and the iliotibial band.

The move: Take your left heel in front of your right hip and drop your left knee to the ground. Fold forward over your left leg.

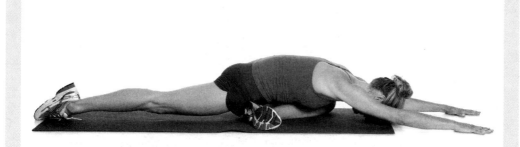

Six Postrun Stretches (cont.)

5. Head to Knee

The payoff: Stretches your hamstrings and calves. Use a strap for assistance if your legs are tight.

The move: Bend your left knee and stretch over your straight right leg.

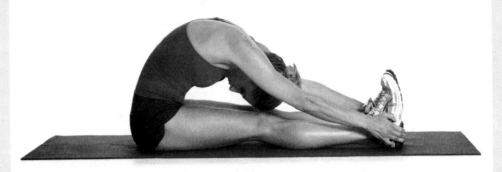

6. Happy Baby

The payoff: Stretches your hamstrings and groin and helps release tension in your back.

The move: Swivel to your back, spread your knees, and hold your hamstrings, lower legs, or feet while keeping your head and tailbone on the ground.

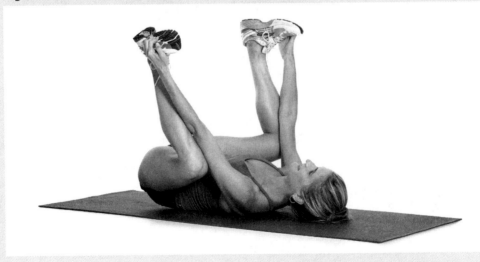

Crossing Over

Here are some general tips to keep in mind to make the most of your cross-training time.

Make it regular. Cross-train when you're healthy and the weather is great. That way, when you're snowed in or injured, you can jump right in and get the benefits cross-training can provide. "It will take a while to build up the quad strength to do an effective bike work-out that would be equivalent to that speed session," says exercise physiologist Scott Murr, PhD, coauthor of *Runner's World Run Less Run Faster,* who codeveloped the popular FIRST marathon-training programs.

Go by feel. Heart rate zone is sport specific, says Murr. For instance, during a running speed session, you may be used to getting your heart rate up to 163 beats per minute, but it might be 10 to 15 beats lower on a bike because cycling is not weight-bearing, you are using a smaller muscle mass, and you don't have to move your arms. It's better to go by feel to gauge your intensity. (See "Measure Your Effort" on page 36.) Tom McGlynn, a three-time qualifier for the Olympic Marathon Trials and a coach at Focus-N-Fly, an online coach-ing service categorizes exertion into an easy effort (65 to 70 percent), an effort where it's harder to chat but sustainable (80 to 85 percent), and a 5-K effort where you can't talk in complete sentences (more than 85 percent).

Be patient and positive. Whenever you do a new activity, it's going to feel awkward at first. Just stick with it, Murr says. "Within four workouts you're going to get more comfortable."

Cross-Training

Runner's World Editor Katie Neitz (page 198) always ran 6 days a week, and even pulled her share of two-a-days. So she was skeptical when, coming back from a stress fracture in her pelvis, she decided to try a marathon training plan with just 3 days of running plus 3 days of pool running or swimming. To her surprise, it worked. "I felt like I was working hard cardio-vascularly, but my legs were getting a rest," says Neitz, 35. "I felt recovered before all my runs." On race day, she ran close to her PR. "It was so nice to finish feeling strong and happy, and I didn't reinjure myself!"

Indeed, cross-training can improve your fitness, prevent and help rehab injuries, let you recover from workouts, and liven up a routine that's starting to feel stale. "It elevates your heart rate, increases blood flow, and prompts muscular strain and cellular adaptation, all without the pounding of running," says Tom McGlynn, a three-time qualifier for the Olympic Marathon Trials and a coach at Focus-N-Fly, an online coaching service.

McGlynn has runners who are training for marathons and half-marathons augment 4 days of running with 2 days of aerobic cross-training (like cycling or working out on an elliptical trainer) and 2 days of strengthening, flexibility, and balance work (like core work, yoga, and Pilates).

That said, McGlynn and other coaches warn that it's important to cross-train right. Whether you're cross-training because you can't run or you're just rounding out your race training, approaching a bike, swim, or elliptical trainer with an "it's better than nothing" approach could leave you feeling bored, unsatisfied, or worse, injured. To get the benefits that will serve you on the road, choose activities that translate to running as closely as possible, approach each activity with a purpose, and perform it at a high-enough intensity that you're taking your cardiovascular and muscular fitness up a notch.

"Not training hard enough is the biggest mistake that most runners who try cross-training make," says exercise physiologist Scott Murr, PhD, coauthor of *Runner's World Run Less Run Faster,* who codeveloped the popular FIRST marathon-training programs. FIRST advocates three weekly running workouts supplemented by 2 days of cross-training by cycling, swimming, or rowing. "Runners like to run. So when they get in the pool or on a bike, they'll exercise for 30 to 40 minutes, but not very vigorously,

— [WHAT WORKS] —————————————

Integrate cross-training into marathon training

Marjorie Patrick, 43, San Diego, CA; associate professor of biology, mom; 6 marathons; 3:46 PR; *Runner's World* **Challenge Race: 2011 Big Sur International Marathon**

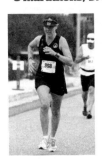

I try to integrate cross-training into my regime—going to the gym, riding a stationary bike, doing the elliptical or some weights. But if I'm not up for the gym, I go out for walks, like walking to work or just around campus. For this last season, I had to cut out the gym due to work and family demands, and I know that my upper body and core muscles are not as strong. I do enjoy the break from training as I think it helps restore my drive to run and gives my body a rest, and I always run faster and better after a break. I truly need to balance the demands of family, career, and running, or I'm not happy. I always strive to run happy. When I don't run happy, when it's not a pleasure, then I need to take a break.

then they get bored and frustrated and quit. It's usually boring because they're not going at the appropriate intensity. If you have a focus for each workout, you're going to do better."

To get the benefits of cross-training, it's also best to start integrating it into your marathon routine before you have to—don't wait until the streets are icy or your IT band acts up. If you make the gym a last resort, you're never going to have a chance to get the aerobic benefits or gains in muscular fitness. McGlynn has runners stick with one form of cross-training—like swimming, elliptical training, or cycling—so that they can become proficient in it. "Unless you've developed the muscles, it's going to be very hard to maintain an aerobic state," he says.

"There's a little bit of a learning curve to effective cross-training," says Murr. "You can't just go in and completely duplicate a planned workout on a bike if you haven't been on a bike in months. Incorporate it into your regular routine early in your training program. Otherwise, the quality of the cross training isn't going to be as high as it could be." Like McGlynn, Murr recommends that you stick to one mode of cross-training—whether it's cycling or swimming—rather than jumping around from one random exercise to another during training.

Cycling

Don't get too obsessed trying to translate bike mileage to time on the bike, says Murr. Just focus on spending the same amount of time cycling as you would running. If you usually go out for a 5-mile run and it takes you 45 minutes, do 45 minutes on the bike. "But make it high quality and go hard," says Murr.

Ideal substitute for: tempo runs, track workouts, active recovery days.

Make it translate: The bike is a great way to train your legs to turn over fast—like you'll want them to do when running. Cycle at a resistance where you can pedal with a higher cadence—simulating a high turnover—that approximates the 170 to 180 strides per minute you should target when running. For runners who cycle, cadence is important. Most runners who cycle tend to "push a big gear" with a low cadence. Cycling is probably more beneficial when runners work on quick pedaling at a cadence of 80 to 100 pedal revolutions per minute (RPM).

Let's say you usually do **speedwork** with 6 × 800 on the track, with 400 meters of jogging as your recovery, and it typically takes you 4 minutes to run 800 meters and 3 minutes to do the 400-meter recovery jog. On the bike, cycle for 4 minutes at a moderate resistance, with the cadence around 95 to 105 revolutions per minute (RPM), then pedal easy for 3 minutes at a reduced resistance, not worrying about RPMs. Then repeat the cycle six times, just as you would on the track.

To replicate a **tempo run,** jack up the bike to a moderate resistance, so that it feels moderately hard, and keep the cadence between 90 and 95 RPMs for the same amount of time you'd spend on a tempo run. If you normally run a 4-mile tempo run and it takes you 27 minutes for the tempo portion, then after a 10-minute warmup on the bike, gradually increase the resistance and maintain a steady cadence—90 to 95 RPMs—for the remaining 27 minutes. If your cadence drops below 80 RPMs, reduce the resistance some.

If you're cycling in lieu of an **easy run**—say to save your legs for the next day's track workout—keep the resistance low and the cadence quick (between 95 and 100 RPMs) for the same amount of time you'd spend running. "What's making it a challenge is not

---

— [WHAT WORKS] ——————————————

Reset your race goals

**John Walter, 61, Ankeny, IA; journalist, father of two, grandfather of one;
2 marathons; 3:48 PR; *Runner's World* Challenge Race: 2011 Big Sur International Marathon**

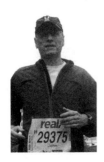

When I turned 60, I decided to resurrect my running life. I ran in the 2009 Des Moines Marathon and started training for the 2011 Big Sur Marathon. The long runs on the weekend became a genuine adventure for me—a physical challenge in an otherwise mostly cerebral, abstract sort of daily life—without having to go to a mountain. I wanted to finish Big Sur without injury, and I began training to finish in 4:30—in the top half of my class. But 6 weeks into the program, I began to develop knee pain. An MRI showed a small meniscus tear and bony edema. So I cross-trained for a month. My cardiovascular condition seemed good. My weight was down, and my knee was numbed by cortisone. Still, I worried about risking a DNF (Did Not Finish) and more knee damage during the marathon. My physical therapist believed I could run it, though not without risk. Everything in my heart was saying to run Big Sur. Even Bart Yasso was on that side of the ledger. But I really needed to weigh the risk of greater damage to my knee and likely a much longer recovery. Maybe it's easier for older runners to take the long view. You look back at a bib you collected in a race more than 30 years ago, and you appreciate what it is to still be running. That's where I wanted to be after Big Sur—still running. The basis for these kinds of decisions are the eternal verities—things like patience, faith, and endurance. Based on my assessment of all that info, I decided not to run the Big Sur Marathon. The risk–reward ratio didn't seem to tilt in its favor. But I stayed on my feet and ran the 9-miler, finishing third in my class—a modest achievement, perhaps, but leaving open a better road to recovery and future marathons, I hope.

INSIDE RUNNER'S WORLD®

WARREN GREENE, 39, BRAND EDITOR, EMMAUS, PA

LESSON LEARNED: FIND RUNNERS TO BE YOUR CAREGIVERS

In 2006, I had surgery to repair a sports hernia, and I developed a sharp pain in my hip. In the 5 years since then, doctors have been trying to figure out why I'm having the pain and how to make it go away. I've been to a sports medicine doctor, a chiropractor, a back specialist, a physical therapist, a massage therapist, and I've even considered acupuncture. None of them could make the pain go away, and countless MRIs gave no hint as to what was causing the problem. But with the addition of core work and fish oil supplements, the pain has been manageable. As frustrating as it has been not to have an answer to why this is happening or some sort of solution to the problem, because I've been able to go to doctors who are runners or who work exclusively with runners, through it all I've been able to keep running. They gave me suggestions for exercises that may help, and they were able to find ways to keep me on the road. They never said, "Well, just stop running." I'm so grateful for the miles I've been able to do. I've been running for 23 years, and I really love the training. I'm used to the fitness, and I really enjoy the camaraderie you get through training—especially now that I have a 4-year-old and a 6-month-old and more commitments in daily life. I got to run the 2009 Richmond Marathon and 2010 Boston Marathon and 2011 Big Sur Marathon with my friends and colleagues. Last summer, I got to do an 11-mile trail run at 6,000 feet with a college cross-country buddy the day before he got married. It was tough, but it was so beautiful out there in the backcountry, and I wouldn't have missed that for the world.

the resistance, but rather the fact that you're spinning your legs fast for an hour," says Murr. "You can get a really good cardiovascular workout without crushing your quads." A word of caution: If you're cycling outside, you still want to maintain a high cadence. Most runners tend to push big gears, which can cause soreness the next day.

The payoff: Cycling will help you strengthen your quads, which will help you climb hills. (Running tends to use the ham-

strings and calves more, and it typically doesn't stress the quadriceps.) Plus, since cycling isn't a weight-bearing activity, injured runners may be able to help maintain their hard-earned fitness by cycling.

Don't get hurt: Use foot straps or clip-in pedals, which allow your legs to go through the full range of motion of pushing the pedal down, pulling it back, pushing up, and pulling the pedal across the top. You'll use more muscles that way and get a better workout. And make sure that your seat is adjusted correctly. When you're sitting on the saddle and your foot is on the pedal at the bottom of the revolution, there should be a slight bend in your knee—your leg should not be straight (if it is, the seat is too high) or bent near 90 degrees (if it is, the seat is too low).

Other tips: A stationary bike is a good way to start. Spinning bikes are great, but because you can't measure the resistance, it's more difficult to duplicate the workout or compare one workout to another, Murr says.

How to Stay Healthy for the First 100,000 Miles

by Amby Burfoot

I consider myself lucky. I'm in my mid-60s, have run more than 100,000 miles, and have had few injuries. You might think that makes me a nonexpert in the field of injury prevention and rehab.

However, consider this: Each of my occasional injuries knocked me off my cherished running regimen, so I focused on getting back in the saddle as quickly and healthfully as possible. Along the way, I took serious note of every trick that worked and every false promise that didn't.

I now have the following modest list of Dos and Don'ts. They're taped to my office wall, just above my computer screen. That way, I see them often and am reminded of them before I make any foolish mistakes. To me, a running-healthy program is more important than a training plan geared toward improving performance. That's because I'm more interested in increasing my years of running than in decreasing my race times. These are the key principles that have kept me running strong.

1. **Rest heals.** And it heals faster when you rest sooner. Don't attempt to run through injuries. At the first signs of an atypical pain or ache, take 3 days off. Then try a short, slow jog. If you still feel that pain, take 7 days off before running again. Still no success? It might be time to consult with the best sports medicine doc in your area.

2. **Use ice and anti-inflammatory meds to erase minor injuries.** Use them immediately for muscle pains and other soft-tissue injuries around the ankles and knees. But stop anti-inflammatory medications after 10 days. Anti-inflammatories are for short-term treatment of specific issues that should resolve quickly. They're not for chronic pain, which requires a more serious exam to discover the underlying cause.

3. **Cross-train for mental and physical fitness.** For many of us, the former is just about as important as the latter. Cross-training works great to reduce or eliminate the right-left-right-left foot-and-leg pounding that occurs when you run. On recovery days, try bicycling and elliptical training. For more serious injury rehab that requires a total break from impact

You can go outside for your bike workout, but it's likely that you're going to be interrupted by traffic, stop signs, and other obstacles.

Swimming

Swimming can be an ideal way to recover from a fatiguing run because it exacts zero impact on your body and requires you to work upper body and core muscles that running doesn't touch. "Getting in the pool and playing and moving for 20 minutes can be a really restorative thing," says Murr, "especially the day after a long run."

shocks, you need to get the weight off your frame. In other words, you need to sit or eliminate gravity. Swimming, aqua jogging, and rowing are the best activities in this situation.

4. **Be careful with stretching and strength training.** Everyone from your best friend to, possibly, your physical therapist is going to suggest stretching and strength training for your injuries. Fine. There may be a time for them—but that time is not while you're still injured. First, get healthy. Then try new routines, but go slow and be cautious when you do. Otherwise, stretching and strength training can cause injuries rather than healing or preventing them.

5. **Be cautious with everything new you try.** Change may bring benefit, but it also entails risk. You're going to be tempted to change your running shoes, change your running form, try hills or speedwork, or maybe change the surface you train on (from roads to parklands and trails). Any of these might prove worthwhile for you, but you'll be tempting fate if you make rapid changes in your fitness regimen. Instead, make changes very gradually.

6. **Patience, patience, patience.** The vast majority of running injuries disappear almost as suddenly as they appeared, but they don't necessarily do this on your schedule. If you have an upcoming race and don't give your injuries a chance to heal, you could be asking for trouble. On the other hand, if you relax a little, stay optimistic, and understand that you'll be running healthy again soon enough, that's exactly what will happen.

7. **Act like an athlete.** Remember: You're an athlete. Act like one. You're probably thinking, "Huh? What's he talking about?" Here's the answer: To get healthy, you must remain focused, disciplined, and consistent. These are the exact qualities that led to your fitness and running success in the first place, and they're the qualities you'll need to get fit and healthy again. Don't whine (excessively; a little is okay), and don't give up. Believe in yourself and your body's incredible capacity to regenerate itself and heal. Stay determined and positive, and you'll be back on the roads again soon.

Ideal substitute for: easy runs, active recovery after a long run or race, workouts during an injury when no weight-bearing exercise is possible.

Make it translate: If you aren't an experienced swimmer, get some lessons. Swimming is so technique-oriented that unless you have a background in it and the upper body endurance that goes along with that, it's hard to get a good aerobic workout, Murr says.

If you do a 20-minute swim workout, for instance, you might have to swim a length, then kick a length, then walk a length. Try to keep moving continuously for 20 minutes.

Once a week, get in the pool, use a kickboard, kick a length, rest for 15 seconds, and then repeat three more times. Be sure to kick from the hip, not the knee. Or get in the pool once a week for 20 minutes of nonstop movement, whether you're kicking or swimming. If you're not used to swimming, this will feel hard. After you're done, showered, and changed, decide how hard the workout was in terms of how you feel.

The payoff: Swimming is a total body workout. Not only is it an aerobic workout, it also works your upper body, lower body, and core, and it can increase your flexibility. Kicking, when done properly, can help increase ankle flexibility, says Murr, so that once you're on the road, you can push yourself farther off the ground with each stride.

Pool Running

Deep-water pool running simulates the arm and leg movements of running without putting any impact on your lower joints. So it's a great exercise if you have an injury like a stress fracture, which requires several weeks with no weight-bearing activities in order to heal. However, because water is denser than air, your legs will turn over more slowly, so you can't get the practice on quick cadence that you can on a bike.

Ideal substitute for: any workout when you're injured and can't do weight-bearing activities (such as when you have a stress fracture).

Make it translate: Ditch the flotation belt, Murr says. If you try to run without a belt, you'll have to work much harder to keep yourself up, and that's going to increase the quality of the aerobic workout itself, says Murr. Then focus on your form. Since it's easy to lean back, it takes a conscious effort to simulate your normal running form. From there, you can mix it up and do intervals, like McGlynn suggests in "The Backup Plan" (starting on page 180).

Elliptical

An elliptical trainer uses the same muscles as those involved in running, allows you to get a good cardio workout, and enables you to burn a fair number of calories. It's great for injured runners who are easing back into running, because it's a weight-bearing activity that doesn't cause the pounding that running does, Murr says.

Ideal substitute for: easy workouts, track workouts, and tempo runs. Also ideal for a runner who is coming back from an injury but can do weight-bearing activities. (Don't use it as a recovery tool, Murr warns, as it uses the same muscles as running and therefore doesn't give your muscles a chance to recover.)

Make it translate: Let's say you're coming back from an injury and want to take time off from running. Start your comeback by doing 1 week on the elliptical at an easy effort. Start doing some running the second week at an easy pace. On week three, add an interval workout on the elliptical. On week four, do intervals on the road. That way, you gradually progress back to fast running.

Don't get hurt: All elliptical trainers are not the same. They have different movement patterns, so try different machines and use the one that works best for your type of body. McGlynn prefers the Arc Trainer because it so closely mimics running—you can swing your arms as you move your legs, just as you do when you run. As a result, "a lot of runners are able to get into that aerobic zone and maintain it," says McGlynn.

Rowing Machine

If you're a healthy runner with no injuries, hitting the rowing machine once a week will give you a great total body and cardiovascular workout. It will strengthen your core, upper body, hamstrings, legs, and glutes. Because rowing requires a lot of upper body endurance and strength, which runners typically lack, even a short workout is going to be difficult. "For most people, there's no such thing as 20 minutes of easy rowing," says Murr.

Ideal substitute for: track workouts and tempo runs.

Make it translate: You're used to measuring your effort by minutes per mile, but most rowing machines (ergometers) display 500-meter pace. In tests with runners who attend FIRST training camps, Murr has found that the average male runner might row at a 2:20 pace (for 500 meters); the average female might hold a 2:45 pace (for 500 meters). Rowing at these paces for 15 to 20 minutes would be challenging for most runners.

Don't get hurt: Because you're flexing your knees more than you do during biking or running, rowing could aggravate any existing knee issues. And if you don't use the proper technique, it's easy to hurt your back. The first few times you get on an ergometer, get a knowledgeable instructor to stand beside you, show you the proper form, and offer feedback, says Murr.

CHAPTER 8

GETTING HURT AND GETTING OVER IT

From IT band syndrome to Achilles tendinosis, there are a myriad of ways to get hurt. But often they share a common cause.

"Without a doubt, the number one catalyst of injury is increasing your mileage, hills, or speedwork too quickly," says ultrarunning champion Nikki Kimball, a physical therapist in Bozeman, Montana.

In many cases, there are also underlying biomechanical problems—weakness in the glutes, hips, and quads; overpronation; and muscle imbalances—which are set off once you start piling on the miles. So in addition to getting to a point where you're pain free, it's also important to do the strengthening work to keep injuries from recurring. "If you don't address the underlying causes, it's not going to go away," says Adam St. Pierre, a 2:54 marathoner and exercise physiologist from the Boulder Center for Sports Medicine.

The Most Common Injuries

Of course, we hope that you stay healthy in your training and you don't have to use the following handy guide. But in case you do hurt yourself, we've outlined some of the most common running injuries, plus how to avoid and recover from them.

Runner's Knee

Called patellofemoral pain syndrome, runner's knee is an irritation under the kneecap that typically flares up during or after a long run or while going down hills and stairs.

What it feels like: You may feel twinges early in the run that go away and reappear postrun. As it worsens, the pain may be on the inside or outside of the knee, which persists even as the day progresses.

What causes it: Weak quads, hips, or glutes, which all can lead to overpronation (excessive inward foot rolling) and cause poor tracking of the knee. Running with too much forward lean can also contribute to runner's knee.

Best remedies: Take extra rest days and cut your mileage by at least 50 percent until you're pain free, says Stephen Pribut, a sports podiatrist in Washington, DC. Avoid running downhill or leaning too far forward when you run, as this can put more stress on your knees. Work on strengthening your quads, which control the tracking of your knees. Pribut suggests straight-legged lifts: Lie on your back and lift one leg straight up until it's at a 30- to 60-degree angle with the floor, and lower it 10 times rapidly. Repeat on the other side to complete 1 set. Do 5 sets, working up to 10 sets.

Best prevention: Strengthen your quads, which help support your knees and keep them tracking correctly. Also, build up your glutes and hips, to strengthen your core and assist your quads. This can also help correct overpronation.

Safe alternatives: Elliptical trainer, swimming, or pool running.

IT Band Syndrome

This is caused by strain of the iliotibial (IT) band, the connective tissue that runs along the outside of your thigh and that stretches from your hip to your shin. When your knee flexes and extends during running, the IT band can rub against the bone, causing friction and irritation.

What it feels like: A dull pain on the outside of your knee; it tends to start a few miles into a run. If it progresses, the pain can radiate up and down your leg, even while walking downstairs or down a hill.

What causes it: Piling on too many miles too quickly can irritate the IT band, as can running on cambered roads. "I think a lot of people aren't used to the distances they've gotten up to," says Pribut. Runners who develop IT band syndrome usually have weak hip abductors, so the IT band becomes overworked and overstressed as the muscles that attach to the band have to take over the function of the weak hip abductors and assist in keeping the hips level. This condition is frequently aggravated by hills.

Best remedies: At the first sign of pain, take a rest day or two, run easy, and cut your mileage in half for about a week. Also, get your shoes checked; you might need orthotics, or a pair that offers more arch support to help correct the pronation. An IT band can be a stubborn injury to heal, because it doesn't have a huge blood supply and it's a tough area to stretch, says Clint Verran, an elite marathoner and physical therapist from Lake Orion, Michigan. He suggests lying on your side on top of a foam roller and rolling back and forth from your knee to your hip 10 times before and after each run, to encourage blood flow to the area, loosen up the tight IT band, and alleviate pain. Pribut recommends using softer rollers, made of white foam, rather than the harder forms that are made with PVC materials. You can get these at sports equipment stores and online. Pribut also suggests doing standing side stretches: Stand with your left foot crossed in front of your right. Lean your upper body to the left with your hands overhead. Lean as far as you can without bending your knees and hold for 15 to 20 seconds. Switch legs and repeat on the other side.

Pribut also suggests strengthening your hip abductors by doing the clam shells or side leg lifts.

To do the **clam shells,** lie on your side, keeping both feet together. Keeping the sides of your feet touching, raise your top knee. Repeat 15 times on each leg.

To do **side leg lifts,** lie on a mat on your side. Keep your top leg straight and your bottom leg slightly bent. Slowly lift your top leg up as far as you can and then return to the starting position. Repeat 10 times on each side to complete 1 set. Start with 5 sets, working your way up to 10 sets.

Best prevention: Add miles and intensity gradually (build your mileage by no more

than 10 percent each week), and work on shortening your stride, Pribut says. If you have a training watch, set the beeper so that it goes off between 70 and 90 beats per minute, and make sure one foot comes down each time the watch beeps. Strengthen your hip abductors with exercises like lateral side steps, side leg lifts (at left), and one-legged squats.

To do **lateral side steps,** wrap a band around both legs above your knees. In a semi-squatting position, walk 10 steps to the right, then walk 10 steps to the left. Work up to 15 steps in each direction.

To do **one legged squats,** stand on one leg with your foot pointing straight ahead. On the standing leg, keeping the knee centered over the ball of the foot, lower into a squat position. Repeat 3 sets of ten squats on each of your legs.

Safe alternatives: Swimming, pool running, and using an elliptical trainer. Hiking and cycling can aggravate IT band syndrome.

Hamstring Strain

Hamstring strains can result from a variety of causes, says Pribut, including overstriding, or bending forward from the waist too much to increase your forward lean. Doing too much speedwork, of even too much hillwork too soon can also cause hamstring strains. "It's important to ease into hillwork, speedwork, and faster running in general," he adds.

What it feels like: Chronic achiness and tightness that forces you to slow your pace and shorten your stride. As it gets worse, the pain can become sharp.

What causes it: Hamstring issues usually arise because these muscles are weak and tight. Often, a strain is due to overextending your legs while trying to gain speed, which is known as overstriding.

Best remedies: Run easy, and shorten your stride. Avoid stretching your hamstring while it's sore, which could repull it, says Pribut. When it feels better, work on strengthening your hamstrings. Skip speedwork for 3 to 5 weeks.

Best prevention: When you return to speedwork, avoid workouts where you're running at a 5-K or 10-K pace, as shorter, higher-speed intervals can aggravate your hamstrings. Stick to workouts with longer intervals, like marathon-pace intervals, then half-marathon pace, progressing to shorter, faster (5-K and

Dr. Pribut's Shoe Pushdown Test

Shoes that bend in the wrong place can lead to plantar fasciitis. To make sure you've got a running shoe with the proper rigidity, press the shoe at a 45-degree or greater angle on a countertop, as shown. The shoe should bend at the ball of the foot. It shouldn't bend before that point, or further back. The shoe on the left flexes at the correct part of the sole. The shoe on the right flexes too far back.

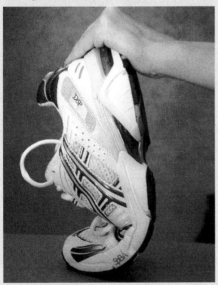
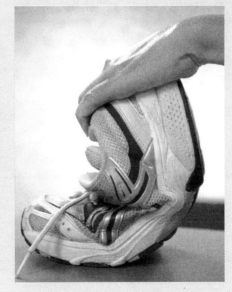

Photos courtesy of Dr. Steven Pribut, DPM

What it takes to . . .
Train for a marathon with epilepsy

Jamie Laposta, 35, Sierra Vista, AZ
Technical editor/writer for a government contractor on Fort Huachuca, AZ, mother of two
Runner's World **Challenge Race: 2011 Big Sur International Marathon**

Running empowers me. It gives me back the life I had before epilepsy, and it gives me back the courage and part of the confidence that epilepsy could have taken away. It's very scary to hear that you have this illness that you can't control—that you're going to have it for the rest of your life. When I was first diagnosed, doctors told me to stop running, saying that it would be too hard on my body, so I did. But I continued having frequent seizures, and all medications failed to control them. Eventually I found doctors and the right mix of medications that would allow me to run and train for a marathon. When I began training, my daughters rode their bikes with me just in case I had a seizure. Now I'm able to run on my own. I let my family know the route I am taking and how long I expect to be gone. I always wear a medical identification bracelet. The medication causes fatigue and suppresses my appetite, so I can't run in the mornings, and I have to be aware of my food intake. I used to love going further out in the country and trail running, but now I stay on the roads, in more populated areas. On days when I have seizures, I can't go out and run because I'm exhausted. And sometimes I am too exhausted to run the next day. Every day I have no idea what's going to happen—whether it's going to be a good day or a bad day, and whether I'm going to have a seizure or not. Knowing that despite all that, I still have the strength and determination to slather on the sunscreen and lace up my running shoes is monumental. It feels like I'm taking back control of my life.

10-K) intervals only after 2 to 3 weeks of successful injury-free running at the lower speed levels.

Safe alternatives: Swimming or the elliptical trainer. Avoid cycling, which can put stress on your hamstrings.

Plantar Fasciitis (PF)

An inflammation of the plantar fascia, a band of tendons and ligaments that run from your heel to your toes. When put under too much stress, it stretches too far and tears, which causes inflammation.

What it feels like: A dull ache or bruise along your arch or on the bottom of your heel, which usually hurts the most first thing in the morning and at the beginning of a run. Most of the time it will go away 4 to 5 minutes into a run.

What causes it: Overpronation and wearing worn-out shoes are the most common causes of plantar fasciitis, says Pribut. A sudden increase in hillwork, speedwork, or running on the forefoot can also set off plantar fasciitis, as can a sudden change in your gait. Long periods of standing can worsen the problem. Those with high arches are more at risk for PF, and often it's worsened by wearing shoes with no arch support (like flip-flops) or walking around barefoot, says Verran.

Best remedies: You don't have to stop running—just stick to flat surfaces and avoid speedwork and hills. "If it goes away after 4 to 5 minutes, or is achy the next day, it's okay to run," says Pribut. "If it's so bad that you feel you shouldn't run, don't run." Make sure you have rigid shoes, which reduce the strain on the plantar fascia. To check, do "Dr. Pribut's Shoe Pushdown Test" (see page 175) to make sure the shoe bends at the ball of the foot. For women, shoes with heels will help reduce the strain on the fascia, says Pribut. Ice the area twice a day, says St. Pierre, by rolling your foot over a frozen water bottle for 5 to 10 minutes at a time. He also recommends massaging it with a golf ball to increase blood flow to the area. Stretch your calves with wall stretches for 10 to 30 seconds on each side, and repeat that 10 times, says Pribut. Also, strengthen your intrinsic foot muscles with toe curls. If you reduce your mileage, check your shoes, do the stretches, and don't feel better within 3 weeks, see a doctor. It might be a good idea to talk to him or her about custom orthotics.

Best prevention: Avoid wearing flip-flops or open-backed shoes that offer no support for your heels. Replace your running shoes every 300 to 500 miles. Stretch your calves as part of your regular routine; if your calves are tight, it will force the Achilles to pull on your foot and cause overpronation, which can cause more strain on the fascia. Strengthen your glutes, which can help prevent pronation.

Safe alternatives: Pool running and swimming. Cycling or using an elliptical trainer can help you maintain fitness, but only if you can do those activities without pain.

Achilles Tendinopathy

The Achilles tendon connects the two major calf muscles to the back of the heel. Under too much stress, the tendon tightens and becomes irritated.

What it feels like: It may start as a dull ache. As it progresses, it may hurt to stand up on your toes, and you may develop severe pain and swelling—even when you're not running.

What causes it: Overuse, speedwork, and hills can all lead to Achilles problems. Some research shows that there's a genetic link as well. A mushy shoe can also be the culprit, says Pribut. If your heel pushes into the ground at the same time that your calf muscle is firing, you can overstretch the tendon. Sometimes tendon tweaks can even be caused by a single misstep—one that you may not even remember—that irritates the tendon.

Best remedies: Running through Achilles tendinopathy can be risky; the problems can be long lasting. Cross-train and rest for a few days. If you catch a minor strain early, a few days off might be sufficient healing time. If you keep running as usual, you could develop a serious case that may take 6 months to go away.

Best prevention: Avoid aggressive calf stretching and wearing flip-flops and high heels, all of which can irritate the Achilles.

Safe alternatives: Pool running, swimming, and biking. Avoid elliptical trainers, which can strain the calf muscles and the Achilles.

Shin Splints

This condition, also called medial tibial stress syndrome, is characterized by a pain that results when small tears occur in the muscles around your shinbones.

What it feels like: Tight, aching pain when running that fades after a warmup and after you stop running. It can feel painful and tender to the touch.

What causes it: Shin splints are common among new runners and those returning after an extended layoff, and they often strike at the beginning of training or after building up mileage too quickly. "Sometimes it's just the introduction to this new force that your shins just aren't ready for," says Verran. Overpronation, running on cambered roads, and wearing worn-out running shoes can also lead to shin splints.

Best remedies: When the first twinges of pain strike, take a rest day, then slowly ramp up your mileage by no more than 10 percent each week. Ice your shins for 10 to 15 minutes immediately after running. If the pain continues through the end of your run and radiates over a wide area, it could be a stress fracture; see a doctor for a bone scan to rule one out. If shin splints don't fade within 2 weeks, see a sports podiatrist, who might prescribe orthotics.

Best prevention: The easiest and best way to avoid shin splints is to increase mileage gradually, run on soft surfaces as much as possible, and make sure your shoes offer the fit your feet need. Building strength in your quads and glutes will help absorb the shock better, says St. Pierre. You might also work on increasing your stride rate. Shorter, quicker strides (above 160 strides per minute) will decrease the impact forces from each stride and prevent and alleviate shin splints. Make any changes gradually.

Safe alternatives: Cycling, pool running, and swimming. Avoid the elliptical trainer.

Stress Fracture

Unlike an acute fracture that happens as the result of a fall, stress fractures develop from cumulative strain on the bone. In runners, they most often occur in the foot (in the metatarsal, right below the toes) or in the shins.

What it feels like: Pain may begin and get worse as you run. If it goes untreated, it may become uncomfortable just to be on your feet.

What causes it: Overtraining, overstriding, and excessive impact. Having a loud and uncontrolled stride. If you increase the duration, intensity, or frequency of your running too soon, your bones can't repair themselves fast enough to keep up. Stress fractures are more common in women than men, usually due to nutritional deficits, low estrogen levels, and inadequate calorie intake.

Best remedies: Expect to take 3 to 4 months off from running. The amount of rest you'll need depends on the severity of the fracture and its location. If you ran through the pain for a while before you realized you had a fracture, your recovery could take longer. Stop all impact exercise.

Best prevention: Gradually build up your mileage, and run on soft surfaces. "Get off the concrete; even asphalt is better," says Pribut.

Safe alternatives: Swim and pool run. Avoid all impact exercise until directed by the doctor.

The Backup Plan

Tom McGlynn, a three-time qualifier for the Olympic marathon trials and coach at Focus-N-Fly, an online coaching service, designed this 8-week cross-training program for injured runners.[1] With this plan, you'll spend 3 weeks building up the intensity of your cross-training, then 3 weeks maintaining that level of activity, and during the last 2 weeks you'll reintroduce running. (Only need to take 2 weeks off? Just do weeks 7 and 8 of the plan.) But don't hit the roads again without approval from your doctor. And in a time crunch, prescribed physical therapy exercises take precedence over aerobic workouts. If your injury ever feels worse on a day after cross-training, stop doing that activity.

The Workouts

Elliptical Trainer: Swing your arms (don't hold on to the bars).

The Backup Plan

WEEK	MON	TUES	WED	THURS	FRI	SAT	SUN
1	No workout, light stretching or yoga	Physical therapy/ strength and flexibility work	30–60 minutes cross-training (65 percent effort)	Pool running intervals (80 percent effort for 30 minutes)	30–60 minutes cross-training (65 percent effort)	Elliptical "long run" for the same length of time as a normal long run	Off
2	Pool-running intervals (80 percent effort for 30 minutes)	30–60 minutes cross-training (65 percent effort)	Spin class (80 percent effort for 30 minutes)	30–60 minutes cross-training (65 percent effort)	Pool-running intervals (80 percent effort for 30 minutes)	Bike for the same length of time as a normal long run	Off
3–5	Elliptical intervals (80 percent effort for 30 minutes)	Pool-running intervals (80 percent effort for 30 minutes)	Spin class (80 percent effort for 30 minutes)	30–60 minutes cross-training (65 percent effort)	Elliptical intervals (80 percent effort for 30 minutes)	Bike for the same length of time as a normal long run	Off
6	Elliptical intervals (80 percent effort for 30 minutes), followed by 10-minute run: 1 minute running/ 1 minute walking	Pool-running intervals (80 percent effort for 30 minutes)	Spin class (80 percent effort for 30 minutes), followed by a 10-minute run: 1 minute running/ 1 minute walking	30–60 minutes of cross-training (65 percent effort)	Elliptical intervals (80 percent effort for 30 minutes), followed by a 10-minute run: 1 minute running/ 1 minute walking	Pool run for the same length of time as a normal long run	Off

WEEK	MON	TUES	WED	THURS	FRI	SAT	SUN
7	Elliptical intervals (80 percent effort for 30 minutes), followed by a 12-minute run: 2 minutes running/ 1 minute walking	Pool-running intervals (80 percent effort for 30 minutes)	Spin class (80 percent effort for 30 minutes), followed by a 12-minute run: 2 minutes running/ 1 minute walking	30–60 minutes cross-training (65 percent effort)	Elliptical intervals (80 percent effort for 30 minutes), followed by a 12-minute run: 2 minutes running/ 1 minute walking	Bike for the same length of time as a normal long run	Off
8	Elliptical intervals (80 percent effort for 30 minutes), followed by a 15-minute run: 4 minutes running/ 1 minute walking	Pool-running intervals (80 percent effort for 30 minutes)	Spin class (80 percent effort for 30 minutes), followed by a 15-minute run: 4 minutes running/ 1 minute walking	30–60 minutes cross-training (65 percent effort)	Elliptical intervals (80 percent effort for 30 minutes), followed by a 15-minute run: 4 minutes running/ 1 minute walking	Pool run for the same length of time as a normal long run	Off

Elliptical "intervals" (45 to 60 minutes): 5-minute warmup; 8 to 14 × 2 minutes hard/ 2 minutes easy; 5-minute cooldown. Maintain average effort above 80 percent of max for 30 minutes during interval portion of workout. Elliptical "long run" (60 to 120 minutes): 10-minute warmup; continuous cycle of 7 minutes hard/3 minutes easy; 10-minute cooldown.

How to Gauge Intensity

- **60 to 75 percent effort:** An easy, conversational run
- **80 to 85 percent effort:** Harder to chat, but a run that's sustainable for longer times
- **More than 85 percent effort:** Like a 5-K; no talking in complete sentences

Pool Running: Run as you would on land—bring up your knees, pump your arms. Pool-running "intervals" (45 to 60 minutes): 10-minute warmup; 3 to 5 cycles of 10 × 50 seconds all-out/10 seconds easy. After each cycle run easy for 2 minutes. Cool down for 10 minutes. Maintain average heart rate above 80 percent of max for 30 minutes during interval portion of workout. Pool "long run" (60 to 120 minutes): 10-minute warmup; continuous cycle of 10 minutes hard/2 minutes easy; 10-minute cooldown.

Biking: Experienced cyclists can hit the roads. Otherwise, stick with a stationary bike or spin class. Bike "intervals"/spin class (45 to 60 minutes): 1- to 3-minute climbs; recovery for 50 percent of the interval time. Maintain average heart rate above 80 percent of max for 30 minutes during interval portion of workout. Biking "long run" (60 to 120 minutes): 10-minute warmup; continuous cycle of 10 minutes hard/ 2 minutes easy; 10-minute cooldown.

Muscle Cramps

Though *Runner's World* Challenger Frank Troilo has finished 12 marathons, lost 25 pounds, qualified for Boston, and run a personal best of 3:14, there's one challenge that he can't seem to elude when he runs 26.2 miles: muscle cramps. In hilly races, on flat stretches, on cool days and hot days, they always seem to plague him after mile 20.

"It always starts like a tightness right in the middle of my hamstring, and then just expands to the whole muscle," says Troilo, 45, a father of two from Media, Pennsylvania.

At the 2010 Boston Marathon, Troilo was reduced to a walk in the final 4 miles. "I just felt the time slipping away."

Troilo is hardly alone. Go to the final stretch of any marathon or half-marathon and you'll see runners clutching their calves and hamstrings, their contorted expressions betraying the physical pain and disappointment they feel. Though muscle cramps are one of the most common problems among runners, their cause is the subject of great debate.

"We are still trying to figure out where the muscle cramps originate," says Kevin Miller, PhD, a professor of athletic training at North Dakota State University. "We just don't have a great understanding of it. The most likely scenario is that each individual is different. In some people, dehydration sets it off, and in others it might be fatigue. Likely it's due to some combination of both."

Some say that these spasms stem from a whole-body electrolyte deficit, which is what happens when runners don't take in enough salt to replace the sodium lost in sweat and then develop a measurable sodium deficit. (Sodium helps the body retain and distribute water.) That's why these kinds of cramps tend to happen any

When to See the Doctor

A little muscle soreness just goes along with the training process; it's a natural part of pushing yourself farther and faster than you've ever gone before. But it can be difficult to know which pain to run through and which pain should send you running to the doctor.

General muscle aches and soreness can often be resolved by taking an extra rest day or by substituting easy cross-training for running. But sometimes aches and pains require more serious treatment. And those who are in training for marathons and half-marathons often delay seeing the doctor much longer than they should, not wanting to go through the hassle of making the appointment and—above all—not wanting to receive the prescription, "Just stop running and it will go away."

"In general, people wait too long to come to the doctor," says Clint Verran, an elite marathoner and physical therapist in Lake Orion, Michigan. "A lot of times, by the time they come into my office they're just so broken, and their training has already been negatively affected."

Here are some surefire signs that you should go running to a physical therapist, sports medicine doctor, orthopedist, or podiatrist before you hit the road.

1. **Your pain is asymmetrical.** If you have a pain on one side of your body but not the other, it's probably something to check out, says Nikki Kimball, a champion ultrarunner and physical therapist from Bozeman, Montana.

2. **Your pain persists for more than 72 hours.** You want most injuries to go away between 3 days and a week after they begin, says Stephen Pribut, a sports podiatrist in Washington, DC. You should rest, cut your mileage, and cross-train at the first sign of pain. But if pain still persists, make an appointment. "You're not supposed to be running in pain," he adds.

3. **Your pain hurts when you're not running.** If you rest, cut your mileage, and the area hurts even when you're standing or walking around, it's best to see the doctor. "If an ache or pain persists in your daily life and normal daily activities, that's a sign that it's a little more serious," says Verran.

4. **Your pain is sharp and limited to one small spot.** "Muscle soreness is okay; anything localized should be checked out," says Kimball.

5. **Your pain is getting worse.** If you rest and cut your mileage and the pain is getting worse, see the doctor. "I try to remind people that running is supposed to be fun," says Verran. "You want running to be a lifelong habit. And if you get to the point where you're running through pain all the time, it's not going to be a lifelong habit."

Help Your Doctor Help You Diagnose and Treat Your Injury

1. **Describe the symptoms.** What were you doing when the pain started? How long did the pain last initially? Often the problems arise from overuse; some problems arise from a single trauma.

2. **Tell the doctor what relieves the pain or makes it worse.** Runner's knee might hurt when you climb the stairs, while a stress fracture might hurt anytime you put weight on it.

3. **Identify the progression.** Has the pain changed at all from when you first noticed it?

4. **Explain what you've done.** How have you responded to the pain? Did you cut down your mileage, take a pain reliever, or run through it?

5. **Talk about your past.** Describe any injuries or unrelated medical conditions that you've had in the past and how you treated them.

6. **Bring your shoes.** Wear patterns on the tread can often clue doctors in to underlying problems. Your doctor may also want to watch you run and evaluate your gait to detect issues like overpronation. Make sure to bring both your new and old pairs of shoes, says Stephen Pribut, a sports podiatrist in Washington, DC.

7. **Bring your running log.** In your running log, keep track of your mileage, when you bought your running shoes, what type of surface you're running on, races, and PRs, says Pribut. "That can be very helpful when trying to diagnose the injury."[2]

time there's an extensive amount of sweat loss—particularly in hot and humid conditions. "You end up with a mismatch between how much sodium you're losing and how much you're taking in," says Michael F. Bergeron, PhD, director of the National Institute for Athletic Health and Performance at Sanford USD Medical Center in Sioux Falls, South Dakota.

These spasms tend to start off in a small area or muscle group, but they can readily spread throughout your body. The cramps might begin in your calves and gravitate to your hamstrings, arms, stomach, and beyond.

Other researchers say that cramps are caused by muscle overload and fatigue, and some sort of disruption in the neuromuscular process that controls muscle contraction. Factors that might contribute to this could include some sort of genetic predisposition, exercising at a higher intensity for longer than what the athlete is accustomed to, or muscle damage before a race—perhaps by not tapering adequately, says Martin Schwellnus, professor of sport and exercise medicine at the University of Cape Town in South Africa.

Often, these cramps are relieved by changing biomechanics or stride.

Everything from plyometrics to pickle juice has been proposed as a remedy for muscle cramps. But stretching is the one foolproof strategy that has been proven to relieve the irritating condition when the muscle cramps are related to fatigue and overload.

"Stretching will break a cramp right away," says Miller. "It will also force you to stop and rest, which can alleviate fatigue."

Prevent a Cramp

Want to avoid cramping? Find some easy strategies below.

Know your risks and prepare accordingly. The best way to prevent cramps is to know your risks before you head out to run, says Schwellnus. If you get cramps often, there may be medications or over-the-counter drugs that may be contributing to them. To fend off fatigue during a race, be sure to train at the intensity that you'll be racing, taper properly, and know that you're at a higher risk of cramping when you're racing in hot and humid conditions.

Stay hydrated—but also maintain an adequate sodium balance. Bergeron recommends hydrating adequately and taking in enough salt, particularly before and after your runs. Use the sweat test (see "Hydration: Take It Personally" on page 96) to determine your own hydration needs.

Try plyometrics. Bounding, jumping, and hopping drills called plyometrics can strengthen muscle spindles, small nerves located between muscle fibers. Some theorize that muscle cramps can occur when these spindles get fatigued, so exercising them can help increase their endurance.[3]

Stopping a Cramp

Here are three stretches to help your cramps subside.

Calf stretch. Take a step forward with your noncramping leg. With your cramping leg's foot flat on the floor and pointing straight forward, slowly transfer your weight onto your front leg until you feel the stretch in your cramping calf. Hold for 20 seconds. Release and repeat.

Quad stretch. Reach back and grab the foot of your cramping leg. While standing upright (don't lean forward), pull your knee back and up toward your buttocks until you feel a stretch in your quad. Keep your standing leg straight and your thighs touching. Hold for 20 seconds. Release and repeat.

Hamstring stretch. Stand with most of your weight on your slightly bent, noncramping leg. Place your cramping leg in front of you so that it is straight and only your heel is touching the ground. Squat down slightly and point the toes of your cramping leg up and back toward your head. Hold for 20 seconds. Release and repeat.

What it takes to . . .
Be a Boston qualifier with rheumatoid arthritis

Linda Nollette, 47, San Jose, CA
Mother of three
Experience: 4 marathons; 3:49 PR
Runner's World **Challenge Race: 2011 Big Sur International Marathon**

I was diagnosed in February of 2006. I just assumed, based on all the reading I did, that I would go into remission and my life would come back. But it didn't. I realized that sitting on the couch, watching Oprah, and feeling sorry for myself really wasn't doing anything. I gained a lot of weight and was not feeling good about myself.

My husband was training for his first Ironman, and I started thinking that maybe I could, too—I swam in high school and college, and as a master, but I hadn't really done anything else. I needed something to motivate me. I signed up for an Ironman in September 2008 and ran a half-marathon 3 weeks later, finishing in 2:15. Then I went and did my first marathon. I finished in 3:59 and qualified for Boston. I did two more marathons, three Ironmans, and then had the race of a lifetime at Big Sur. Everyone said to add 20 minutes to your expectations for Big Sur because it's a hard course, and I chose not to. I ran a 3:49, a personal best by 10 minutes. And I'm hooked. My doctor is surprised that I can do this, and she still isn't thrilled about it. But the joint changes haven't been anything extreme—nothing more than the natural progression they would expect with someone who wasn't running. While I know that I'm damaging my joints, the good things that I'm doing for my muscles, tendons, ligaments, and weight—and my head—really outweigh that. Running helps keep everything in focus. I'm able to sleep better at night. So I think it's an integral part of my treatment. Running isn't a cure, but it's helped me manage arthritis. There will probably come a time when I won't be able to run. I don't know if that will be tomorrow. But I do know that it's not today. It's become a lifestyle. It's fun and it's addicting, and I truly believe that it's helping me.

Overtraining

Meleah Shank was feeling strong in the fifth week of training for her first Boston Marathon. She was logging her runs, teaching her spinning classes three times a week, and preparing for a half-marathon tune-up, logging an average of 50 miles per week. The week before the half, her kids got sick. She canceled her spin class but continued to train hard, and she came home from the Surf City

Half-Marathon with a 1:39 personal best. But she also came home with another not-so-welcome reward: a fever and a cough that developed into pneumonia 4 days later.

"My immune system was already hanging on by a thread," says Shank, a mother of two from Lake Forest, California. "By the end, I had pushed it to the brink and compromised my whole foundation."

It took about 10 days of no running to feel good enough to run again, another week to get back to running comfortably, and yet another week of getting back to the level of fitness she felt she was at before she got sick.

"That bout of sickness showed me how powerful my body can be in giving a signal to slow down," says Shank. "I got the message after that!"

Shank had a close encounter with overtraining, a condition that afflicts an estimated 10 percent of all runners. When you get too little recovery time, your training plateaus and you get sick.

"It's an imbalance between training and recovery that leads to a long-term loss of ability to train and compete at the levels you're used to," says Jack Raglin, a sports psychologist at Indiana University.

And often it doesn't even come from training too much, says Kristen Dieffenbach, a sports psychology consultant and psychologist and assistant professor at West Virginia University. "There may just be a hole in your recovery because you're not getting enough hydration, nutrition, or rest."

Most athletes underestimate the importance of rest and recovery in the training process, says Stacy Sims, PhD, an exercise physiologist and nutrition scientist at Stanford University.

It's during recovery that your body adapts to the stresses of training so you can get fitter and faster. Your muscles and neuromuscular systems get stronger, reaction time quickens, and your body adapts so that it can overcome the acute training stress more easily next time and it won't release as much cortisol (the stress hormone), so that you'll be more relaxed if you get exposed to that stress again, Sims says.

"If you're constantly exercising, your body never has a chance to fully adapt to that stress and get stronger," she says. "If you're not feeding it well during recovery, getting enough protein, getting sleep, and getting massages, you're not going to get the benefit of your training or see your body perform to its potential."

Unfortunately it's easy to write off symptoms of overtraining—irritability, fatigue, elevated heart rate, loss of appetite, and inability to sleep—as par for the course when you're pushing your body to run farther and faster than you've gone before.

But there are a few key distinctions. With overtraining, says Raglin, you might put in the same amount of effort as before but get subpar

Are You Overtrained?

Jack Raglin, a sports psychologist with Indiana University, developed a questionnaire to detect overtraining. Take this quiz once a week—or once a day, during periods of hard training. A score of 40 or more means that you should rest more and run less. A score of 15 or less suggests that you're balancing your training and recovery well. A score that falls in the middle isn't of immediate concern, but should be monitored.[4]

1. How is your mood today?
Very, very good (–2 points)
Very good (–1 point)
Good (0 points)
Average (1 point)
Bad (3 points)
Very bad (5 points)
Very, very bad (7 points)

2. How many hours did you sleep last night?
More than 9 (–1 point)
8 or 9 (0 points)
7 (1 point)
5 to 6 (3 points)
Less than 5 (5 points)

3. Last night I slept:
Same as normal (0 points)
1 hour more than normal (1 point)
2 or more hours more than normal (3 points)
1 hour less than normal (1 point)
2 hours less than normal (3 points)
3 or more hours less than normal (5 points)

4. Have you been sick the past week?
Yes (5 points)
No (0 points)

5. How would you rate yesterday's workout?
Very, very easy (–3 points)
Very easy (–1 point)
Easy (0 points)
Average (1 point)
Hard (3 points)
Very hard (5 points)
Very, very hard (7 points)

6. How do your muscles feel?
Very, very good (–3 points)
Very good (–1 point)
Good (0 points)
Tender, but not sore (1 point)
Sore (3 points)
Very sore (5 points)
Very, very sore (7 points)

7. Do your legs feel "heavy"?
No (0 points)
A little (1 point)
Somewhat (3 points)
Very (7 points)

results. You might feel fatigued when you wake up in the morning, before you even start your workout, feel your heart rate skyrocket during an easy run, or be winded just by walking up the stairs. And you may not feel like you even want to work out. "It's multiple days in a row of feeling like you just can't stand the thought of training," adds Dieffenbach.

The problem is that when most people have these symptoms, they panic and do the opposite of what they should do. "They think, 'Oh my gosh, I'm falling behind, I've hit a plateau,' and they redouble their efforts and add another workout or more repeats," says Raglin. "That's exactly the wrong thing to do."

Trying to push through overtraining is a losing proposition, experts say. If you continue to deprive your body of the recovery time it needs, it will lead to a cascade of other symptoms. Loss of appetite, for example, could lead to not getting enough calories to fuel your workouts and to even more fatigue and injury. "You just have to stop or reduce your training or make adjustments to allow your body to recover," says Raglin.

How long does it take? There is no one definitive answer to this, the experts say. It largely depends on whether you were injured and how deeply you were fatigued. Sims recommends at least 4 to 5 weeks of low-intensity exercise before returning to running, while simultaneously keeping track of variables like heart rate, perceived exertion, and sleep quality.

Once you do get some rest, you'll feel stronger and faster when you come back to training. Shank certainly did. After her bout with overtraining, she ran a 3:40 personal best at the Boston Marathon and went on to run a 3:49 negative split at the Big Sur Marathon just 13 days later.

Time to Rest

If you spot the signs of overtraining, consider implementing some of the following strategies.

Take a few days off. Give yourself 2 or 3 days off, and see how you feel. Take the test on page 188. "If you're not feeling rested, you're not going to perform well in training anyway, so you should keep resting," says Raglin.

Keep a training log. In addition to the miles that you log and the pace you maintain, take notes on how you feel before, during, and after your workouts. Rate your level of fatigue and how heavy your legs feel. Note whether you have a loss of appetite. "Keep really good records," says Dieffenbach. "Hindsight will be your best teacher."

Be active. While you're taking time off from running, don't feel like you have to go on bed rest. Go on a bike ride or take a hike. "Do something physical so you're not going crazy,"

Runner's Rehab

The following moves, suggested by Chicago physical therapist Annie O'Connor, corporate director of musculoskeletal practice at the Rehabilitation Institute of Chicago, will help you build leg, core, and rotational strength, and can help prepare your body to return to running. Only do exercises that do not affect your injured body part, unless instructed otherwise by your doctor. And be sure to check with your doctor before doing any of the exercises below.[5]

Power runner. Stand with your hands behind your head. Lift up your left knee, while simultaneously rotating your torso and bringing your right elbow forward to touch your knee. Return to the starting position. Tap your left toe on the ground and power back up. Continue to perform the move for 15 seconds and then switch sides. Work up to a minute on each side, varying your speed each day, moving slowly one day and more quickly the next.

Reverse lunge with a twist. Take a big step back with your left leg, keeping your arms down at your sides. As you lower into a lunge, turn your torso to the right. Return to starting position. Lunge back with the other leg and twist. Continue to alternate sides, doing 5 lunges on each side. Gradually add reps as you feel stronger.

Plank to side bridge. Start in a plank position, supporting yourself on your forearms. Turn your body by pivoting on your feet and shifting to one arm. Remember to turn your body as if it is a log, keeping your hips and shoulders aligned. Lift your arm up to the sky. Hold the position for 10 seconds, then lower yourself back to plank position. Put your weight on the opposite arm and repeat the move on the other side. Try to do 6 to 10 repetitions, holding each position for 10 seconds.

High-knee skipping. Don't try this until you're almost ready to resume running. Find an open space and start skipping. Thrust your arms and knees upward, and alternate, lifting your right arm with your left foot and your left arm with your right foot. Continue for 15 seconds. Increase to 1-minute intervals.

says Raglin. "Physical activity is a source of satisfaction and pleasure, and you don't want to feel like you have to deny yourself that. Just don't turn it into training." Sims suggests exercises like yoga and aquajogging—activities that don't trigger rushes of adrenaline or cortisol. "You've got to take your body out of that constant state of fight-or-flight."

Coping with Injuries

For Maggie Smith, running has been the one constant while she juggled her duties as a sergeant in the army, a wife, and mom of a toddler. "Running gives me a clear head, allows me to feel in control of something, and enables me to sort through issues that seem impossible," says Smith, 31,

Return to Running

The biggest mistake runners make is coming back from an injury too soon and reinjuring themselves, says Craig Souders, DPT, Lehigh Valley Health Network in Bethlehem, Pennsylvania. Here's his plan to help you get back to running. All of these runs should be done at an easy, comfortable, conversational pace, and they should be pain free. "Running faster won't help," says Souders. "The goal is to get your injured part used to the physical demands of running. Faster running comes after you have ramped up to 100 percent of your previous total training time."

MISSED DAYS	WHAT TO DO
1 to 4 days	Don't worry. Just pick up the training schedule where you're supposed to be. Start extra slow on your next run to shake out the sluggishness.
5 to 7 days	Run 50 percent of the mileage that you had planned for 3 days, followed by 3 days of running 75 percent of the mileage planned. Then, if you're pain free, continue at 100 percent of the mileage planned.
2 weeks	Drop your mileage by 50 percent for 7 days; back off your target pace by 2 percent. Then start building back gradually toward the mileage on the plan. Expect that it will take 3 to 4 weeks to regain your fitness.
3 weeks	Drop your mileage by 50 percent for 10 to 14 days; run 4 percent slower, then start building again. Consider readjusting your race goals.
28 days or more	Rethink your race goals. Enter a race that's further down the road, or resolve to use the marathon as a "training run" without a time goal. To build back up, for a period of time equal to one-third of the days you took off, run for 33 percent of the total time that you'd normally run. Then for one-third of the days you took off, run for 75 percent of the total time that you'd normally run. After that you can run for the full amount of time you'd normally run. If you've taken off 6 weeks or longer, you'll need more time to build back up to your previous mileage.
1 long run	On your next long run, run 80 percent of the mileage on the plan, then try to do the full mileage of the next long run. On both runs, be sure to take it at an easy pace.
2 long runs	On your next long run, complete 60 percent of the mileage on the plan. On the following long run, complete 80 percent of the mileage. Then get back on track.
3 or 4 long runs of 2 hours or more	Rethink your race goal. Enter a race that's later in the year, or resolve to use the marathon as a "training run." Don't run for a race goal.

→RW CHALLENGER PROFILE:
Christine Yarosh

Christine Yarosh has run 17 marathons with a 3:28 personal best, and she's logged thousands of miles to prepare for them. But the amount of time and sweat she's put into being able to run those miles isn't anything that could be measured on a finish-line clock.

In 2005, on the last mile of a 100-mile bike ride, she swerved to avoid hitting a dog and went headfirst over the handlebars. She fractured both wrists, sprained both ankles, and injured her left hip and shoulder. She lost range of motion in her left ankle and tore ligaments in her hip.

Then there was knee surgery and hip surgery, and then surgery on her other knee. And then there was Achilles tendonitis and piriformis syndrome, and then the femoral stress fracture that accompanied her on all 26.2 miles of the 2010 Toronto Marathon with the *Runner's World* Challenge. And then there was another knee injury that came from compensating on her gait due to the stress fracture.

It has taken a massage therapist, a physical therapist, a biomechanist, a sports medicine doctor, a chiropractor, and an acupuncturist for Yarosh to stay on the road, not to mention the unwavering support of her husband, Rick Slawsky.

A cynic might ask, "Why bother?" but for Yarosh, retiring from running wasn't an option. "Running gives me mental clarity," says Yarosh, 46, who lives in Austin, Texas. "Sometimes I'm focused on my breathing and my pace, but mostly I'm reflecting on the things going on in my life, solving problems, or planning something."

What's more, "It is the hub of so many

a seven-time marathoner with a personal best of 3:22.

So when she was diagnosed with a stress fracture in her left ankle and told she couldn't run, "I bawled my eyes out," she says. "I felt 'fat,' I felt lazy, I felt weak, and I felt silly. I was a runner, so if I couldn't run, what the heck was I going to do to maintain my sanity?"

Indeed, as Smith learned, when you get sidelined by injuries, whatever physical pain you might feel pales in comparison to the emotional blow. All the miles that you've logged and speed sessions you've slogged through feel like a waste. And if you rely on running for stress relief or it's a core part of your identity, you're left reeling.

"Runners are pretty goal-oriented and not happy about having their path blocked," says Jim Taylor, a San Francisco–based sports psychologist.

Many of the bad feelings that go along with injury are also influenced by brain chemistry,

things in my life," she says. She shares it with her husband. It offers her community, gives her focus, and is the underpinning of her charity work with groups like Medals4Mettle.

To be sure, Yarosh learned some pretty tough lessons on the road to recovery. She learned to focus on her abilities, rather than her limitations. When swimming was all she could do, she took classes and joined a masters swim group. When thoughts of "I'll never run again," crept in, she learned to be flexible and accept that nothing lasts forever—not the logy feeling of not being able to run *or* the unlimited PRs. And she learned to take it one step at a time, not trying to short-cut recovery time or to let a positive or negative experience carry her thoughts away for better or worse.

"I've learned that good runs don't mean that I'm out of the woods," she says, "and bad ones aren't the start of a downward spiral."

And most important, she's learned that running doesn't have to be any less enjoyable—even at a different pace.

"I do tend to appreciate the ability to run more now than when it was a given," she says. "Even if it's a bad run, I feel good to have accomplished it."

Yarosh hasn't abandoned hope of reaching big running goals—like running a 2:59:59 marathon or completing the 56-mile Comrades Ultramarathon in South Africa. But for now, she's focusing on 30- to 45-minute runs and on building up to 30 to 40 miles per week without breaking down.

Exciting? Maybe not. "But it's reasonable and attainable and I do feel good about the effort," she says.

says Shawn Talbott, a Salt Lake City, Utah, nutritional biochemist who has completed more than 100 marathons and triathlons. Running—or any exercise, for that matter—naturally filters out cortisol, the stress hormone, and provides a short-term hit of endorphins, the feel-good chemicals that block pain. Without your daily run, the cortisol builds up in your body, causing fatigue, anxiety, and depression. Plus you miss out on the endorphins, says Talbott. Add the mount-

ing stress and guilt about missing your runs, "and that gets you into a cycle of feeling worse and worse."

Taylor says that when runners get injured, they go through the same series of emotions—denial, anger, depression, and acceptance—that accompany any loss. Getting over the denial is often the toughest part. "The reality is that the sooner they accept there's an injury," says Taylor, "the sooner they can get better."

The good news is, just because you're out

doesn't mean you have to be down. There are ways to cope with an injury that can help your body and mind heal.

"As an injured runner, you have to understand that you do have choices and you need to act on them," says Stan Beecham, a sports psychologist based in Atlanta, Georgia. "That in itself is pretty empowering."

Treat rehab like your training. "The worst part for runners is feeling like they're just falling behind, losing fitness, and being schlubs," says Taylor. So apply the energy and discipline you devote to your training to your rehab routine. Work with your physical therapist to map out a plan—just like you do with your training plans for races—so that you can have a focus and a goal for each day and feel good about checking it off when you're done. "That will make you a better runner, make you feel like you have some sense of control and that things are going in the right direction," says Taylor.

Focus on what you can do, not what you can't. Reframe yourself as an athlete, not just as a runner. Join a gym, go to a spinning class, do anything you can to get moving. "You've got to focus on 'What can I do now?'" says Beecham. "Stress your body enough to get the psychological benefits of exercise," he says. That will keep the endorphins flowing and the stress hormones at bay. Indeed, Smith started swimming and biking while she couldn't run and found that she gained much more total body strength. "I had to stay in shape," Smith says. "My cross-training goal became a drive for strength, and I was able to meet it by trying new types of cardio training," she says. Though she has three more marathons on her to-do list this year, her main goal is to stay healthy. "Keeping plans to run helps me through those injuries," she says. "It gets me focused on healing so that I can get back on the road or trail."

Learn from it. There's usually a good reason for an injury: the wrong shoes, overtraining, muscle weakness, or problems with your gait. It's important to find out what that reason is and address the issue. "That way, you can increase your confidence that you're not going to get injured again," says Taylor. On the other hand, "if you just look at it as an inconvenience, you're going to stay stuck, or worse, repeat the same mistake," says Beecham.

Stay connected. It helps to stay engaged with your running community even while you're injured, says Beecham. Ride your bike alongside your buddies on training runs, or take your turn as support crew. Keep reading your running books and magazines, and plan races for the future, when you're healed. This will help reinforce your sense of identity as a runner. When Katie Livingood learned that she had a stress fracture just a few days before her marathon, she started reading everything about running, preventing injuries, and training smart—buying books and visiting the *Runner's World* forums almost every day. "I planned my next race almost obsessively—what I was going to wear, and my fueling plan—and I became a big cheerleader for my running friends," says Livingood, 29, of Jenks, Oklahoma. "Surrounding myself with people who had made successful running comebacks helped me build the 'If they can do it, so can I' mentality."

The Art of the Comeback

Craig Souders, DPT, Lehigh Valley Health Network in Bethlehem, Pennsylvania, sees many of the same cases over and over again: injured marathoners he rehabbed weeks ago wobbling into his office after reinjuring themselves.

Often, after a layoff, runners try to pick up where they left off. Or worse, they try to accelerate the pace and distance in their remaining workouts in an effort to catch up with their training plans and cram for the race. That, Souders says, is a recipe for disaster.

"Your heart and lungs may be in great shape, and you may feel like you can go out and run for 2 hours, but you must remember that you're

(continued on page 198)

— **[WHAT WORKS]** —

Cut back on mileage in order to go the distance

Scott Francis, 44, Danville, CA; chief technology officer for Premier Retail Networks; father of two; 1 marathon; 3:53 PR; *Runner's World* Challenge Race: 2011 Big Sur International Marathon

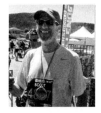

My body seems to have some kind of flare-up when I push new weekly training loads. About 4 weeks into training for my first marathon, in Big Sur, my IT band flared up. It felt as if someone were inserting a knife right in between my femur and tibia. I dropped my mileage significantly—cutting 50 percent or more of the week's mileage. I focused on completing the easy runs rather than the quality work, and even cut those easy runs very short. The first few times, I ran until I could feel a little irritation starting, then walked home. I iced and took ibuprofen like crazy. About 6 weeks later, I fully recovered. It cost me a pretty serious cutback, but I was running well and in good shape. Treating the symptom and cutting back a bit allowed me to push ahead and conquer that boundary to find the next. I guess that's running. And age. I feel fitter, stronger, and faster than I ever have. And I finished the race in 3:53.

On Shifting Gears

by Bart Yasso

The way I see it, you walk into the woods for 8 years of running, where you're just getting into the sport and you're getting faster and running farther, and no matter what age you are, you're continuously improving. But at some point, you start walking out of the woods. Maybe it's because of injury or illness or age or pregnancy, but you stop getting faster. Or maybe you have to stop running altogether, or limit your running dramatically. A lot of people just hit the point where they can't run. And at that point, you have to ask the question, "Do I give up for good? How do I handle it?"

For me, that walk out of the woods started in June 1997, while climbing Mount Kilimanjaro. I had my second flare-up of Lyme disease, which made my vision blurry, my joints swell, and my legs throb, and made me feel thoroughly exhausted.

Up until that point, I had been doing 100-mile training weeks; I'd run a 2:40 marathon, I'd run 146 miles across Death Valley, done Ironman Triathlons, and completed more than 1,000 races. Running was my livelihood. It had given me focus and a direction I hadn't found any other way. And as race promotions director of *Runner's World,* the sport was literally my life. I was flying all over the country to race 50 weekends of the year. And now, because of a chance bite by a deer tick, there was a chance that it could all be taken away.

When I first contracted Lyme disease, I couldn't run at all. I was struggling to walk, let alone run. I was just worried about trying to get healthy. I knew that it was going to affect me for the rest of my life. It was really traumatic. I knew that if I had any shot of recovery, I'd have to take it easy and rest like the doctor ordered. After 3 weeks, I started feeling like my old self again, and the inflammation in my joints subsided. Still, I took it slow, running 2 or 3 easy miles every other day. My body responded to the familiar motion, and I regained my endurance.

I was able to lead the 3-hour pace group at the Chicago Marathon. But after that and other bouts with Lyme disease, I slowed down.

It's hard to stop running when you get hurt or sick, especially when you're on a roll and feeling good and getting faster, and your running is at an all-time high, and then—bam!—you pull a hamstring or have a knee problem. I meet guys who say, "I'd race if I could run faster," but I think that's crazy and is the worst attitude to have.

Every runner wants to be fast, and every runner wants to be fast forever. I had the same aspirations. But reality is a little bit different. We all slow down at some point. If I would have given up when I slowed down, I would have missed out on so many opportunities and adventures and encountering all these great people and great stories.

When the slowdown comes, don't freak out and get crazy about it because, in the big picture, we're very fortunate that we're physically able to do this. Most of our injuries will go away and we'll learn from them. Maybe your body gave you a signal that you shouldn't have run, but you went out anyway, so instead of a rest day, you have to take 6 weeks off. You've got to make the best of a bad situation. Stay as fit as you can by doing cross-training.

These days I run less than 10 miles a week. Where before I might have gone on a 40-mile bike ride, now I only do 20.

I take as my role models guys like Amby Burfoot: He was one of the top runners in the country, and now he's doing 4-hour marathons and he's just happy to be out there. And I admire my wife, Laura. When she slowed down, she never said, "I'm outta here." They just kept it fun, and kept the passion in it. And that's what it's all about.

And I don't enjoy running any less now that I'm slower. It's very different to go from winning races and being a top age-group runner to blending into the back of the pack. But as I do, I'm just happy to be out there. I don't feel sorry for myself that I used to be up front.

If I could get out there and do what I used to do, that would be the ultimate. But I don't think it's ever going to happen.

With the problems I have, I know that I don't have a lot of running left in my legs. So now it's a matter of doing races I've never done before, or running unusual races that sound fun. I did the 2010 Comrades Ultramarathon, a 56-mile race in South Africa that is the toughest footrace in the world. Since then I did the Kauai Half-Marathon in Hawaii, the first ever Jerusalem Half-Marathon in Israel, and I did a nighttime trail run that started and ended in the dark, just because I'd never done anything like that before.

I just love to be a part of the sport. I still have fun doing it. I've never lost my enjoyment of just being out there. So when I'm out there having fun, it doesn't matter what part of the pack I'm in.

At the 2011 Big Sur Marathon, everyone was asking me whether I was running the race. I wasn't even remotely thinking about it. I had my years to race in Big Sur. I was so happy to be able to run it when I did, but those years are gone. I don't pout or feel bad about it.

Instead, I dwell on how lucky I am. If I didn't do all of that stuff that I did in my younger days, then I would have never had the opportunity—ever. I've had a pretty cool career, and I'm very grateful to be out there trying to spread the word about the power of our sport and how it can change lives.

So for me, it's still worth it to be a part of the game. If the joy of running and just being out there is what you thrive on, it doesn't matter how fast you are. We're all runners: That's the bottom line. And we've all got to be happy with our running ability. You just have to go out and give it your best.

coming back on your weakest link and you need to think about how much that newly rehabbed part can handle," says Souders. "The problem is that the muscles, ligaments, tendons, and bones have to handle the impact of running."

The key to returning to running safely, and staying healthy and injury free, is to take it slow. Follow the chart in "Return to Running" on page 191, and while you're coming back, do strengthening exercises that will help you develop the muscles you'll be calling on when you're back on the road. (See "Runner's Rehab" on page 190.)

Just as important as taking it slow is a willingness to adjust your goals for the racing season. If you rush your recovery, you risk "taking a relatively minor injury that should clear up in a few weeks and turning it into a chronic, season-long nuisance," says Souders. "It's better to heal completely and build gradually. The goal is to get back to sustained training, not sporadic training."

INSIDE RUNNER'S WORLD ®

KATIE NEITZ, 35, SENIOR EDITOR, EMMAUS, PA

LESSON LEARNED: DON'T RUSH A COMEBACK

I ran throughout my pregnancy, and after my baby was born, I took about 6 weeks off. I was eager to get back on the roads again, so as soon as I got the okay from my doctor, I was back out there. I wanted to lose the baby weight and get into a routine that I identified as sane and normal. For years, I had started most days with some sort of exercise. And here was this baby who completely turned my life upside down. My nights turned into days. I was really tired, nursing was challenging, and so I was physically and emotionally drained. I looked forward to my daily workout because it was a chance to do something familiar and to feel strong. I was up to about 9 miles within about a month of coming back. But I was doing a lot of these runs while pushing the jogger stroller. I think that helped do a number on my pelvis, which was still healing from delivery, because I developed a pelvic stress fracture. Recovering from a stress fracture (especially one in your pelvis) is no fun. It means no running and lots of cross-training for about 8 weeks. So I hit the pool and the yoga mat, and I learned some good core and pelvic strengthening exercises at physical therapy. And within 8 weeks, I was running again. I signed up for a marathon and did a 3-day-a-week training program, just to be sure that I wasn't overdoing it. Four months later, I ran a successful marathon.

Rediscovering Speed:
How to Add Fast Running Back to Your Routine

After getting up to 100 percent of the distance in the chart "Return to Running" on page 191 and getting comfortable running easy and pain-free, you can add quality workouts to your schedule to reactivate dormant fast-twitch muscle fibers and increase your ability to run fast. Here's a guide from Ed Eyestone, an exercise physiologist, coach of the Brigham Young University Cross-Country team, and "Fast Lane" columnist for *Runner's World*.[6]

INTRODUCE	WHEN	HOW
Strides	After 2 weeks easy running	Do eight to ten 100-meter strides twice a week at the end of your easy run. Build speed to 80 to 90 percent effort for 40 meters, maintain for 30 meters, then diminish it through the final 30.
Tempo runs	After 3 weeks easy running	Do a 6-minute surge in the middle of a 30-minute easy run once a week. Increase duration by 2 minutes every time you do a tempo run.
Intervals	After 6 weeks easy running	Once a week, run speed sessions of 5-4-3-2-1 minutes of hard running, followed by equal amounts of easy running. Gradually increase the duration until you can run 10-5-3-2-1 comfortably.

Enduring Questions

What day of the week should I do strength work?

It's best to do strength training on the same day as a hard workout, like a speed session or a long run. "The best thing is to finish your run, get some quick fuel and fluid, then do the strength workout," says McGlynn. That said, not a lot of people have the time for that, as hard workouts are already hard enough to squeeze in. The next best thing, he says, is to fit in two strength sessions each week and just avoid doing them on the days before your long runs and speed sessions. That way,

you're not sore the next day, when you want to go fast or long.

I take over-the-counter pain relievers before my long runs. Is that okay?

While using a pain reliever after a run to reduce soreness is fine, if you have to pop a pill to relieve pain to get through a run, it's better to rest instead and see a doctor to get to what's causing the pain, experts say. Using a pain reliever to mask pain could only make the cause of it worse. Plus, there's evidence that nonsteroidal anti-inflammatory drugs (NSAIDs, such as ibuprofen and naproxen) can cause muscle damage and impair kidney function when taken in excess before or during a run, says David Nieman, DrPH, of the North Carolina Research Center and Appalachian State University. In studies of runners at the 100-mile Western States Endurance Run, Nieman found that the habitual users (those who used the daily maximum recommended dose of 1,200 milligrams per day) ended up with up to 50 percent more inflammation and oxidative stress than those who didn't use NSAIDs. Plus, their kidneys weren't clearing creatinine as well as those who used no ibuprofen. To top it all off, those who used ibuprofen had the same level of muscle soreness after the race as those who didn't, and there was no difference in the rate of perceived exertion or pain between the people who used ibuprofen and those who didn't. "We found that ibuprofen is not helping diminish muscle soreness," says Nieman, "it is just making runners more inflamed and causing kidney issues." If you have to use anything, aspirin may be a better alternative, as long as it doesn't upset your stomach, Nieman says. "I think athletes should just leave ibuprofen alone," he adds. "The better bet is to manage your training and exercise so that you can keep pain and discomfort under control." That means follow your training program, build your miles gradually, and don't go into races unprepared. Also, eat more fruits and vegetables. The antioxidants in fruits and vegetables help the body fight oxidative stress.

I feel sore for 2 days after a long run. Is it okay to run then?

Delayed onset muscle soreness (DOMS) peaks 24 to 48 hours after a hard workout or a race and tends to dissipate within a week. It is normal to feel sore any time muscles are worked in a new way, like in speedwork, races, or long runs, or after any new workout or if you're racing faster, or longer, or on hillier terrain than you've run before. These new activities can cause microtears in your muscles, which is what causes the soreness, says Carol Torgan, an exercise physiologist in Bethesda, Maryland. As your muscles repair themselves, they grow stronger and more resistant to the fatigue. It's fine to do an easy run while you're feeling that DOMS, but hold off on intense workouts for a few days. If the soreness lasts longer than a week or there's pain or swelling, see a doctor.[7]

How do I relieve a side stitch?

Side stitches—sharp pains just below the rib cage—feel like cramps, but they're a different problem. Some say that they happen because of pressure on the diaphragm muscle (located just below the lungs), which can partially cut off oxygen flow to the muscle. This can also happen because abdominal muscles push up against the diaphragm or a too-full stomach pushes down on it. As you increase your fitness, side stitches should subside. If you get a side stitch, stop and walk and breathe slowly and deeply from your belly for 30 seconds. Raise your arms straight up to the sky, then bend at the waist directly away from the stitch to form a C shape with your body.[8]

Is it okay to run when I have a cold?

If you're just sniffling and sneezing, it's fine to go out, but if you're running a fever of 100.4°F or higher, stay in, says sports medicine doctor Darrin Bright, a 3:02 marathoner and medical director for the Columbus (Ohio) Marathon. Running high mileage has been shown to suppress the immune system and make you more susceptible to the common cold, which is why runners so often get sick in the 3 to 4 weeks before race day. If you have a fever, your ability to regulate heat is disrupted and you'll be more susceptible to heatstroke or heat exhaustion. If you're feeling a tightness in your chest or you have trouble breathing, then it's best to stay in until you're feeling better. Make sure you hydrate well when you have a cold. If you're heading to a race, avoid taking any decongestants. Many of them are stimulants, which affect your ability to regulate your temperature and set you up for heat illness. If you are put on antibiotics, be sure to talk with your doctor about your running plans. A certain class of antibiotics called fluoroquinolones (which are sold under names like Cipro, Levaquin, Floxin, and Noroxin) have been shown to increase the risk of Achilles injuries, even for weeks after you're done taking the medication.

When is the best time to get a massage—before or after a race?

Massage releases tight areas, breaks up scar tissue, and helps flush lactic acid and other waste products out of the muscles, says Mike Blackmore, a Eugene, Oregon–based massage therapist. Getting a light massage immediately after a race can help reduce postrace soreness, move fluid through your tissues and keep them hydrated, and encourage blood flow to your legs, which will help reduce soreness and encourage nutrient flow to your glycogen-starved muscles. If you've never had a massage after a race, be sure to let the therapist know. He or she will make sure that the pressure is appropriate for you. Getting regular massages throughout your training can

help keep you running efficiently and injury free, adds Blackmore. "A solid training plan that includes massages can reduce recovery time from hard efforts so the next effort produces the desired results," he says. During training, the best time for a massage is 2 to 4 days before or after a hard workout (like a speed session or a long run), says Vicki Huber Rudawsky, a two-time Olympian and massage therapist in Wilmington, Delaware. You might head to a massage therapist 4 or 5 days before a race, so you're not sore for your big event. After a race, wait 5 to 7 days. Look for a massage therapist who has experience working with long-distance runners. Ask for referrals from your running buddies or a local running store. Look for someone who is licensed by the state and certified by a national certification board for therapeutic massage and bodywork. There are different forms of massage. A sports massage can go deep into the muscles, help smooth out knots, and release tight IT bands. Myofascial release is a slow application, where the therapist holds tension in a particular area and waits until the body responds and the area releases, says Rudawsky. Active Release Technique (often referred to as ART) is a technique where the therapist uses his or her hands to evaluate the tightness and movement of the muscles, fascia, tendons, ligaments, and nerves, and he or she then puts tension on the tissue while it's directed through specific movements. ART is often helpful for those muscle imbalances and repetitive stress injuries that runners often cope with. Talk with your therapist about which type is most appropriate for you.

PART IV

PUTTING IT ALL TOGETHER

The hay is in the barn.

That's certainly what *Runner's World* Challenger Mike Gross thought 3 weeks before the 2011 Boston Marathon. He was in shape to meet his 2:40 goal; he was hitting his Yasso 800s right on target, and he felt better than he had in years. But within 24 hours of finishing his last long run, he developed a scratchy throat, runny nose, and congestion. He skipped some workouts and took others easy, but on race day, he finished more than 30 minutes off his goal and ended the day in the medical tent.

"All that training had to get thrown away," says Gross.

Gross's story is a lesson: No matter what happens during the monster months of training, for better or for worse, anything can happen on the big day. And that's not always a bad thing. *Runner's World* Challenger Carrie Parker went into the 2011 Blue Nose Marathon in Nova Scotia after a "brutal training season," expecting nothing but a tough finish. Between sickness and unrunnable weather, she'd lost nearly 2 weeks of training. Still, she ended up finishing with a personal best of 4:35, a 7-minute PR.

"I was just ecstatic," says Parker, a technical analyst at the New Brunswick Department of Education in New Brunswick, Canada. "I felt so proud of myself that I had managed to do what I did after all that I'd been through."

Some things, like weather and illness, are beyond your control. But the good news is that there is plenty that you can do in the weeks before go-time to make or break your race.

In this section, you'll find everything you need to know about how to handle the critical weeks before the race, how to race well, and what to do after you cross the finish line to keep your mind and body healthy, strong, and ready to run again, whether the race results were what you wanted or not.

CHAPTER 9

BEFORE THE RACE

Fourteen days before the Big Sur marathon, Pam Franklin was, by anyone's measure, well prepared. After all, she'd poured 4 months and more than 400 miles into training. But there she was, just 4 miles into her 13-miler—her second to last long run—struggling to make it up a hill.

"Man, am I screwed," she remembers thinking. "I wonder if I should just cancel the trip?"

Indeed, while the taper might seem like it should be a breeze compared to the long runs and track work, for most runners, it's the toughest part of training. As the big day draws closer, you start to question every mile you ran or missed. Hip pains, raging IT bands, and twinges in your back start to crop up. And to top it all off, the fact that you're running fewer miles makes you worry that you're losing fitness.

But research has shown that reducing mileage volume and intensity before the race can boost your time on race day. In a June 2010 study in the *Journal of Applied Physiology*,[1] researchers found that runners improved their performance by 3 percent when they dropped their mileage in the 3 weeks before their race.

The runners kept up their easy runs and intervals, but limited their moderately hard efforts, such as tempo runs. During the taper, the runners maintained their VO_2 max and the fast-twitch fibers in their calf muscles got bigger, stronger, and more powerful. The overall capacity of their muscles and cardiovascular systems rebounded.

"We overload these fibers when we're training, and when we pull that stress back, they recover and come back stronger and more powerful," says Scott Trappe, coauthor of the study and director of the Human Performance Laboratory at Ball State University in Muncie, Indiana. The study showed that "if you can back off the volume considerably, you're not going to lose any cardiovascular fitness, plus your muscles are going to recover in a way that is advantageous to your performance."

People often make the mistake of running too much in those final 3 weeks, says Joe McConkey, coach at the Boston Running Center. The last long run of training, which tends to be 20 to 22 miles, takes more out of people than they think, he says. "There's nothing to be gained from added intensity."

If you know what to expect as you back off of your training, you'll be better equipped to survive the taper and arrive at the starting line feeling rested and ready to run your best. Here are some of the most common mental and physical troubles that tend to crop up, plus how to deal with them.

Taper Trouble

Your knee, IT band, or hamstring starts to ache.

While scientists don't know exactly what causes these aches and pains, they concede that reducing mileage after months of maximum effort introduces a new stress to the body and the mind. And because you've poured so much

Amby's Advice

If there's a more important part of your training program than the prerace taper, I can't imagine what it might be. Without the right taper, all of your hard-earned fitness can go down the drain faster than spoiled milk. None of us is that wasteful. We want to train, and then we want to see our training pay off with a strong race effort.

time and energy into this event, you're on high alert for any subtle changes in how you feel. Shawn Talbott, a Salt Lake City, Utah, nutritional biochemist who has completed more than 100 marathons and triathlons, likens these feelings to a type of withdrawal. "When you're training every day, you're getting a consistent dose of endorphins, stress hormones, glucose, and blood and oxygen supply to the muscles, lungs, and brain," he says. "When we taper, we reduce the delivery of these compounds to our muscles, tendons, and ligaments—so we feel these physical twinges."

Solution: McConkey says that although those random twinges don't usually amount to much, he advises people to get anything they're worried about checked out. "You've got to chase every tail," he says. "We don't want people worrying about things if they don't have to." If nothing else, it will give you one less thing to stress about. If you're nursing an injury, it's okay to rest or cross-train—and run less—even more than the taper calls for, says Trappe. As long as you're moving, your fitness for the race won't be affected.

Your confidence sinks.

You start to worry that you won't be able to finish, much less meet your time goal.

Solution: Get a reality check. Review your training log. Look at all of the miles you logged, the speed sessions you gutted out, and the number of days when you went through with your run despite a strong desire not to.

"Look at evidence about yourself and your preparation, and focus on the joy that goes along with it," says Harvard psychologist Jeff Brown, author of *The Winner's Brain*. And remember that there's no perfect way to train, says Stan Beecham, a sports psychologist from Atlanta, Georgia. "What you may have done to prepare for this race may not have been perfect, but nobody else probably trained perfectly either." In the week before the race, McConkey has his runners spend 5 minutes each night visualizing success for themselves by creating a movie reel of the race. "See yourself in the morning waking up, dealing with the logistics, and getting to the race. Visualize how you want to look and feel—excited, but relaxed and confident." And don't forget to see yourself taking on the tough stuff, like heat, wind, and hills. "Just get your mind relaxed and ready so that when the starting gun goes off, you're in the right mind-set," says McConkey. "Remind yourself of all the work you've done. There's nothing to be gained from worrying or putting in extra intensity."

You have the urge to cram in miles.

You're used to longer runs at higher intensities, and the reduced volume feels like it's not enough to even qualify as exercise. So you want to sneak in just a few extra speed sessions and miles.

Solution: Stick to the training plan. And this is not the time to start yoga or Pilates or any other new activity. Pour the energy and time you'd normally spend running into cleaning, connecting with friends and family you haven't seen during training, or catching up on gardening and housework. Have structured activities in place that are mentally engaging but not physically taxing, says Brown. "Don't pick up kayaking or do something that's risky for you," he says, "but it should be something that you can get into," like going to a movie with your running buddy. This is also a great time to volunteer or spectate at a race. You can feel like a part of the excitement without risking injury.

You feel sluggish.

It's natural to feel fatigued and stiff during the taper. During this time, your body is storing more carbohydrates and water, which can leave you with the same feeling you might have after consuming a big meal.

Solution: Throw a few race-pace miles into your shorter runs to reinforce your confidence in your ability to hold that pace. If you've been practicing your race pace throughout the training, this pace should feel easy. Or throw five to seven strides into some easy runs to boost your heart rate and get your fast-twitch muscle fibers firing. But remember, if you let yourself rest, you will feel energized for race day. Trappe says that when he feels like this, "I remind myself that I'd rather feel crappy today, during the taper, than on race day."

You gain a pound or two.

This is common. Water gets stored, along with the glycogen, when you eat high-carbohydrate foods. It can also make you feel bloated and heavy. Plus, the extra fluids you might be drinking to stay hydrated can also add on pounds.

Solution: Don't weigh yourself, and don't go on a diet. "People think because they're running less, they should eat less, and then they're not topping off their stores for the race," says McConkey. "That extra pound or two going into the race will serve them better than the weight loss, in terms of energy stores. They're better off keeping up their standard diet." In the final 3 weeks, eat 60 percent carbs, 10 to 15 percent low-fat protein (such as chicken, fish, lean meats, beans, and legumes), and 25 to 30 percent fat, says *Runner's World* Challenge sports nutritionist Pamela Nisevich Bede. "Runners have busted their butts for months," she says. "They shouldn't throw all that work away by cutting back in the few days leading up to a race!"

You get a cold.

This is very common. A 1995 study published in *Thorax*[2] showed that endurance athletes are at increased risk for upper respiratory

---

The Lowdown on Carb-Loading

A lot of folks think that the term carb-loading means downing a box of pasta the night before the race. Unfortunately, many find out the hard way that this is a recipe for a sleepless night and a feeling of being bloated and waterlogged as the starting gun fires.

There's a saner approach. Carb-loading involves gradually reducing your mileage (through the taper) and gradually increasing your carbohydrate intake in the days before a race. This helps load up your body's fuel tank so that when the starting gun goes off, your muscles are fully loaded but your stomach isn't stuffed.

Give yourself a week before race day to carb-load. Focus on spending your calories on carbs. Simply make sure each meal has some carbohydrate in it—such as a bagel, bread, pasta, rice, or cereal. (See "Race Week Carb-Loading Plan" on page 248.)

If you want to be precise about it, there have been proven formulas for carb-loading success: In the 7 days before the race, have 2.3 grams of carbs per pound of body weight. In the 1 to 3 days before, have 3.6 to 5.5 grams per pound of body weight. (If you're training for a half-marathon, you can do a mini carb-load: In the 2 days before the race, aim for 2.5 to 4 grams of carbs per pound of body weight.)

It's best to practice this at some point during your race preparation (such as before a long run), rather than testing it out on race week. Carbs tend to promote water retention. If you experience this during training, it won't be one more worry to add to your list during race week!

tract infections during the heaviest times of training—and in the 1 to 2 weeks after a marathon or similar event.

Solution: Rest as much as you can, get 8 hours of sleep each night, stay hydrated, and as long as you don't have trouble breathing, or a temperature, it's okay to keep running. Studies haven't shown whether exercise makes symptoms better or worse. Eat a well-balanced diet to keep your pool of vitamins and minerals high.[3] Be extra vigilant about washing your hands. Avoid putting your hands near your eyes and nose, because that can introduce new viruses to your body. Avoid sick people and large crowds when you can. If your symptoms do not improve, see a doctor.

Don't Go Out Too Fast!

Far and away the biggest mistake that most runners make is going out too fast, either because they have unrealistic time goals or they don't know their pace, says Sean Coster, coach and director of Run Portland, an Oregon-based running club. Follow these tips to make a smart start.

Practice, practice, practice. Practice your goal race pace as much as possible during training so that on race day it feels natural. Coster recommends that marathoners try a 14- to 18-mile run at goal pace 3 to 4 weeks before the race. Those doing a half-marathon might try an 8- to 10-mile run at goal race pace about 3 weeks out from the race.

Do a tune-up. About a month before your goal event, run a shorter event to test your fitness. If you're training for a half-marathon, run a 10-K about 4 weeks before the race. If you're targeting a marathon, do a half-marathon tune-up. Plug your finishing time into a finish time prediction calculator like the one at runnersworld.com/tools to help you figure out whether your goal time for your big race is realistic.

Ignore the pack. Run the first 2 to 3 miles 10 to 15 seconds slower than goal pace, with the idea that you'll finish strong. Don't try to "bank" time by going out faster than your goal pace. If you do that, you risk burning out early. As everyone around you dashes off at the start, you may fear that you'll be the last person to finish the race, but chances are you won't be. Just let those folks go, and focus on getting into a rhythm that feels comfortable for you. There's a good chance that during the final miles, you'll see all those people who passed you early!

Listen to your body. During the race, tune in to signals like how hard you're breathing, how tired your muscles are feeling, and whether you have clenched up any areas of your body (such as your jaw or shoulder) that you can relax. "It may feel ridiculously slow," says Coster. "But when you get up to the 20-mile marker, it's very humbling how heavy your legs are and how much work its takes to support your body. Even a slow pace is going to feel challenging to maintain for your final 10-K." If it's your first race, it's a good idea to figure out what your base effort translates to in terms of finishing time so that you can set a realistic goal. Avoid using music, as it can distract you from paying attention to your effort and evaluating your pace.

CHAPTER 10

THE BIG DAY

Even for seasoned racers, the days before a marathon or half-marathon can be stressful. With all the hope and hard work that you've invested in your goal event, you want to arrive at the starting line feeling calm, healthy, and ready to run your best. Here are some things you can do to stay on track in the critical days and hours before the starting gun fires and to help you recover after you cross the finish line.

Race Week Rules

Don't do anything new. Race week isn't the time to try new shoes, exotic foods, cool new gear you see at the expo, or anything else that you haven't used on several training runs. Stick with the fuel and gear that work for you. If you absolutely must buy something at the expo—a cute outfit or a bargain pair of shoes—wait until after the race to wear it.

Double-check logistics. A week before the race, reconfirm your hotel reservations, race registration, and any travel arrangements. Figure out how you're getting to the starting line and, if you're driving, where you'll park. Often, there are road closures on race morning. These are typically outlined on the race Web site. Decide where you're going to eat the night before the race, and make a reservation. You don't want to

become panicked racing around town in search of a place that serves pasta. For suggestions on good runner-friendly restaurants and hotels, check the race Web site or call the convention and visitors' bureau in the area.

Review the course. Take a look at the course map and elevation chart before race day; check out the video course tour on the race Web site, and if you can, drive the course in the days before the event. Get to know the landmarks and the terrain. Pick out the spots where you're going to need to push yourself harder, and map out a strategy to get through those tough spots.

Pack early. Start setting aside your race gear at least a week before the race. Check the weather forecast, but pack clothes for any conditions, just in case a freak storm or heat wave blows in. It will likely be cold at the start, so be sure to pack clothes that you can throw off once you warm up. (These clothes are typically donated to charity.) Even if you're racing locally, it's best to pack a bag with your gear, clothes, and fuel. That way, it's all in one place and you're not searching around frantically on race morning.

Get some sleep. The closer to the race you get, the tougher it may be to get some shut-eye, as you'll likely be anticipating the big day. But it's best to get as much sleep as possible—at least 8 hours a night—and nap if you can. "Try to prioritize sleep early in the week, when you're not feeling anxiety and nervousness," says Cheri Mah, a researcher at the Stanford University Center for Human Sleep Research. Her research on athletes of all sports shows that extra sleep impacts reaction time, mood, and energy levels. "Recognize that sleep is an important part of your training," she says. "Unfortunately, it's typically one of the things that we sacrifice first."

Don't overdo the expo. Plan to pick up your race number as soon as the expo opens. Browse, but give yourself a time limit there, and stick to it. All the walking and bucking the crowds can drain you and leave your feet aching. It's tempting to linger and bask in the excitement of the race, but you want to conserve your energy for the race, so you can make the most of all the hard work you did in the previous months.

INSIDE RUNNER'S WORLD®

NICK GALAC, 28, ASSOCIATE PHOTO EDITOR, EMMAUS, PENNSYLVANIA

LESSON LEARNED: NO MATTER HOW EXPERIENCED YOU ARE, ALWAYS RUN YOUR FIRST MARATHON OR HALF-MARATHON WITHOUT A TIME GOAL

I ran track and cross-country in college, so I thought I was superspeedy and could just bump up to the marathon, no problem. I trained for months, ran my four 20-milers, and was running my Yasso 800s at 2:52, so I thought I could just break 3 hours without the blink of an eye. At the 2007 Philadelphia Marathon, conditions were great, and I crossed the half-marathon mark in 1:28, on pace to achieve my sub-3-hour finish. But at mile 15 my quads, hamstrings, and abductors cramped up, and I had to walk and shuffle the last 11 miles. Until you do the marathon, you just don't know how the full 26.2 miles is going to feel. In the end, I am still happy to have finished a marathon. But looking back, if I wouldn't have had a goal time, I might have been able to run the entire marathon at a controlled pace and finished without walking or cramping.

Don't eat anything new. You know your body best, so in the days leading up to the marathon or half-marathon, stick to foods you've eaten before and that you know your stomach can easily digest. For some runners that means avoiding high-fiber foods, high-fat foods, and dairy. Eating high-carb foods, such as pasta, rice, and potatoes, will ensure your glycogen stores are stocked for race day.

Watch alcohol and caffeine consumption. If you normally avoid alcohol and caffeine, then don't drink them the night before or day of the race. However, if you're accustomed to drinking alcohol, one drink the night before likely won't hamper your running. Similarly, if you normally drink coffee before a long run, then you can drink it before the race.

Put your hands on your bib and chip. The night before the race, attach your chip to your shoes and fasten your bib to your clothes. You must have those two supplies at the starting line. Don't show up without them!

Make a meeting place. Designate a spot to meet up with family and friends after the race, and give them a range of time for when you'll come in. Many races offer "athlete tracking," which allows people who "follow" you to get emails or cell phone alerts as you pass certain mile markers during the race, giving them a better sense of when to expect you. Suggest an immovable landmark that you can all identify ahead of time. However you feel when you cross the finish line, you're going to want to get postrace hugs and congratulations.

Race Day Reminders

Sure, the race is about running. But logistics, fuel, and gear can have a big impact on how well you perform.

Don't overdress. It will probably be cool at the start, but wearing more clothes than you need can make you sweat and slow you down. Dress for 20 degrees warmer than it is outside. To stay warm at the start, bring clothes that you can throw off after the first few miles. (To find out how to dress for any running conditions, check out the "What Should I Wear?" tool at runnersworld.com/tools.)

Give your bladder a break. The morning of the race, stop drinking 1 hour before the start. This way you'll avoid pit stops early on. The longest lines occur 20 to 30 minutes before the race starts, so go earlier or later to beat the rush.

Line up early. You don't want to be rushing to the starting line, so don't wait for the last call to get there. It's best to line up about an hour before the starting gun goes off. This will give you a chance to hit the bathrooms, do a last-minute check to make sure you have your fuel and gear, and try to decompress. Don't go any earlier; the extra wait may only make you nervous.

Line up in the correct corral. Many races have signs showing you where to stand according to your predicted pace. It's best to stand near the appropriate sign. If you line up too far back, you could get frustrated trying to weave your way around a wall of slower runners. Hang around a faster crowd, and you run the risk of going out faster than

Packing List

At most marathons and half-marathons, you'll have the option of taking a bag to the start and checking it to pick up at the finish line. Most races have very reliable services, but just in case, it's best not to put anything in the bag that you can't live without. Some things that you should consider packing include:

ID. Put your name, address, cell phone number, bib number, and e-mail address clearly on the outside of the bag, just in case something happens to it. Some races require you to use the plastic or mesh bag that they provide, with your bib number clearly marked. Others will allow you to check a bag of your own. Check the race Web site for the specific requirements.

Trash bag. At big point-to-point races, like the New York and Boston marathons, runners often spend hours waiting for the start. A heavy-duty trash bag can provide a nice seat so you don't have to plop down on wet grass. If it's raining at the start, you can use the trash bag as a raincoat (just rip a hole in the bottom for your head and on the sides for your arms).

Extra tissue or toilet paper. The only thing worse than waiting in a long porta potty line is getting to the front and realizing that there's nothing to wipe with.

Reading material. If you have a long wait before the race, it's best to pack some magazines or a book to keep your mind occupied. This can keep you from obsessing about the race. The less mentally taxing the material, the better. *War and Peace* will probably be tough to engage in, and it may not offer the lift you need.

Extra race fuel and drink. Sometimes energy gels can slip out of your hands, or your favorite flavor of sports beans will fall out of your fuel belt. So bring extras just in case, plus the water and sports drink that you prefer. Many races offer refreshments at the start, but it's best not to expect it and then be disappointed and stressed when you get there.

Dry, clean clothing. After the race, you'll cool down and chill quickly. Best to have something warm and dry to change into. Include a fleece and a change of shoes (you might try comfortable after-sport shoes like sandals or flip-flops, which will give your feet a chance to breathe). You might want to pack a hat and gloves, if it's cold out. Also include a towel or baby wipes to wipe your face.

Postrace refueling. There are always snacks at the finish line, but whatever the race provides may not sit well with you. It's best to have the snack that you know works for you. For maximum recovery, choose something with a 4:1 ratio of carbs to protein. This will help restock your spent glycogen stores and repair broken-down muscle tissue. You might try an energy bar or other packaged food that won't spoil, spill, or get ruined in transit.

your goal pace and burning out early, or getting trampled and passed, which can deflate your confidence.

Start your watch when you cross the starting line. At bigger races, it could take up to 10 minutes just to cross the starting line. Using your watch will help you keep track of your personal time without having to do math when you see the time clocks on the racecourse.

Fix it sooner, not later. If your shoelace is becoming untied or you start to chafe early in the race, take care of it before it becomes really painful later in the race. If you need to tie a shoe, address a side stitch, or readjust some gear, step to the side of the road; don't stop midpack, as you could create a pileup. (See "Handling Midrace Mishaps," page 217.)

Give everyone else some space. In a long-distance race, there's no need to stay right on another runner's shoulder. Runnersworld .com executive editor Mark Remy, author of *The Runner's Rule Book*, often cites the "Heimlich maneuver" rule to personal space: "If you're close enough behind another runner to perform the Heimlich maneuver on him or her, then you are too close to that runner," he jokes. "Unless he or she is choking on something, of course. In which case you're exactly where you want to be."

Stay aware of your surroundings. Beware of runners who may not be aware that you're approaching, either because they're listening to music or have a laserlike focus on their training watches. If you're closing in on a water station or you need to step to the side, make sure to warn them with a simple shout-out like "On your left!" or "Excuse me!" or "Coming through!" Likewise, if you must race with music, keep just one earbud in and keep the music low enough that you can hear what's going on around you.

Mastering the Mental Game

You've probably heard it many times before: Racing 13.1 miles—or 26.2—is as much of a challenge for the mind as it is for the body. After all the hard work you poured into training, it's important to not let pessimism, fear, or fatigue get the best of you. On the course, you've got to be your own cheering section, and talk back to those negative voices and doubts. "If you give too much credence to negative thinking, it will slow you down and make your shoes heavy," says Brown. Remember that marathon training involves running more than 500 miles, and half-marathon training runs you more than 200 miles. The race day—covering just 26.2 or 13.1 miles—is a victory lap. There are things you can do to stay focused during the race.

Problem: You feel overwhelmed by the distance you still have to run

Solution: Break it down

Studies have shown that about two-thirds of the way through any race—whatever the distance—runners tend to hit the wall. At that point, the newness has worn off; the starting gun fired ages ago, and the finish line still feels like it's a very long ways away, says Kate Hays, a Toronto-based sports psychologist and cofounder of the Toronto Marathon Psyching Team. Anticipate that you're going to hit this tough mental stretch, and prepare for it. Make sure you're fueling enough that you keep your energy levels stable and even throughout the race. And break the marathon into segments, like two 10-milers and a 10-K for the marathon,

(continued on page 218)

Bart's Tips on Nailing the Negative Split

I firmly believe in the negative split—that is, running the second half of the race faster than the first half. People think it's impossible, but it's not. Here are a few tips to help you pull it off.

Start slow. Head out 10 to 15 seconds per mile slower than goal pace, and take walk breaks early on. That way, you're storing energy that you can use later on. It should feel so easy that it's crazy. In a half-marathon, you should be running so easy that you feel like you could go the whole 26.2. In a full marathon, you should be running easy enough that you feel like you could run 150 miles at that same pace.

Stay in your own zone. The hardest part of the negative split is that you're so amped up: The music is blaring, someone's singing the national anthem, and you've trained hard for months to prepare for this. You feel like you want to charge out of the start like they just released you from prison. And you don't want to go easy when it seems like everyone is passing you. Ignore everyone else. Just stick to your own race plan. All those people who passed you? You'll pass them late in the race.

Listen to your body. Music players and training watches like Garmins can be great, but in a race, you really want to tune in to how you're feeling—how easy or labored your breathing is, how your muscles are feeling—to monitor your own pace. With a Garmin, it's way too easy to start stressing about your splits at each mile. Remember that it's the finishing time that counts. The individual splits along the way don't mean a thing.

Take the hills at an even effort. Your pace is going to be slower uphill and faster downhill, but you want to maintain the same level of effort both ways. If you kill yourself to stay on pace on the way up and then let yourself free-fall on the way down, you're going to zap the strength and energy you'll need later in the race. Any time that you lose on the way up you'll make up on the way down.

The Water Stop

In theory, grabbing a cup of water from a table should be a simple proposition. But if you've participated in any major race, you know that getting through a water stop requires both agility and grace. If you're not careful, you could end up getting the fluid up your nose, missing the water cup entirely, or causing a pileup.

Know where the stations are. Check the race Web site ahead of time so you know where the stations are. Have a plan for which ones you'll hit and when.

Make the time. You may hesitate to stop at water stations for fear of losing precious time, but the few seconds you spend stopping are way less than what you'll lose if you get dehydrated and have to slow way down later. Have a hydration plan, and stick to it. (See "Hydration: Take It Personally" on page 96.)

Make your way over slowly. You don't want to cut off another runner or cause a 10-person pileup. Slowly ease over to the water stop. Watch for slowing or stopped runners.

Skip the first table. Everyone will make a mad dash for the water at the first table, so aim for the second table or beyond. Race volunteers are usually good about calling out which tables have which drinks.

Watch what you drink. If you just took an energy gel, you'll want water. If the race serves a brand or flavor of sports drink that doesn't sit well with you, make sure you don't go for it. Call out "water" or "sports drink" to confirm with the volunteer before you drink.

Watch your step. It's easy to slip on the waxy water cups on slippery pavement. Watch your footing as you rejoin the pack.

Sip, don't swig. Avoid pouring all the water down your throat at once; it's easy to choke or end up coughing. Or, even worse, you might spill water into your shoes, leaving your feet wet and vulnerable to blisters. Take small sips instead—you'll get more down that way.

Crush the cup. As you grab the cup, pinch the top together to make a spout, which will keep the water from spilling and let you sip without getting the fluid up your nose or taking such a big gulp that you end up coughing it up.

Keep moving. No use going to all the trouble of getting the water if you don't get any of it down. After you get the cup, step away from the water station—so other runners don't plow into you—and slow down or walk if you need to in order to get the water down.

Handling Midrun Mishaps

Here's how to conquer some common running problems when they strike during an all-important race.[1]

Chafing
Recovery Plan: Most races offer Vaseline, adhesive bandages, or sports lubricants at aid and medical stations. Or carry your own. Lip balm is easy to carry and neater than Vaseline, and it can ease the rubbing that leads to chafing.

Muscle Cramp
Recovery Plan: Stop running and apply pressure to the muscle. Press firmly for 15 seconds—don't massage. Then gently stretch the muscle. Repeat the pressure/stretch cycle until the cramp subsides. Walk at first, then slowly increase your pace.

Blister
Recovery Plan: In a short run or race, keep going. If it becomes painful enough to throw off your gait, cover it with an adhesive bandage or moleskin at the next aid station. But if an aid station or home is miles away, adjust your laces. Tightening them could stop heel slippage; loosening them could take pressure off a hot spot.

Side Stitch
Recovery Plan: Notice which foot is striking the ground when you inhale and exhale, then switch the pattern. So if you were leading with your right foot, inhale when your left foot steps. If that doesn't help, stop running and reach both arms above your head. Bend at the waist, leaning to the side opposite the stitch until it subsides.

Stumble and Fall
Recovery Plan: Get up and assess your injuries. Road rash or minor scrapes can be patched up later, but heavy bleeding needs immediate treatment. Running might feel difficult at first because you'll be shaken up. Take a deep breath, do an honest assessment of yourself, and if you are all right, refocus on your goals and keep running.

Stiffness After a Pit Stop
Recovery Plan: Keep your breaks brief—2 minutes at most. Walk while taking water rather than coming to a complete stop. Start back up slowly; don't resume your prior pace right away.

or two 5-milers and a 5-K for the half-marathon. Just focus on achieving a goal for whatever segment you're in. New York City running coach Mike Keohane encourages his runners to just take it 10 minutes at a time, or to take walk breaks to get a drink or an energy gel. "It makes the distance more doable," he says. "And because you know you're getting a break, you have something to look forward to."

Problem: You start to fatigue
Solution: Distract yourself

When you start to think, "I'm tired," or "I want to quit," remember that everyone around you is hurting more than you are. "The worst thing you can do is start thinking that you're feeling worse than everyone else," says Stan Beecham, an Atlanta-based sports psychologist. "Once you start down that road, you're giving yourself permission to back out." Beecham recommends that you have an inspiring affirmation or mantra to sync with each footfall, to keep yourself going. Ideally, you will have tested it out during training. "You make mantras effective by using them over and over," he adds. He likes the mantras "This is my time" and "The longer I go, the stronger I get." John Stanton, founder of The Running Room, an Edmonton, Alberta–based network of running stores, reminds runners in the later stages of a marathon to think of someone who is struggling with a health issue. "All of a sudden the heavy legs and heavy breathing don't seem that bad," says Stanton. "You remember that your health is a gift."

Problem: You feel discouraged
Solution: See your success

Having images that are personal and easy to conjure up, and that elicit positive emotions, can be helpful, says Harvard psychologist Jeff Brown, author of *The Winner's Brain*. Replay the "highlight reel" of the greatest moments of your running career—your last PR, the first time you ran 10 miles, and how you feel when your training is clicking along. "Float" was the word that one of Brown's clients used to get up Heartbreak Hill, for instance. Some people like the images of themselves chugging along and moving forward like a train. Beecham encourages runners to envision themselves as vessels. "Over the course of the race you want to imagine pouring yourself completely into it," says Beecham. "You want to feel totally empty when you cross the finish line."

Problem: You feel demoralized because people are passing you
Solution: Draw strength from the spectators and the other runners

That runner who just whizzed by? He's showing you what's possible, and how fast you can run, says Beecham. "Think that these people are there to help you, not work against you," he adds. By the same token, encouraging others and accepting encouragement from the sidelines can also give you a boost. Soak in the roar of the crowd, and let them fuel you to a peak performance. Make eye contact with cheering spectators, and say thank you when they yell, "Good job!" "Don't say anything to yourself that you wouldn't say to your running buddy," says Don Garber, head coach of the Sports Backers Training Team, which trains runners for the Richmond Marathon. "You wouldn't tell him, 'You're running horribly, and you're going to die.' So don't say it to yourself, either."

Problem: The PR you had your heart set on slips away
Solution: Stay flexible with multiple goals

Have at least three goals for the race. Have an A goal for your banner day—if the weather is perfect and you got plenty of sleep the night before. Make sure that this goal is based on a realistic assessment of your training and fitness. Set a B goal that will leave you feeling like you gave it all that you had, even if the temperatures are soaring and your stomach is a mess. Finally, set a "process" goal—one that isn't attached to the time on the finish line clock. You might have a goal of fueling on schedule every hour. Or you might have a goal of running even splits—running each mile at about the same pace. Write out these goals before your race. This will help you stay calm and focused when you hit the tough spots. (See "Setting Smart Race Goals" on page 11.)

Problem: You want to quit
Solution: Remember why you run

Not just today, but every day. Knowing that you've lost weight, adopted a healthy lifestyle, found a whole group of new friends through running, or are raising money for charity can help you stay positive through the tough patches, says Brown. Wear something that you can glance at during the race to remind yourself of that, or write a reminder on your hand with a permanent marker.

CHAPTER 11

BEYOND THE FINISH LINE

After you cross the finish line, your work isn't done. The steps you take after you get your medal will have a big impact on how quickly you bounce back. Here are some key things you need to do in order to ensure that you feel good beyond race day.

Keep moving. Get your medal, food, and water, and keep walking for at least 10 minutes to prevent blood from pooling in your legs and to gradually bring your heart rate back to its resting state. Though your legs will be tired, sitting too soon can make you stiff and tight, which can delay recovery.

Refuel. Within 30 minutes of finishing, refuel with carbs and sources of lean protein. If you can't eat postrace, pack a recovery drink in your gear bag. Within a few hours, try to eat a regular healthy meal with carbs and protein. (See "Postrace Refueling" opposite.)

Get warm. Change out of the clothes you ran in, and get into dry clothes as soon as possible. After you cross the finish line, your core temperature will start to drop fast, and keeping sweaty clothes on will keep you cold.

Take an ice bath if you can. If you're near a hotel room or home, take an ice bath. (See "Ice Baths" on page 135.) Uncomfortable as they sound, these have been proven to reduce inflammation, swelling, and muscle soreness, and they can help you feel better, sooner.

Do the postrace recovery squat. This move, suggested by *Runner's World* contributor Sage Rountree, gently stretches your back, hips, quads, and calves; it encourages fresh blood to pump into these muscles, and it requires no equipment.[1]

• Squat wide over toes that point slightly outward, or take a tighter squat with your toes facing straight ahead. Either way, keep your knees in line with your ankles.

• Use your hands to help support you—they can rest on the ground behind you or in front to stop you from toppling forward. If you are feeling really wobbly, wait until you can find a stable item to hold on to, such as a fence post or chair. Lean away from your support as you drop your hips and heels toward the ground.

• Take a few slow, deep breaths. When you are ready to stand, move slowly, keeping your head up. If you need assistance, have a friend or race volunteer pull you up.

Get a massage. It's best to wait 24 to 36 hours after a race to get a massage. Once race-induced muscle soreness has subsided (2 to 6 days), a deep-tissue massage can help release tension. It is okay to get a light massage after the race if it's offered—just make sure the practitioner steers clear of any strained areas.

Celebrate your success. Sure, the medal is a great token of your accomplishment, but

Postrace Refueling

In order to recover quickly—regardless of whether you are taking the next month off or have another race right around the corner—it's important to refuel and rehydrate within 30 minutes of crossing the finish line.

Try to replace water and electrolytes lost through sweat by drinking 16 to 24 ounces of fluids as soon as possible after finishing. If you're racing in a hot or humid environment or if you are a salty sweater, be sure to choose sports drinks to help replace the electrolytes you lost through sweating. Continue to sip fluids throughout the day. The color of your urine can indicate whether you're rehydrated; it should be pale yellow. If it's darker, like the color of apple juice, you need more fluids.

Aim to eat 15 to 25 grams of protein and 0.7 grams of carbohydrates per pound of body weight. (For example, a 120-pound runner would need about 82 grams of carbs. A 165-pound runner would need 113 grams.) This might include:

• Peanut butter and jelly on whole grain bread with a glass of low-fat milk

• Greek yogurt, a serving of fruit, and low-fat granola

• Whole grain bagel topped with peanut butter and honey

• Cup of oatmeal made with skim milk and topped with chopped nuts and a banana

• Turkey sandwich on whole grain bread alongside a serving of pretzels

• 16-ounce sports drink with a slice of cheese pizza and baby carrots

• Grilled chicken sandwich alongside a serving of fruit

• Energy bar, a serving of fruit, and a serving of pretzels

What it takes to . . .
Get through a race when an unforeseen disaster strikes

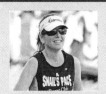

Amy Katz, 40, Irvine, California
Real estate accountant
Experience: 32 marathons; 3:37 PR
Runner's World Challenge Race: 2009 Chicago Marathon

Three times I've had training go well, only to have some unforeseen disaster pop up on race day. Leading up to the 2010 Boston Marathon, I ran a couple of strong half-marathons, got through my long runs and marathon-pace runs, plus I did plenty of hill work to prepare for the course. But the night before the race, I got the stomach flu. On race day, I just tried to put it out of my mind, but quickly knew that I wasn't doing very well, so I just tried to make it as long as I could. I wanted to finish and get that medal—no matter what. I was walking a lot, and going very slowly, and everyone on the sidelines could tell that I wasn't doing so great, so they were cheering really hard for me. I talked to other runners and realized that they were also struggling, and that helped put my own woes in perspective. It brought me back to when I first started running, and I never even thought about goal times—I just wanted to finish. And I was really proud of myself for sticking it out. With racing, you just have to think about the big picture. It's important to realize that there are races every single weekend, and one race isn't the be-all and end-all. During a training season you're gaining fitness, and no matter what, it's going to pay off, even if you have a bad race. After Boston, I recovered very quickly. (The slow pace and the walking took very little toll on my body.) Less than 2 weeks after the marathon, I ran my fastest 5-K in over a year. I ran three more 5-Ks in the 3 months after that, also in fast times.

it's also great to have some reward planned that you can look forward to during the race. Maybe it's a big meal at your favorite restaurant with family and friends; maybe it's a day at the spa or a package of massages. No matter how you feel about your race performance, you trained hard for months, committed to this goal, and just covered a distance that most people will always dream about one day covering. Make sure to celebrate the occasion.

The next day, get going. As sore as you might feel the day after the marathon, it's important to do some sort of low-impact activity like swimming, cycling, or working out on the elliptical trainer. The movement will increase circulation to your sore muscles and help you bounce back sooner. Just keep the effort level easy.

Moving On

After a perfect training season leading up to the 2011 Boston Marathon, *Runner's World* Challenger Mike Gross was sick, and beside himself. "I was a mucus factory," says Gross, a veteran of 20 marathons. "It was not fun."

On race day, he stuck to his goal. But by 10-K into the race, he had to back off the pace. By the 23-mile mark, he was walking and jogging. After he crossed the finish line, he spent 90 minutes in the medical tent, throwing up and getting rehydrated with the help of an IV.

"I was really bummed about the whole thing," says Gross, a father of three and an engineer from Holland, Pennsylvania. "All those workouts went so well, and it's amazing how it can all just go down the tubes."

From weather to work to sleep, as Gross found out, the day of the race has many factors you can't control. Falling short of your goals—whether because of unrealistic expectations or an unforeseen sickness—can discourage any runner racing any distance. But the investment that goes into marathon and half-marathon training can magnify the disappointment.

Still, it's important to keep perspective.

"It's just one day out of 365," says Don Garber, head coach for the Sports Backers Training Team, which trains runners for the Richmond Marathon. "It could turn out to be a great day, or not a great day. But you can't put your whole self-esteem on one morning. It's just one piece of the puzzle."

Here's some help for getting over a bad race:.

1. Wallow a bit, then move on. Acknowledge that you're going to go through a natural grieving process that's going to include denial, anger, bargaining, and acceptance, says Harvard psychologist Jeff Brown, author of *The Winner's Brain.* "You lost time with your family due to training, maybe there were missed opportunities at work," he says. Talk with some running buddies about it. Journal for a few weeks, if you need to. Cry to get rid of the loss.

2. Find a positive. Whatever the time clock says, you spent the morning doing something good for your health, and you spent months training for a goal. Even if you didn't meet your goal, there are probably many positive outcomes that you reaped even before you arrived at the starting line. Did you lose weight? Get into a habit of exercising regularly? Did you get stronger and meet new people?

3. Learn from it. Did you go out too fast? Blow off your fueling plan? No matter how your race went, there's something you can learn from it. Reflect and see if there's something you could change. Were your race goals

→RW CHALLENGER PROFILE:
Gary Resnick—Running Through Cancer

When Gary Resnick crossed the finish line of the Big Sur International Marathon in 4:07, he stumbled around, astounded. "I just couldn't believe how fast I ran," says Resnick, 49, a father of three. "My legs felt so good that I couldn't believe I ran 26.2 miles. It was just a perfect day."

Anyone would have been happy with that time—especially if they'd run the Boston Marathon 13 days earlier, as he had, in 4:19. But for Resnick, the fast finish at Big Sur was just one more step in the most improbable comeback of his life.

Two years earlier, he was diagnosed with stage three pancreatic cancer and given a 5 to 10 percent chance to live. One year earlier, when the cancer came back in his sacrum, the large triangular bone at the base of the spine, he was downgraded to stage four; his chances for survival shrank to 1 percent.

Again and again, he insists, it was the running that saved him. It was bleeding after a 13-miler, after all, that first led him to the doctor and the tests that uncovered the cancer.

It was running the 8-mile round-trip to chemotherapy once a week that made him realize that he could probably do more than the doctors predicted.

And it was running his two best times—a 1:38 in the 2010 Queens Half-Marathon and a 4:00 at the 2010 Boston Marathon—with active untreated cancer—that proved to him that he could beat the odds. Above all, it has been the daily training runs that have helped

realistic? Talk to your running buddies, who have seen you in training, know how important this reality check is, and can offer guidance and perspective. Gross says that while he knows he couldn't have prevented getting sick, maybe if it had been a different race, he would have modified his race goals.

4. Set new goals. After devoting months to your training it's easy to feel aimless and lost once the day is over. You don't need to sign up for a race right away, but it's good to set up another meaningful goal. Maybe you'll aim to run 5 days a week, keep your weekly mileage at a certain level, or meet a yearly mileage goal, just to keep yourself on track. Or maybe you'll focus on something you didn't have time for while you were in training. Take that yoga or spinning class you've always wanted to check out, or go on vacation. Take advantage of the high level of fitness that you developed for the race to try something new. Gross took about 4 weeks off and was already reg-

him stay focused, calm, and positive, even in the face of such an uncertain future.

"Running has saved my life, mentally and physically," he says. "If I wasn't running, they would have never found the cancer. So I feel like the luckiest man alive."

Though he ran in high school, Resnick restarted his running life in June 2008 at the age of 46, the day after retiring as a trader on the New York Mercantile Exchange. Over the next 6 months he gained strength, speed, and endurance, and by December he had lost 55 pounds. After a 13-mile training run, he found blood, saw the doctor, and began his journey through two surgeries, 21 radiation treatments, and 650 hours of chemotherapy. Since he was diagnosed, he has run five marathons and 15 half-marathons.

Now, Resnick incorporates running into his daily life every chance he gets. When he went to meet his family at a baseball game, he ran the 18 miles from home to the stadium. He runs to dinner at his brother-in-law's house 17 miles away.

"The minute I started running, I started to feel much better," he says. "It kept me healthy and busy, and it made me not think about cancer."

Resnick had three marathons planned for 2011, and one day he'd like to run marathons in Maui, Kauai, and at the Great Wall of China— any chance to use his passport, which has never been stamped.

"It's been 30 months since I was diagnosed—which is a very long time—and to be running and doing what I am gives me hope," he says. "And that's all I want."

---

istered for the New York City Marathon that fall. "Having another goal on the calendar helped a lot," he says.

5. Get some perspective. Four months for a marathon and 2½ months for a half-marathon is a long time to train. Just getting to the starting line is an accomplishment. Don't take your good health for granted. Realize that most people in the world won't ever do this. Over time, Gross recognized that he'd just had a bad day, and everyone has

them. "If it's not there, you can't force it or fake it," he says. "Not every race has to be the Boston qualifier or the Olympic Trials." And remember why you run in the first place. "We focus on the athletic aspect," says John Stanton, founder of The Running Room, an Edmonton, Alberta–based network of running stores, "but it's the mental payback we get—the camaraderie and the uplifting feeling—that keeps us coming back." And Stanton reminds us that's why all marathons and most half-marathons have finishers medals.

"It's to recognize that there's a champion of some sort in everyone."

As for Gross, his 7-year-old son helped him keep a broader view of things. When Gross explained that he was disappointed that he didn't get the time he wanted, his son asked, "Did you get the same medal?" When Gross said yes, his son asked, "Can I wear it?"

Racing Again

Whether you ran the race of your life or crashed and burned, it's tempting to sign up for another race right away to capitalize on the fitness you've built over the past few months. But should you?

Most experts caution that it's best to wait. Step to the line too soon, and you may end up getting injured because you haven't given your body a chance to recover from the race and the months you spent working hard to prepare for it.

Many coaches suggest that runners wait at least 4 weeks after a marathon or half-marathon to race again, and preferably even longer, to let the musculoskeletal system recover. "There's a lot of tissue damage," says Sean Coster, coach and director of Run Portland, an Oregon-based running club. "Muscle fibers and the connective tissue have to work very hard to keep you weight bearing for as long as a marathon or a half-marathon.

You've got to give the body a chance to repair that." He recommends that first-time marathoners wait at least 6 months before trying a second marathon. "You need a full training cycle to progressively build back up," he says.

It's important to give your body time to rest, gradually build up mileage, and taper again for a second-chance effort. "People always think that they're a lot more ready than they are," says Patti Finke, an exercise

BART SAYS...

Some people like to just do marathons and half-marathons a lot. That's fine, as long as you pick a few races to go all out and peak at and others to do for fun. You have to be comfortable with not racing all out when everyone around you is running as fast as they can, and you have to have a plan for each race. If you're running on the edge of death at every race, you're going to get injured and burnt-out. See how you feel after the race. If you don't feel like you hurt yourself or wiped yourself out, then you may be ready to run again. And if you set a PR, in either time or distance, you've taken your body to a realm that it has never experienced before. After that, you need to back off and take it easy. If you try to PR every time, something is going to snap or break. So back off while you're feeling good.

physiologist and coach of Team Oregon. Even beyond the physical effort, "it takes a lot of mental energy to race all out. Sometimes you just need some time away from the hard work before you can go out and race again."

The overriding factor should be how you felt during the race. If you ran the race at an easy effort, it should only take a few weeks to bounce back. If it was hot, you bonked hard, or you're nursing an injury, it's best to wait longer.

The more miles you run, the more fit you are, the more quickly you can recover. If you don't run very much (say 30 miles a week or less), it takes a longer time to rebound, and you won't have the endurance to race well again very quickly. "How quickly you get [your physical strength] back varies so much on what your goals are and how much experience you have," she says.

With the right mix of rest and quality work, you can sharpen your high level of fitness and redeem your racing hopes.

Want to Race Again?

If you're healthy after crossing the finish line, with the right mix of rest and quality work, you can sharpen your high level of fitness and race again. If your half-marathon or marathon left you feeling depleted or, worse, injured that's another sign that you should take some time off and try again in 6 to 9 months. Follow the schedules, designed by Team Oregon coach Patti Finke, to make your racing season twice as nice.[2]

Marathon in 4 Weeks

WEEK	MON	TUES	WED	THURS	FRI	SAT	SUN
1	Rest	3 miles easy	Rest	5 miles easy	Rest	Long run 8 miles easy	Rest
2	3 miles easy	Marathon pace run 6 miles with 4 miles @MP	3 miles easy	6 miles	Rest	Long run 12 miles easy	Rest
3	4 miles easy	Marathon pace run 6 miles total, with 4 miles @MP	3 miles easy	6 miles easy	Rest	Long run 8 miles easy	Rest
4 Race Week	2 miles easy	4 miles easy	Rest	4 miles easy	2 miles easy	Rest	Marathon

Want to Race Again? (cont.)

Marathon in 6 Weeks

WEEK	MON	TUES	WED	THURS	FRI	SAT	SUN
1	Rest	3 miles easy	Rest	5 miles easy	Rest	Long run 8 miles	Rest
2	4 miles easy	Marathon pace run 8 miles with 6 miles @MP	4 miles easy	8 miles easy	Rest	Long run 12 miles	Rest
3	5 miles easy	Marathon pace run 8 miles with 6 miles @MP	5 miles easy	10 miles easy	Rest	Long run 16 miles	Rest
4	4 miles easy	Marathon pace run 8 miles with 6 miles @MP	4 miles easy	8 miles easy	Rest	Long run 12 miles	Rest
5	4 miles easy	Marathon pace run 6 miles with 4 miles @MP	4 miles easy	6 miles easy	Rest	Long run 8 miles	Rest
6 Race Week	2 miles easy	4 miles easy	Rest	4 miles easy	2 miles easy	Rest	Mara-thon

MP = marathon pace

Marathon in 8 Weeks

WEEK	MON	TUES	WED	THURS	FRI	SAT	SUN
1	Rest	3 miles easy	Rest	5 miles easy	Rest	Long run 8 miles	Rest
2	4 miles easy	Marathon pace run 8 miles with 6 miles @ MP	4 miles easy	6 miles easy	Rest	Long run 12 miles	Rest
3	5 miles easy	Marathon pace run 8 miles with 6 miles @ MP	5 miles easy	10 miles easy	Rest	Long run 16 miles	Rest
4	5 miles easy	Marathon pace run 8 miles with 6 miles @ MP	5 miles easy	10 miles easy	Rest	Long run 18–20 miles	Rest
5	5 miles easy	Marathon pace run 8 miles with 6 miles @ MP	5 miles easy	8 miles easy	Rest	Long run 16 miles	Rest
6	4 miles easy	Marathon pace run 8 miles with 6 miles @ MP	4miles easy	6 miles easy	Rest	Long run 12 miles	Rest
7	4 miles easy	Marathon pace run 6 miles with 4 miles @MP	4 miles easy	6 miles	Rest	Long run 8 miles	Rest
8 Race Week	4 miles easy	2 miles easy	4 miles easy	Rest	2 miles easy	Rest	Mara-thon

Half-Marathon in 2 Weeks*

WEEK	MON	TUES	WED	THURS	FRI	SAT	SUN
1	Rest	4 miles easy	6 miles easy	4 miles	Rest	Long run 8–12 miles	Rest
2 Race Week	4 miles easy	Half-marathon pace run 3 miles with 1 mile @ HMP	Rest	4 miles easy	2 miles easy	Rest	Race Day

Half-Marathon in 3 Weeks*

WEEK	MON	TUES	WED	THURS	FRI	SAT	SUN
1 Half Marathon	Rest	4 miles easy	6 miles easy	3 miles easy	Rest	Long run 8–12 miles	Rest
2	4 miles easy	Half-Marathon Pace Run 4 miles with 2 × 1 miles @ HMP	4 miles easy	6 miles easy	Rest	Long run 10 miles	Rest
3 Race Week	4 miles easy	Half-Marathon Pace Run 3 miles with 1 mile @ HMP	Rest	4 miles easy	2 miles easy	Rest	Race Day

Half Marathon in 4 Weeks*

WEEK	MON	TUES	WED	THURS	FRI	SAT	SUN
1	Rest	4 miles easy	6 miles easy	4 miles easy	Rest	Long run 8 miles	Rest
2	4 miles easy	Half-Marathon Pace Runs 6 miles with 3 × 1 mile @ HMP	4 miles easy	6 miles easy	Rest	Long run 10–12 miles	Rest
3	4 miles easy	Half-Marathon Pace Runs 4 miles with 2 mile @ HMP	4 miles easy	6 miles easy	Rest	Long run 10–12 miles	Rest
4	2 miles easy	4 miles easy	Rest	4 miles easy	2 miles	Rest	Race

*Follow these schedules only if you have been regularly running more than 40 miles per week.

HMP = half-marathon pace

Acknowledgments

I would like to thank all of the *Runner's World* Challengers. It's been such a joy to work with each one of you, answering all of your questions, and working together with you to help you fulfill your dreams. You are the ones who inspire and motivate me to keep running. Always remember: it's not how far you run, but how far you've come that counts.

—*Bart Yasso*

I'd like to thank Jennifer Van Allen for inviting me to be part of this book. I resisted at first. I thought she should take all the credit, because we were agreed that she would do 99 percent of the work. But she kept insisting that I could make some modest, technical contributions. In the end, I agreed only because she is such a good friend and such a dream collaborator-in-chief.

Ninety-five percent of everything I know about running I learned from John J. Kelley, George Sheehan, Ken Cooper, Dave Costill, Peter Wood, Tom Osler, Paul Thompson, Jim Fixx, Russ Pate, Nancy Clark, Jack Daniels, Peter Cavanagh, Walter Bortz, Tim Noakes, Liz Applegate, Lawrence Armstrong, Bernd Heinrich, Steve Blair, Claude Bouchard, Irene Davis, Joe Vigil, and the hundreds of editors and writers I have worked with in my three-plus decades at *Runner's World*.

The other 5 percent I learned from myself. From my mistakes. There have been many, and they are great teachers.

—*Amby Burfoot*

I am so grateful to Bart Yasso and Amby Burfoot, whose wisdom, warmth, and tireless dedication brought this book and the *Runner's World* Challenge to life. You were willing to take time out of your packed schedules to personally help hundreds of runners reach for their dreams, answering their questions on weekends and in the wee morning hours, being there to run alongside them on the way to the starting line, and at the finish to offer your heartfelt congratulations. You guys are two of the true greats of our sport, and I am honored to call you my mentors and friends, and to work with you on this book. You have taught me so much.

Thank-you to *Runner's World* editor-in-chief David Willey who had the vision behind the Challenge, and unwavering dedication to it year after year. Your belief in the power of our sport to change people's lives —and your willingness to reach beyond the pages of the magazine to make that happen—is what made the Challenge possible. I deeply appreciate all of the opportunities that you have provided, and for your support at every turn. Thank-you Warren Greene for all of your encouragement, unwavering support and patience, and for being so calm in the eye of so many storms. Big thanks to Pamela Nisevich Bede, for generously bringing your encyclopedic knowledge of nutrition to the Challenge and to this project.

Lots of gratitude goes to our deft and patient editors Shannon Welch, John Atwood, and Mark Weinstein, for having such confidence in this project from the get go, and the skill and flexibility to make it happen.

Many members of *Runner's World* poured tons of energy into the Challenge, often behind the scenes. My sincerest gratitude to Lori Adams, Jane and Bill Serues, Maryann Fosbenner, Chris Evans Gartley, Mark Remy, Jeff Dengate, David Cooper, Kevin Knabe, Lois Confer, Demian Faunt, Tish Hamilton, Robert Reese, Meghan Loftus, David Graf, Brian Sabin, Charlie Butler, Christine Fennessy, Joanna Golub, Katie Neitz, Chris Junior, Lindsay Bender, Sue Hartman, Kathleen Jobes, Traci Conrad-Nicholas, Robyn Jasko, and Nicole Burrell.

Thank-you to all of the experts, who allowed us to share the most comprehensive and up-to-date running science with our readers, including Adam St. Pierre, Michael Bergeron, Douglas Casa, Craig Souders, Janet Hamilton, Scott Murr, Patti Finke, David Nieman, Scott Trappe, Jonathan Dugas, Tom McGlynn, Jeffrey Brown, John Castellani, Bill Roberts, Stephen Pribut, and Clint Verran.

Thank-you to all of you *Runner's World* Challengers. You let us in on your dreams, and trusted us to help you achieve them. You continue to inspire and amaze us, and I am so happy to call so many of you my friends.

Finally, thanks to Fred Kirsch, for giving me the courage to become a runner. And much love to Peter, for making my every day so magical.

—*Jennifer Van Allen*

Appendix A: A Guide to Common Running Terms

A

Aid station. Also called a water stop. Any point along the course that offers water and sports drinks, handed out by volunteers. Often, at bigger races, gels, energy bars, and other items are also handed out.

Altitude training. Elite runners train at altitude to increase their number of red blood cells, improving oxygen delivery to their muscles. When you get to altitude, the kidneys secrete more of a hormone called erythropoietin (EPO), which causes the body to create more red blood cells. Runners find they can train harder and perform better for several weeks after they return from about a monthlong stay at altitude. Many elites choose to live at high altitudes and do speedwork at low altitudes. If you're traveling to a race at altitude, plan to run there 4 to 6 weeks before the race. If that's not possible, arriving at altitude just 24 hours before the start is your best bet. You won't acclimate, but you'll limit your exposure to some of the negative effects of the thin air, such as dehydration and disturbed sleep. Start your race slower, and build intensity. Expect race times to be slower. Dehydration can occur at altitude because the air is thinner and dryer, so drink plenty of fluids. Get plenty of rest, and allow 5 to 7 days back at lower altitudes before you race again.

Aquajogging. Running against the water's resistance in the deep end, where you can't touch, provides many of the benefits of running on land. A flotation belt will help keep you upright and give you stability. Keeping your body erect with a slight lean and your gaze forward, run as you normally would on land, with your hands pushing back the water. Your leg action can vary: Do high knees and march in place, bend your knees slightly and move your legs as if you were cross-country skiing, or do a more long-striding leg extension.

Athena. Races will often have divisions designated as "Athena" or "Filly" for female runners who are over a certain weight. The minimum weight to qualify for that division varies from race to race.

B

Bandit. Someone who is participating in the race unofficially, without having registered or paid for an entry.

Bib. The sheets printed with numbers (called "bib numbers") used to identify each runner in a race.

Black toenails. Lots of downhill running and too-small shoes can cause these, because both cause your toes to slam into the front of your shoe. They typically heal on their own within a few months.

Bloody nipples. These are often caused by chafing, friction caused by the rubbing of the nipples against the shirt while running. They're more common in men and during cold weather, and they can be remedied by covering your nipples with adhesive bandages or nipple guards, which are sold in many specialty running stores.

Body Mass Index (BMI). A simple measure of body fat that can be used to determine whether or not your weight is healthy. BMI is derived by comparing your height to your weight. It can be used by men and women of all ages.

BQ. Shorthand for Boston Qualifying time. Often used to describe a marathon or half-marathon finish time that qualifies a person for entry into the Boston Marathon.

Brick workouts. A workout that includes consecutive biking, then running. Often used by triathletes and duathletes to prepare for their goal events.

C

Carb-loading. The practice of increasing the percentage of carbs in your diet during the 3 to 5 days leading up to an endurance event such as a marathon, half-marathon, or even a long training run. (Note: Carb-loading is not simply eating more of everything.) Carb-loading stores glycogen in the muscles and liver so that it can be used during the race; it is most effective when done along with a taper. Make sure your food choices are carbohydrate-rich, not full of fat. For example, choose spaghetti with red sauce, instead of Alfredo sauce, or a bagel instead of a croissant.

Certified course. Most marathons and half-marathons are certified by USA Track and Field, which ensures that the distance of the race is accurately measured. For any running performance to be accepted as a record or nationally ranked, it has to be run on a USATF-certified course.

Chafing. Bloodied, blistered skin caused by friction that happens after clothing-on-skin or skin-on-skin rubbing.

Chip. A small plastic piece attached to a runner's shoelace that's used to track a runner's progress and record times during a race.

Timing chips are activated once you step over the electronic mat at the start and finish of a race, and at various points in between. At most races, if you forget your timing chip, your race time will not be officially recorded.

Clydesdale. Races will often have divisions designated as "Clydesdale" for male runners who are over a certain weight. The minimum weight to qualify for that division varies from race to race.

Cooldown. A period of light physical activity, like jogging or walking, after a longer or harder run. Done to help bring the heart rate down gradually and prevent the blood from pooling in the legs.

Corral. A sectioned area at the lineup of a race that helps separate athletes into different pace groups. The faster an individual is, the more likely he or she will end up in one of the first few corrals. These corrals are especially important at large races, such as marathons, where elite athletes are running.

E

Endorphins. Brain chemicals long credited with producing a "runner's high," a sense of elation that runners report experiencing. More recent research attributes this to endocannabinoids, molecules created by the body that are said to reduce pain and anxiety and promote well-being.

Ethyl vinyl acetate (EVA). A material used for the midsoles of running shoes. EVA is used in most running shoes because it's lighter and has a more cushioned feel than polyurethane. Different companies embed a variety of air bags, gels, plastic devices, and viscous solutions in their midsoles; these can also affect midsole durability because they replace midsole foam.

F

Fartlek. Speed play, or "fartlek" in Swedish (the concept originated in Sweden), is a speedwork format in which you run faster for however long (or short) you want.

G

Glycogen. The form of carbohydrates that is stored in your muscles and liver and converted to glucose for energy during exercise. The amount of glycogen that is stored depends on your level of training and the amount of carbohydrates in your diet. The glycogen that is stored (so it can be made available for use during a race) is increased during periods of carb-loading.

H

Heat index. A combined measurement of temperature and humidity that shows how hot it feels outside. When humidity is high, it cripples the body's ability to sweat—the body's self-cooling mechanism—so the body retains more heat and it's riskier to be outside. High humidity also increases the risk for conditions like heat cramps, heat exhaustion, and heatstroke. The National Weather Service issues an alert when the heat index is expected to exceed 105° to 110°F for at least 2 consecutive days.

Hill repeats. A workout that includes sprinting uphill fast, then jogging downhill at an easy pace to recover, then repeating the sequence. A workout thought to be an efficient way to build leg strength, speed, and aerobic capacity. Hill repeats reduce your injury risk by limiting fast-running time and because the incline of a hill shortens the distance you have to fall, which reduces impact.

I

Ice baths. Typically taken after long runs, races, and hard workouts, ice baths involve immersing one's legs in ice water for 15 to 20 minutes. The ice constricts blood vessels and decreases metabolic activity, which reduces swelling and tissue breakdown. Once you get out of the cold water, the underlying tissues warm up, causing a return of faster blood flow, which helps flush waste products out of the cells.

Interval training. Technically, this refers to the time you spend recovering between speed segments. But the term is commonly

used to refer to track workouts in general or fast bouts of running.

L

Lactate threshold (LT). Lactate is a byproduct created when your muscles break down glucose for energy. The LT is the speed above which lactate accumulates faster than your body can make use of it. To improve performance, you want to move your lactate threshold higher so you can run faster before lactate begins accumulating in your blood. High-intensity workouts, such as tempo runs, improve your heart's capacity to deliver oxygen and your muscles' ability to use that oxygen and clear lactate from the blood.

Long slow distance runs (LSD). Any run that's longer than a weekly run, which is the foundation of marathon and half-marathon training. These workouts, typically run 45 to 60 seconds slower than marathon pace, help build endurance and psychological toughness that can help you endure race day.

N

Negative splits. Running the second half of a race faster than the first half.

O

Overuse injury. Any injury incurred from doing too much mileage before the body is ready. Examples of common overuse injuries among runners include runner's knee, IT band syndrome, and plantar fasciitis.

Overpronation. Excessive inward roll of the foot, which can cause pain in the foot, shin, and knee.

Overtraining. A collapse in performance that occurs when the body gets pushed beyond its capacity to recover. It can lead to fatigue, stale training, poor race performance, irritability, and loss of enthusiasm for running. Serious overtraining can cause sleep disturbances, hampered immune function, poor appetite, and the cessation of menstrual periods in women.

P

Peak. The highest mileage on the training plan. Typically refers to the longest long run or the week with the highest training mileage.

Periodization. Division of training into periods that emphasize different training goals. Each period builds on the one preceding it so that you are able to reach a peak of fitness. Marathon and half-marathon training plans are divided into microcycles that focus on base building (building cardiovascular fitness and a base of aerobic fitness), strengthening (building long-distance endurance with long runs), sharpening (building speed), and tapering (reducing mileage before the race).

Personal record (PR). Term used to describe a runner's farthest or fastest time in a race. Also called a Personal Best (PB).

Q

Quality workouts. Any workouts that are faster or longer than daily runs. Within the context of marathon and half-marathon training, the term usually refers to workouts such as long runs, speed sessions, and tempo runs, which all require a day or two of recovery.

R

Racing flats. Thin-soled, lightweight shoes (usually weighing less than 7 ounces) used for racing, speedwork on the track, or tempo runs. Racing flats typically have a tight, second-skin fit and can be worn without socks. While some people use racing flats for the track, they're not necessary for most people running marathons and half-marathons.

Recovery. In the context of a speed session, like mile repeats or Yasso 800s, recovery intervals refer to the bouts of easy running between the bouts of fast running. These segments allow you to recover from the hard work and gather the energy and strength needed for the next round of hard work.

Rest. This usually means no running or exercise at all, or light cross-training with an activity like yoga or swimming. When rest follows difficult bouts of work, it lets the body adapt and improve. Rest helps restock glycogen stores, builds strength, and reduces fatigue. Without recovery, the body can't adapt to the stresses of training and get stronger. Rest can also prevent overuse injuries like IT syndrome and shin splints.

Repeats. The fast segments of running that are repeated during a workout, with recovery in between. If you're training for a marathon, you might run 800-meter repeats six times. For shorter races, like 5-Ks, you might do shorter repeats of 400 meters or so at your goal race pace.

RICE. Refers to Rest, Ice, Compression, and Elevation. These measures can relieve pain, reduce swelling, and protect damaged tissues, all of which speed healing. They're most effective when done immediately following an injury. RICE is the standard prescription for many aches and pains, such as strained hamstrings and twisted ankles.

Running economy. This measures the amount of oxygen you need to run at a given sub-maximal pace; it's a gauge of how efficiently your body uses oxygen and how efficiently you run. Like the fuel economy of a car, the less oxygen and energy you need in order to run at a certain pace, the longer you can go without ending up gassed—running out of energy. Some physical factors can impact running economy. If you're over-weight or have a sloppy gait, for instance, you're going to need more oxygen than a leaner person with a cleaner stride would. As you run more, do more speedwork, and improve factors like VO_2 max, weight, and biomechanics, you'll develop better running economy.

Run/walk. Method popularized by Olympian Jeff Galloway, columnist and author of *Runner's World*'s monthly "Starting Line" column. Walk breaks allow a runner to feel strong to the end and recover fast, while providing the same stamina and conditioning as a continuous run. By shifting back and forth between walking and running, you work a variety of different muscle groups, which helps fend off fatigue. To receive the maximum benefit, you must start the walk breaks before you feel any fatigue, during the first mile. If you wait until you feel the need for a walk break, then you've already let yourself get fatigued and defeated the purpose of the walk break.

S

Side stitch. Also called "side stickers." A sharp pain usually felt just below the rib cage (though sometimes farther up the torso). It's thought to be caused by a cramp in the diaphragm, gas in the intestines, or food in the stomach. Stitches normally come on during hard workouts or races. To get rid of a side stitch, notice which foot is striking the ground when you inhale and exhale, then switch the pattern. So if you were leading with your right foot, inhale when your left foot steps. If that doesn't help, stop running and reach both arms above your head. Bend at your waist, leaning to the side opposite the stitch until the pain subsides.

Specificity. Training should be relevant and appropriate to the sport for which you're training in order to maximize performance. Long runs, for instance, as opposed to cycling, are specific training for marathons and half-marathons because they prepare your muscles for the specific activity that you'll be doing during the race: covering a long distance for hours at a time.

Speedwork. Also called intervals or repeats, speedwork refers to any workout run at a faster-than-normal pace. Often done at a track. Done to increase cardiovascular fitness.

Splits. The time it takes to complete segment of the total distance that will be run. If you're running 800 meters, or two laps around a track, you might check your split after the first lap. If you are running a marathon, you might check your split after each mile to shoot for an even pace throughout the race.

Streaker. Typically refers to someone who has completed a race multiple years in a row.

Stride rate. The number of times your feet hit the ground during a minute of running. This measurement is often used to assess running efficiency. Having a high stride rate—say 170 steps per minute or more—can reduce injuries and help you run faster. Typically the number used refers to the number of times both feet hit the ground. So for a person with a stride rate of 170, the right foot and the left foot would each have hit the ground 85 times.

Strides. Also called striders or "pickups," these are typically 60- to 100-meter surges that are incorporated into a warmup or a regular workout. Strides increase heart rate and leg turnover; they get your legs ready to run hard. Strides are run near 90 percent of maximum effort for 20 seconds at a time with easy jogging in between.

Supination. The insufficient inward roll of the foot after landing. This places extra stress on the foot and can result in iliotibial band syndrome, Achilles tendinitis, and plantar fasciitis. Runners with high arches and tight Achilles tendons tend to supinate.

Sweat test. According to experts, this is the best way to get an estimate how much liquid to take in during a run or race: Weigh yourself nude before a timed training run, and then again after. Calculate your sweat rate and use this to determine your fluid needs during a run or race.

T

Taper. The period of reduced mileage 3 weeks before a marathon and 1 to 2 weeks before a half-marathon. It allows the body to recover from the stresses of training and rest for the race. The ideal taper reduces mileage but keeps in some intense training (like speedwork) to keep the fast-twitch muscle fibers firing.

Technical clothing. This typically refers to clothing made of synthetic fibers that wick moisture away from the skin. These fibers do not absorb moisture, like cotton does, and they help prevent uncomfortable chafing. *Runner's World* highly recommends technical clothing for marathon and half-marathon training and racing.

10 percent rule. Don't increase mileage or intensity by more than 10 percent from one week to another. This is a classic injury-prevention rule meant to prevent a runner from doing too much, too soon, and getting injured.

Track. Most tracks are 400 meters long. Four laps, or 1600 meters, is approximately equivalent to 1 mile. Many runners use the term "track" to refer to a speed session done on a track. Given that they're flat, traffic-free, and have measured distances, tracks are ideal for speed sessions such as mile repeats and Yasso 800s. Many schools allow the public to use their tracks outside of school hours.

U

USATF. USA Track and Field (usatf.org), the governing body of track and field, long-distance running, and race walking in the United States. This nonprofit organization selects and leads Team USA to compete at the Olympics, World Championships, and more than 12 other international events each year. It also certifies racecourses for accuracy, validates records, and establishes and enforces rules and regulations of the sport.

Ultramarathon. Any race of a distance greater than 26.2 miles.

V

VO_2 max. A measurement of the maximum amount of oxygen that can be consumed per minute while exercising. VO_2 max is determined by genetics, gender, body composition, blood chemistry, age, and training. Runners with a high VO_2 max often find it easier to run faster because their hearts can deliver more oxygen to their muscles. There are many ways to boost VO_2 max, including speedwork, which forces the heart to pump blood at a higher rate. Beginners can raise their VO_2 more than experienced runners, who will have to work on their running economy as well if they hope to get faster.

W

Warmup. A period of walking or easy running or any light activity that is done for 10 to 15 minutes before a workout. It gradually increases heart rate, breathing rate, and blood flow to the muscles, and it prepares the body for more vigorous work. A good warmup allows the body to work more efficiently and helps prevent muscle pulls and strains.

Wall. Typically refers to a point when a runner's energy levels plummet, breathing becomes labored, and negative thoughts begin to flood in; this often happens at mile 20 of a marathon. Experts say that it usually happens two-thirds of the way through any race, no matter the distance. Hitting the wall often occurs because you've run out of fuel and need carbohydrates (like a sports drink or an energy gel) that the body can convert into glucose for the muscles to use. For any run of more than 75 minutes, runners should have some carbs every 45 to 60 minutes to avoid hitting the wall.

Wind chill. How cold it really feels when you're outside due to the wind. As the wind grows stronger, it draws heat from the body and drives down the skin temperature.

Y

Yasso 800s. Invented by Bart Yasso, chief running officer of *Runner's World,* this workout has become famous for both predicting marathon finishing times and building fitness. The workout is 8 × 800 meters, with a 400-meter recovery in between. Run each 800 in the same amount of time—in minutes and seconds—that you are targeting for a marathon. So if you want to run a 4-hour marathon, you'd try to run each 800 in 4 minutes.

Appendix B: Meal Plans and Carb-Loading Plans

If weight loss is your goal, nutritionist Pamela Nisevich Bede recommends women eat 1,500 calories per day and men eat 2,000 calories per day. The following 3-day meal plans reveal the smart food choices that will keep you satisfied, trim you down, and keep you running strong.

1,500-Calorie Plan

DAY 1: 1,516 calories (135 g protein, 198 g carbs, 27 g fat, 33 g fiber)

Breakfast
Egg Sandwich and Grapefruit

- 1 large egg
- 1 slice reduced-fat cheese
- 1 whole wheat English muffin
- 1 tablespoon reduced-fat vegetable oil spread
- 1 medium grapefruit

Coat a nonstick skillet with cooking spray and place it over medium heat. Add the egg to the pan and scramble until it's almost done. Top with the cheese and heat until the cheese melts. Toast the English muffin and top it with the reduced-fat vegetable oil spread (optional). Top with the egg and cheese and serve with the grapefruit.

Lunch
Chopped Chicken and Turkey Salad

- 1 cup romaine lettuce
- 1 cup iceberg lettuce
- 1/4 cup chopped bell pepper
- 1/2 cup chopped carrots
- 1/2 cup chopped tomato
- 2 tablespoons crumbled feta cheese
- 3 ounces grilled chicken breast, chopped
- 3 ounces grilled turkey breast, chopped
- 2 tablespoons reduced-fat Italian dressing

In a large bowl, combine the lettuce, pepper, carrots, and tomato. Top with the cheese, chicken, and turkey. Add the dressing and toss to coat. Serve with cranberry juice cocktail.

Dinner
Grilled Chicken over Pasta with Spinach and Marinara

- 2 cups cooked whole wheat spaghetti
- 1/2 cup pasta sauce
- 3 ounces grilled chicken breast
- 2 tablespoons shredded part-skim, low-moisture mozzarella cheese
- 2 cups steamed spinach

Place the pasta in a large bowl. Warm the sauce and drizzle it over the pasta, topping with the chicken. Sprinkle the cheese on top and serve with spinach on the side.

DAY 2: 1,530 calories (112 g protein, 202 g carbs, 38 g fat, 30 g fiber)

Breakfast
Whole Grain Treat

2 low-fat, frozen whole grain waffles

1 tablespoon peanut butter

1/2 cup fresh blueberries

1 cup slice banana

8 ounces brewed green tea

1 teaspoon honey

Prepare the waffles according to the package directions and spread the peanut butter on them. Top with the blueberries and banana. Serve with the green tea, mixed with honey.

Lunch
Salad and Sandwich

Side Salad

1 cup romaine lettuce

1/4 cup chopped green pepper

1/2 cup chopped tomato

1/4 cup crumbled feta cheese

2 tablespoons reduced-fat Italian dressing

Sandwich

2 slices 100 percent whole wheat bread

3 ounces sliced turkey breast

1 slice low-fat cheese

2 leaves romaine lettuce

1 tablespoon reduced-calorie mayonnaise

1 teaspoon mustard

To make the salad: In a small bowl, combine the lettuce, pepper, tomato, and feta cheese. Top with the dressing, and toss to coat.

To make the sandwich: On one slice of bread, pile the turkey, cheese, and lettuce. Top with the mayo, mustard, and the remaining slice of bread.

Dinner
Grilled and Seasoned Tilapia

1 large sweet potato, baked with skin on

6 ounces grilled tilapia (or other mild fish)

1 teaspoon herbs and spices (your choice)

8 stalks asparagus

1 tablespoon low-fat margarine

1 teaspoon brown sugar

8 ounces skim milk

Preheat the oven to 400°F. Bake the sweet potato for 45 minutes, or until soft.

Preheat the broiler or grill. Sprinkle the fish with your desired herbs and spices. Broil or grill until the fish is flaky and fork tender—about 3 minutes per side. Steam the asparagus to your desired level of firmness (3 to 4 minutes), and slice it into 1/4-inch pieces.

Serve the fish and asparagus with the sweet potato, topped with the margarine and brown sugar, and a glass of milk on the side.

DAY 3: 1,580 calories (85 g protein, 243 g carbs, 30 g fat, 27 g fiber)

Breakfast
English Muffin and Yogurt

- Whole grain English muffin
- 1 tablespoon margarine
- 6 ounces low-fat light yogurt
- 1 orange

Toast the English muffin and spread the margarine on top. Serve with the yogurt and orange on the side.

Lunch
Stuffed Pita Pocket

- 1 whole wheat pita pocket
- 1 tablespoon hummus
- 3 slices lean deli meat
- ½ cucumber, sliced
- 2 medium tomato slices
- Shredded lettuce
- 1 pear, large

Spread the inside of the pita pocket with the hummus, then stuff with the meat, cucumber, tomato, and lettuce. Serve the pear on the side.

Dinner
Big Sur

- 2 slices whole wheat bread
- 2 teaspoons Dijon mustard
- 2 tomato slices
- ¼ avocado, sliced
- 1 ounce Gouda cheese
- 1 ear corn on the cob, boiled
- 8 ounces skim milk

Preheat oven to 350°F. Spread each piece of bread with mustard and layer the tomato, avocado, and Gouda on the slices, dividing equally. Place the slices on a baking sheet and bake until the Gouda begins to melt and the sandwich is warmed through, 5 to 10 minutes.

Serve with the corn on the cob and milk.

2,000-Calorie Plan
DAY 1: 1,990 calories (101 g protein, 248 g carbs, 66 g fat, 29 g fiber)

Breakfast
Omelet

- **1 tablespoon canola oil**
- **½ cup liquid egg substitute**
- **¼ cup shredded reduced-fat cheese**
- **3 ounces grilled chicken, chopped**
- **¼ cup chopped bell pepper**
- **½ cup chopped tomato**
- **1 teaspoon reduced-fat margarine**
- **1 slice whole wheat bread, toasted**
- **1 cup blueberries**

Coat a skillet with canola oil and place it over medium heat. Add the egg substitute to the pan and cook until the eggs are almost set. Spoon the cheese, chicken, pepper, and tomato into the center of the omelet. Using a rubber spatula, fold one half over the other. Slide the omelet out of the pan and onto a plate. Spread the margarine on the toast and serve with the omelet and blueberries on the side.

Lunch
Tuna Melt

- **1 whole wheat English muffin**
- **½ can water-packed tuna**
- **2 slices tomato**
- **2 ounces (approximately 2 slices) low-fat cheese**
- **1 medium piece fresh fruit**
- **½ bell pepper, sliced**
- **2 tablespoons hummus**

Preheat the oven or toaster oven to 350°F. Layer each half of an English muffin with equal amounts of the tuna, tomato, and cheese. Place each half on a baking sheet and bake until the cheese begins to melt, 5 to 10 minutes. Serve with the fruit on the side and green pepper strips dipped in hummus.

Dinner
Fiesta Dinner

- **1 cup vegetarian low-fat canned chili with beans**
- **¼ cup chopped tomato**
- **¼ cup chopped yellow bell pepper**
- **¼ cup chopped orange bell pepper**
- **2 tablespoons Spicy Ranch Dressing**
- **2 ounces baked blue corn tortilla chips**
- **8 ounces fat-free milk**

Heat the chili according to the package directions. In a small bowl, combine the tomato and bell peppers and toss with the dressing. Serve with the chili, tortilla chips, and milk.

DAY 2: 2,000 calories (89 g protein, 299 g carbs, 50 g fat, 39 g fiber)

Breakfast
Gourmet Oatmeal

1 packet instant plain oatmeal

¼ cup chopped dried fruit

1 medium banana

8 ounces skim milk

8 ounces black tea

Prepare the oatmeal according to the package directions, using skim milk. Once the oatmeal has thickened, add more milk if desired and top with the dried fruit and sliced banana. Serve with the remaining milk and tea.

Lunch
Turkey Wrap

1 whole wheat tortilla wrap

1 tablespoon low-fat mayonnaise

4 ounces deli-style turkey breast

2 fresh lettuce leaves

½ cup chopped celery

2 slices medium tomato

6 medium raw baby carrots

1 medium fresh peach

8 ounces calorie-free sparkling water, flavored

Place the tortilla flat on a plate and spread it with the low-fat mayonnaise. Layer the turkey, lettuce, celery, and tomato slices in the wrap, and fold it up. Serve with the baby carrots, peach, and sparkling water.

Snack
Fiberful Snack

1 cup bran flakes cereal

2 tablespoons pecans

1 medium banana, sliced

1 cup skim milk

Top the cereal with the pecans and banana. Add the milk and serve.

Dinner
Fettuccine Primavera

1 cup cooked fettuccine pasta

½ cup marinara sauce

1 cup cooked mixed frozen vegetables

1 teaspoon grated Parmesan cheese

1 cup fresh honeydew melon

8 ounces fat-free milk

Cook the pasta according to the package directions. Heat the marinara sauce and toss it with the pasta and mixed vegetables. Sprinkle the cheese on top. Serve with the melon and a glass of milk on the side.

DAY 3: 2,015 calories (77 g protein, 305 g carbs, 54 g fat, 40 g fiber)

Breakfast
Bagel

- 100 percent whole wheat bagel
- 1 tablespoon low-fat cream cheese (Neufchâtel)
- 1 cup fresh berries (blueberries, raspberries, blackberries)
- 8 ounces brewed coffee or tea

Slice and toast the bagel, and top it with the cheese. Serve the berries on the side and tea to drink.

Lunch
Peanut Butter and Jelly Sandwich

- 2 tablespoons creamy peanut butter
- 2 tablespoons all-fruit strawberry spread
- 2 slices 100 percent whole wheat bread
- 1 large apple
- 10 strips green bell pepper
- 2 tablespoons hummus
- 10 ounces fat-free milk

Spread the peanut butter and strawberry spread on the bread to make the sandwich. Serve with the apple, bell pepper strips dipped in hummus, and a glass of milk on the side.

Dinner
Chicken Salad

- 1 large apple
- 3 ounces grilled chicken breast
- 2 cups fresh spinach leaves, washed and chopped
- 1 tablespoon light dressing of your choice
- 6 ounces lemon-flavored iced tea
- 1 medium oatmeal raisin cookie

Chop the apple (with the peel) into bite-size pieces. Place the chicken and chopped apple on top of the spinach. Add the dressing and toss. Serve the iced tea on the side and the cookie for dessert.

Race Week Carb-Loading Plan

Eat according to this plan for the 3 days leading up to a marathon.

If you are looking to carb-load but don't want to follow a set plan, simply make sure each meal has some carbohydrate in it—a bagel, bread, pasta, rice, cereal, or fruit. The goal for the days leading up to the race is to eat a diet high in carbohydrates, moderate in protein (meat, cheese), and low in fat (so you can "spend" your calories on carbohydrates).

3 Days Before the Race

Breakfast

2 whole wheat pancakes topped with ½ cup canned fruit (drained)

12 ounces English tea mixed with ½ cup fat-free milk and 1 teaspoon honey

Nutrient Analysis: 310 calories, 10 g protein, 4 g fat (1 g saturated fat), 58 g carbs, 3 g fiber

Snack 1

Sandwich: 2 slices whole wheat bread, 1 table-spoon light mayo, 2 ounces roasted turkey, 2 ounces chicken breast, 2 romaine lettuce leaves

2 ounces pretzels (approximately 40 small braided) dipped in 6 ounces light low-fat yogurt

Nutrient Analysis: 710 calories, 40 g protein, 15 g fat (3 g saturated fat), 104 g carbs, 7 g fiber

Lunch

1 chicken taco: 3 ounces grilled chicken, 1 medium (6-inch) whole wheat tortilla, ½ cup shredded lettuce, ½ cup reduced-fat shredded Cheddar cheese

1 ounce baked tortilla chips dipped in ¼ cup salsa

16 ounces lemonade

⅓ cup dried mixed fruit

Nutrient Analysis: 920 calories, 50 g protein, 21 g fat, 133 g carbs, 7 g fiber, 9 grams saturated fat

Snack 2

1 cup fat-free pudding topped with ½ cup each of blueberries, raspberries, and blackberries

Nutrient Analysis: 330 calories, 7 g protein, 2 g fat, 72 g carbs, 4 g fiber

Dinner

6 ounces grilled salmon

1 cup wild rice topped with 1 teaspoon light vegetable oil–based spread

1 cup steamed cauliflower and broccoli medley

1 cup berry cobbler

Nutrient Analysis: 715 calories, 41 g protein, 12 g fat (3 g saturated fat), 111 g carbs, 9 g fiber

Total Daily Nutrient Analysis: 2,985 total calories, 148 g protein (20% of total calories), 51 g fat (16% of total calories), 478 g carbs (64% of total calories), 30 g fiber, 16 g total saturated fat

2 Days Before the Race

Breakfast

1 cup cooked oatmeal, made with $\frac{1}{2}$ cup fat-free milk and 1 medium banana, sliced

16 ounces coffee with $\frac{1}{4}$ cup fat-free milk

1 whole grain medium bagel ($3\frac{1}{2}$ inches in diameter), toasted and topped with 1 tablespoon apple butter

Nutrient Analysis: 800 calories, 25 g protein, 6 g fat, 163 g carbs, 10 g fiber

Snack 1

1 medium piece of fresh fruit

8 ounces sports drink

6 ounces fat-free Greek fruited yogurt

Nutrient Analysis: 525 calories, 32 g protein, 15 g fat, 65 g carbs, 7 grams fiber

Lunch

Salad: 3 cups fresh spinach, 3 ounces grilled chicken breast, 2 tablespoons dried cranberries, 2 tablespoons low-fat French dressing

1 cup couscous sprinkled with 1 tablespoon shredded Parmesan cheese

1 cup hearty minestrone soup with 5 saltine crackers

16 ounces water with lemon to drink

Nutrient Analysis: 640 calories, 34 g protein, 13 g fat, 98 g carbs, 9 g fiber

Snack 2

1 cup raw vegetables and 1 ounce whole wheat pretzels dipped in 2 tablespoons peanut butter and 2 tablespoons hummus

1 cup skim milk blended with 2 tablespoons fat-free chocolate syrup, 1 tablespoon peanut butter, 1 medium banana, and 1 cup crushed ice

Nutrient Analysis: 700 calories, 25 g protein, 15 g fat, 117 g carbs, 7 g fiber

Dinner

Sandwich: 2 slices whole grain bread, 3 ounces rotisserie chicken, 2 teaspoons brown mustard, 2 slices romaine lettuce, $\frac{1}{2}$ cup sliced roasted red pepper

1 cup cooked green beans topped with 2 tablespoons vegetable oil–based spread

1 medium baked potato topped with 2 tablespoons light sour cream and $\frac{1}{2}$ cup low-fat cottage cheese

12 ounces fat-free milk to drink

Nutrient Analysis: 715 calories, 41 g protein, 12 g fat (3 g saturated fat), 111 g carbs, 9 grams fiber

Total Daily Nutrient Analysis: 3,380 total calories, 157 g protein (18% of total calories), 61 g fat (16% of total calories), 554 g carbs (66% total calories), 42 g fiber

1 Day Before the Race

Breakfast

1 cup cooked oatmeal, prepared with water according to package instructions. (Adjust water amount according to desired consistency.) Top with ¼ cup raisins or dried fruit and 2 table-spoons brown sugar.

Nutrient Analysis: 668 calories, 24 g protein, 6 g fat, 130 g carbs, 7 g fiber

Snack 1

1 cup apple-cinnamon flavored O's cereal topped with 1 cup fat-free milk and 1 medium banana, sliced

Nutrient Analysis: 310 calories, 11 g protein, 2 g fat, 62 g carbs, 3 g fiber

Lunch (aim to eat your largest and most carb-rich meal at lunch the day before a race)

2 cups spaghetti topped with 1 cup marinara sauce and ½ cup steamed broccoli

2 slices whole wheat bread topped with 1 table-spoon vegetable oil–based spread (optional)

8 ounces lemonade

Nutrient Analysis: 980 calories, 25 g protein, 26 g fat, 163 g carbs, 17 g fiber

Snack 2

15 animal crackers dipped in 1 tablespoon peanut butter

1 medium piece fresh fruit

Nutrient Analysis: 310 calories, 6 g protein, 12 g fat, 45 g carbs, 3 g fiber

Dinner (aim for a light, mild dinner the night before a race)

1 whole wheat pita stuffed with 2 ounces lean deli meat (such as lean roast beef, turkey, or chicken), ½ cup shredded lettuce, 2 slices tomato, 2 table-spoons fat-free honey mustard

1 ounce baked potato chips

1 soft chocolate-chip granola bar

½ cup unsweetened applesauce

16 ounces sports drink

Nutrient Analysis: 740 calories, 22 g protein, 11 g fat, 139 g carbs, 6 g fiber

Total Daily Nutrient Analysis: 3,008 total calories, 88 g protein (12% of total calories), 57 g fat (17% of total calories), 539 g carbs (71% of total calories)

Appendix C: The Workouts

Since 2008, *Runner's World* contributing editor Bob Cooper has been interviewing top athletes across the world about their favorite workouts and sharing them with *Runner's World* readers each month in the training section. Below you'll find more than two dozen of these workouts that you can integrate into your marathon and half-marathon training. Substitute any of these workouts for your weekly speed sessions or integrate them into you strength training, as appropriate.

Core Builder

Why Maintain form when you're fatigued

Who Recommends It Alysia Johnson, 24, of Berkeley, California, US 800-meter champion and bronze medalist in the 800 at the 2010 World Indoor Championships

Do this series twice a week.

Russian Twists: Holding a medicine ball, sit with your legs bent and feet together on the floor. Raise your feet off the floor. Keeping your legs still, twist your torso to your left, then to your right. Do 20 reps.

Medicine-Ball Push-Ups: Start in the push-up position, with both hands on a medicine ball. Do one push-up with both hands on the ball. Then do one with one hand on the ball and one on the floor. Switch hands and do another push-up. Alternate like this for 15 reps.

Inch Worms: Start in the push-up position. Inch your legs forward until your butt is pointed skyward. Walk your hands forward until you are back in the push-up position. Do 1 push-up. Repeat 10 times.

Treadmill Step-Down Long Run

Why Speed reminder

Who Recommends It Michelle Frey, 28, of Minneapolis, winner of the 2010 City of Lakes 25-K in 1:31:15

Warm up with a 20-minute jog. Then run intervals on the treadmill of 15 minutes, 10 minutes, 10 minutes, 5 minutes. Start at about half-marathon race pace and do each interval a little faster, finishing at 5-K pace. Recover between efforts with a 5-minute jog. "This teaches me to push myself progressively harder, even as my legs are getting more and more fatigued," says Frey. "It breaks up the monotony of treadmill running when cold weather and bad footing keep me indoors."

Tempo Test

Why Build mental toughness

Who Recommends It Mo Trafeh, 25, of Duarte, California, winner of the 2010 US 15-K Championships (Gate River Run) by nearly a minute, finishing in 42:58

After a 25-minute jog, run 7 to 10 miles at slightly slower than half-marathon race pace. Finish with a 10-minute slow jog. "I do this workout on a gently rolling dirt road, so it's tough work running that pace," says Trafeh. "It builds the physical capability and mental toughness to tolerate running at a fast pace for an extended time, and it gets me in great shape to race any distance of 10-K or longer."

Minute Man

Why Get reacquainted with speed

Who Recommends It Sergio Reyes, 29, of Palmdale, California, winner of the 2010 US Championships (Twin Cities) Marathon in 2:14:02

In the second half of a midweek run, set your watch to beep every minute. With each beep, alternate running hard with running easy. The hard segments should be run at 5-K pace or slightly faster; the easy segments should be performed at your easy-run pace. "I usually do 8 to 20 hard minutes," says Reyes. "The workout provides relief from pace and distance constraints, letting you just run freely, while putting some speed in your legs."

Mile Repeats

Why Get race-ready

Who Recommends It Scott Bauhs, 24, of Mammoth Lakes, California, winner of the Rock 'n' Roll Half-Marathon in 1:02:39

Bauhs performs this workout 5 days before a half-marathon. After a 20-minute warmup jog, run 1 mile at 5 to 10 seconds faster than goal race pace. Jog or walk for 4 minutes. Repeat the sequence four times. "This pace should feel smooth and controlled, while still raising your heart rate," says Bauhs. If your goal race is a 10-K, run three repeats; if you're targeting a 5-K, run two repeats. Finish with a 10-minute jog.

The Drop-Down

Why Build speed

Who Recommends It Brent Vaughn, 26, of Boulder, Colorado, winner of the USA Cross-Country Championships in San Diego.

After a 20-minute jog and four strides, hit the track for 2 × 1000 meters at 5-K pace, then 2 × 400 meters at mile pace (or 40 to 60 seconds faster per mile than 5-K pace), then 2 × 250 meters all-out. Between repeats, do a slow jog of the same duration as the first repeat. Between each set of repeats, jog one lap. Finish with a 20-minute jog. "This gets you used to turning your legs over at a pretty good clip, which should make 5-K pace feel easier," says Vaughn. "It also improves your finish-line kick."

10-K Simulation

Why Develop a strong finish while tired

Who Recommends It 1996 Olympic marathoner Linda Somers Smith, 50, of Arroyo Grande, California, who set four US 45–49 records (including a 33:39 10-K and a 1:13:31 half-marathon) in 2010 and qualified for her seventh Olympic Marathon Trials in 2010 by placing second at L.A. in 2:36:39

After a 20-minute jog, run 2 × 800 meters at 5-K pace, do a 4-mile out-and-back run from the track a bit slower than half-marathon pace, and finish with 2 × 800 at 5-K pace. Jog one lap after each 800. "I call it a 10-K Simulation because it mirrors that race distance and effort," say Somers Smith, "with an emphasis on running the last two 800s hard when you're tired. By mixing both 5-K speed and near-half-marathon pace, it boosts fitness for those race distances, too."

On & Off

Why Develop speed

Who Recommends It Paige Higgins, 27, of Flagstaff, Arizona, who ran the 2009 World Championships Marathon in 2:37:11

Higgins does these "On & Off" runs twice-monthly year-round: After 15 to 30 minutes of easy running, do 10 to 20 repeats of 1 minute "on" and 1 minute "off." Run the "on" segments at a quick, strong—but not exhausting—pace, and jog the "off" segments. "It's an especially practical workout in the winter, because you can do it anywhere—on a road, track, or treadmill," says Higgins. "The objective is to get some turnover and speed in your legs, which is important even for the marathon, without depleting them of strength."

10-K Tune-Up

Why Race-pace reminder

Who Recommends It Molly Huddle, 25, of Providence, Rhode Island, winner of the 2009 US 10-K and 10-Mile Championships

Warm up with 20 minutes of easy running, then do four 6-minute repeats at about 10-K race pace, with a 2-minute slow jog between each, on roads or a grass field. Cool down with another 20 minutes easy running. "This is the most beneficial and challenging of the 'effort' workouts I do in the off-season," says Huddle. "Because you can't measure the distance or pace, you have to learn to tune in to the effort level. That's good practice for racing a 10-K."

Treadmill Test

Why Learn to finish fast

Who Recommends It Kristin Price, 28, of Raleigh, North Carolina, winner of the 2009 Pittsburgh Marathon and USA 10-K Trail Championships

Gradually increase your speed for the first mile to a comfortably hard pace, or about marathon race pace. Then increase your speed by one-tenth mile per hour every half-mile until you've been on the treadmill for about 45 minutes. Finish with a half-mile jog. "Continually increasing your speed until you're hitting a quick pace is a mental and physical test, simulating the challenge of hitting negative splits in a half-marathon or marathon," says Price. "Besides making outdoor workouts seem easy by comparison, this workout will increase your stride turnover."

The Mix

Why Save time

Who Recommends It Nick Arciniaga, 26, of Fountain Valley, California, eighth-place finisher at the 2009 New York City Marathon (2:13:46)

This dual-purpose workout combines tempo runs with speedwork. Run 3 miles at slightly slower than 10-K race pace. Jog for 2 to 5 minutes. Then run 4 × 400 meters at 1-mile to 5-K race pace, with 1 to 3 minutes of recovery between efforts. Finish with a 10- to 20-minute jog. "The tempo portion helps you find your race rhythm and builds endurance," says Arciniaga. "The track portion challenges your speed when your muscles are fatigued, simulating what happens late in a race."

Triple-Decker

Why Learn race pace

Who Recommends It Lauren Fleshman, 28, of Eugene, Oregon, winner of the Reebok Grand Prix 5000 and XTERRA Trail Run National Championships in 2009

After a 15-minute warmup, do 5 × 400 meters at 5-K race pace with 200-meter recovery jogs. Jog 400 meters, then run 1-K (2½ laps of the track) at 5-K pace. Jog 400 meters. Repeat the 5 × 400 meters, then cool down. "It's a good workout to transition to track," she says. "It teaches your body to run race pace at increasing levels of fatigue."

Short & Sweet

Why Develop speed for short races

Who Recommends It Lindsey Gallo, 28, of Arlington, Virginia, whose outdoor mile of 4:27.91 was the fastest of the year among women in 2009

Jog 2 miles and do four strides to warm up. Then run 800 meters at 5-K race pace, jog for 1 minute, run 200 meters at a very hard pace, and jog for 3 minutes. Repeat this sequence up to four times. "This workout gets you accustomed to the intensity of the pace demanded by a short race like the mile or 5-K," says Gallo. "It's a good indicator of the kind of shape you're in for a 5-K and a great way to improve your finishing speed."

Core Curriculum: The Plank

Why Strengthen entire core to stabilize the trunk for running

Who Recommends It Lee Marks, University of Colorado's assistant strength and conditioning coach. He has worked with runners like steeplechaser Jenny Barringer, who set an American record at the 2008 Olympics.

Lie in plank position with your forearms on the ground and your elbows under your shoulders. Hold for 30 seconds, rest for 30 seconds, and repeat. It works the abs thoroughly, says Marks. "It forces you to contract the entire core, lower abs, and obliques."

Single-Leg Squats

Why Strengthen hip-, knee-, and ankle-stabilizing muscles

Who Recommends It Terrence Mahon, head coach of Team Running USA, in Mammoth Lakes, California, which includes his wife, 2008 Olympic 5000 runner Jen Rhines

Stand on one leg, with the other leg bent behind or in front of you, lifted off the ground. Slowly lower your body 4 to 6 inches toward a squat position. Slowly return to the standing position. (If you feel any pain or tightness in the leg you're working, don't bend as deeply.) Aim for 10 reps on one leg, then repeat with the other leg. This exercise strengthens each leg individually, which helps prevent muscle imbalances that can lead to injury, Mahon says. "When you run, 85 percent of your weight is carried by one leg," he says. "This exercise helps each leg to quickly stabilize with each step."

Ladder Step-Down

Why To build speed and endurance

Who Recommends It Pete Rea, elite athlete coach for the ZAP Fitness team

Caitlin Tormey did this workout on a treadmill when she was training for the 2008 More Half-Marathon (1:20:13).

After warming up, run intervals of 7, 6, 5, 4, 3, 2, and 1 minute, taking each hard interval slightly faster than the previous one, progressing from marathon pace to 5-K pace. After each speed segment, recover by running easy for half as long as you spent running hard. Cool down with a slow jog. "This hits a wide range of pace and effort levels," says Rea, "from the speed-based endurance needed for a 5-K to the anaerobic-threshold work needed for the marathon."

Long and Short Hills

Why To build aerobic capacity early in the training season

Who Recommends It Tom McGlynn, a three-time qualifier for the Olympic Marathon Trials and a coach at Focus-N-Fly, an online coaching service. He trains Jim Sorensen, 41, who holds the masters world record for 1500 meters (3:44:06).

Run three times up a moderately steep hill that takes about 5 minutes to climb, making each ascent slightly faster. Jog or walk down. Then run faster uphill for 30 to 45 seconds; do this four to six times, with each repeat faster than the one before it. "Hills are aerobically intense without putting too much strain on the muscles and joints," says McGlynn.

Two-by-Six Fix

Why Tune up for the marathon

Who Recommends It Coach Kevin Hanson, whose Hansons-Brooks runners Desiree Davila and Mike Reneau did this tune-up 3 weeks before their first-American finishes at the 2008 Chicago Marathon

After a warmup, do two 6-mile runs, each at 5 seconds per mile faster than your marathon goal pace. Walk or jog for 10 minutes between them. "You're trying to teach your body to run fast while it's tired, before beginning the marathon taper," says Hanson. "So don't ease up on your training before this workout."

Mile Repeats

Why Build strength

Who Recommends It Kelly Jaske, 32, who did these workouts before placing second in the 2009 US Half-Marathon Championships

After a warmup, run 2-mile repeats at 10-K pace. Recover for 3 minutes in between. Every time you do the workout, increase the pace, cut the recovery time, or add 1 mile, up to a maximum of six repeats. "I did five of these workouts in the 2 months leading up to the half-marathon," Jaske says. "They teach you that when your body says, 'Stop,' you can say no."

Aerobic Power Intervals

Why To jump-start your season

Who Recommends It Dathan Ritzenhein, who placed second at the US Olympic Marathon Trials (2:11:06)

At a track, run 5 × 2-K (5 laps) at a little faster than threshold pace (about half-marathon race pace). Recover with a 2-minute slow jog between each repeat. Warm up and cool down with a 15- to 20-minute jog. Ritzenhein follows his warmup with a series of drills, including bounding, high knees, and butt kicks, as well as 8 to 10 strides. "This workout is a good introduction to faster-paced running when I'm coming out of an easy phase," he says.

No-Rest Intervals

Why To make race pace feel easier

Who Recommends It Marlene Atwood, a USATF-certified coach in the Atlanta area

Run 400 meters (one lap) at 30 seconds slower than your per-mile goal pace for the 5-K or 10-K, then 400 meters at 30 seconds faster than goal pace. Continue alternating between these moderate and fast speeds for a total of 3 to 4 miles. For example, if your goal 5-K pace is 7-minute miles, run a 7:30-paced lap, then a 6:30-paced lap, then a 7:30, and so on. Do a warmup and cooldown before and after. "This strength-building workout forces you to sustain a high level of effort from start to finish," says Atwood, "which will help make race pace feel less demanding."

Tempo Hill Runs

Why To prepare for a hilly race

Who Recommends It Tina Klein, an elite masters racer and coach. Her athletes do this workout four times during their 10-week buildup to the Peachtree Road Race on July 4, a 10-K with four significant climbs, including the near-mile-long Cardiac Hill.

Every 2 to 3 weeks, replace your weekly tempo run with a "tempo hill" workout. Find a 20- to 25-minute route that has two to four moderately tough climbs that will take you at least 3 minutes each to crest. After a 10-minute warmup, run the route at a pace that keeps your heart rate at about 80 percent of your maximum (you can talk only in short sentences). Your pace will slow on the uphills and speed up on the downhills; that's fine, because the goal is to sustain the effort, not the pace. Finish with 10 minutes of easy running. "In addition to building strength and speed, this 40- to 45-minute run prepares your mind and your body for hilly events," says Klein.

Lane-Change Miles

Why To pick up the pace

Who Recommends It Russ Hart, coach of the Cornbelt Running Club in Davenport, Iowa, which hosts 11,000 runners annually for the Bix 7-Mile road race on July 26

Two to 3 weeks before race day, Hart's runners do this variation on mile repeats, which requires gradual acceleration: After a 2-mile warmup, run four laps: do the first at a 10-K race pace on the inside lane, the second in lane 2, the third in lane 3, and the last in lane 4—with each lap run at the same time, meaning you'll need to pick up your pace by 2 seconds per lap to cover the extra few steps. "You'll start out at an aerobic pace, but you'll move into anaerobic territory by lap four," says Hart. Do two to five intervals of four laps, with at least a 400 recovery in between. Variation: Do just one of these, but keep extending to lane five, six, and so on until you can no longer hit the same time for each lap.

Breaking Down the 10-K

Why To build strength and confidence

Who Recommends It Michael Gaige, a coach in Portland, Maine, who heads the training program for the Beach to Beacon 10-K

Gaige has runners train for the distance with this workout: Start with a 2-mile warmup, then run 5 × 1200 meters, with a 400-meter recovery jog between repeats. Finish with a 1½-mile cooldown. "Early in training, run the 1200s at a comfortably hard pace," says Gaige. "In the final 2 months, run them at 10-K goal pace or slightly faster."

High-Intensity Long Run

Why To build fatigue-resistance at your goal marathon pace

Who Recommends It Brad Hudson, an elite running coach based in Eugene, Oregon, and coauthor of *Run Faster from the 5-K to the Marathon*

Hudson's athletes do this workout 6 to 8 weeks before a marathon: Warm up by running 2 miles at an easy pace. Then run 1 mile 10 seconds faster than your marathon pace, followed by 1 mile 45 seconds slower than marathon pace. For example, if your goal marathon pace is 8 minutes per mile, run a mile in 7:50, followed by a mile in 8:45. Repeat this pattern six times, for 14 total miles (including the warmup).

"This workout does a good job of building specific endurance for long races," says Hudson, "but it's more manageable—physically and mentally—than doing a long run at race pace."

Dress Rehearsals

Why To learn marathon goal pace

Who Recommends It Coach Jenny Hadfield, author of *Marathoning for Mortals* and blogger at runnersworld.com

The runners whom Hadfield trains for the Chicago Marathon practice their marathon goal pace in two "dress rehearsals." Six to 7 weeks before the race, they run 3 miles at MGP midway through a long run. Three to 4 weeks before the race, they run 5 MGP miles near the end of a long run. "You need to be close to perfect, so running these miles any faster or slower than MGP defeats the purpose," she says.

Long-Run/Tempo-Run Combo

Why To simultaneously improve on endurance and race pace

Who Recommends It Paul Pilkington, who has coached 2008 US Olympic steeplechaser Lindsey Anderson

After 8 miles at a conversational pace, do four 20-second "strides," then run 4 miles at a pace that's about 15 seconds per mile slower than your 5-K pace. Return to a conversational pace for the final 3 miles. "Adding tempo-paced mileage to long runs," says Pilkington, "gives you a mental break from doing the same pace for the entire distance."

Predator Run

Why Simulate the increasing effort of a race

Who Recommends It Scott Simmons, coach of the American Distance Project, an elite running group that includes US road-race star Justin Young

After a 2-mile warmup, run at a pace that's comfortably hard: 15 to 45 seconds off your goal race pace. Gradually speed up until you're running moderately hard at midrun and then very hard—no slower than goal race pace—at the end. "Your fatigue increases steadily from aerobic to anaerobic running, just as it does in a race, so it's an excellent race simulation," says Simmons. "They're called predator runs because predators must accelerate to catch their prey." Do 3 miles if you're training for a 5-K, 6 miles for a 10-K, 6 to 10 miles for a half-marathon, or 6 to 13 miles for a marathon.

Appendix D: The Training Plans

In the next section you'll find some of the half-marathon and marathon training plans for beginner, intermediate, and advanced runners that we used in the *Runner's World* Challenge program. Look at each plan, and determine which plan best fits your goals and needs. Make sure that the days of running, the weekly mileage, and long runs are in line with your ability and fitness level and your schedule. Follow the instructions for the workouts listed with each plan. The plans do not include training paces. To determine your pace for each of the workouts, use the training calculator at runnersworld.com/tools.

Good luck!

Beginner Half-Marathon Plan

This 10-week plan is ideal for first-time half-marathoners or beginner runners who log an average of 15 to 25 miles per week. Each week of training includes 4 days of running and 3 days of rest. The weekly mileage starts at 13 miles and peaks at 23 miles. The long runs start at 5 miles and peak at 10 miles a few weeks before the race.

WEEK	MON	TUES	WED	THURS	FRI	SAT	SUN	TOTAL
1	Rest/XT	2 miles	Rest/XT	4 miles	Rest/XT	2 miles	5 miles LSD	13 miles
2	Rest/XT	2 miles	Rest/XT	5 miles	Rest/XT	2 miles	6 miles LSD	15 miles
3	Rest/XT	2 miles	Rest/XT	5 miles total, with 3 miles @ HMP	Rest/XT	2 miles	7 miles LSD	16 miles
4	Rest/XT	2 miles	Rest/XT	6 miles total, with 4 miles @ HMP	Rest/XT	2 miles	7 miles LSD	17 miles

Beginner Half-Marathon Plan (cont.)

WEEK	MON	TUES	WED	THURS	FRI	SAT	SUN	TOTAL
5	Rest/XT	4 miles	Rest/XT	3 miles	Rest/XT	3 miles	4 miles LSD	14 miles
6	Rest/XT	2 miles	Rest/XT	7 miles total, with 3 miles @ HMP	Rest/XT	3 miles	8 miles LSD	20 miles
7	Rest/XT	2 miles	Rest/XT	6 miles total, with 4 miles @ HMP	2 miles	3 miles	9 miles LSD	22 miles
8	Rest/XT	2 miles	Rest/XT	6 miles total, with 4 miles @ HMP	2 miles	3 miles	10 miles LSD	23 miles
9	Rest/XT	2 miles	Rest/XT	8 miles total, with 6 miles @ HMP	2 miles	2 miles	9 miles LSD	23 miles
10	Rest/XT	2 miles	Rest/XT	5 miles total, with 3 miles @ HMP	Rest/XT	2 miles	Race Day	22.1 miles

Key

All miles should be run at a comfortable, conversational pace unless otherwise noted. To figure out your half-marathon and 10-K paces, use the training calculator at runnersworld.com/tools.

REST/XT: Take a rest day, or do moderate cross-training with a no-impact activity like yoga or swimming.

LSD: This is a long slow distance run to build endurance. These should be done at an easy, conversational pace, 1 to 2 minutes slower than your goal race pace.

HMP: Half-marathon pace. This is the pace that you hope to maintain during the race. To figure out your half-marathon pace, you can do a 1-mile time trial. Go to a 400-meter track or any stretch of road that's 1 mile long. After a 10-minute warmup, time yourself while running four laps (1 mile) as fast as you can. Cool down with 10 minutes of walking and jogging. Plug that time into the training calculator at runnersworld.com to find out what a realistic half-marathon time and pace should be.

Intermediate Half-Marathon Plan

This 10-week plan is ideal for runners with some experience who regularly log an average of 25 to 30 miles per week. Each week of training includes 4 to 5 days of running and 2 to 3 days of rest. The weekly mileage starts at 21 miles and peaks at 30 miles. The long runs start at 8 miles and peak at 13 miles a few weeks before the race.

WEEK	MON	TUES	WED	THURS	FRI	SAT	SUN	TOTAL
1	Rest/ XT	4 miles	Rest/ XT	5 miles total, with 3 miles @ HMP	4 miles	Rest/ XT	8 miles LSD	21 miles
2	Rest/ XT	5 miles	Rest/ XT	Mile repeats 5 miles with 2 × 1 mile	4 miles	Rest/ XT	8 miles LSD	22 miles
3	Rest/ XT	5 miles	Rest/ XT	5 miles total, with 3 miles @ HMP	4 miles	Rest/ XT	9 miles LSD	23 miles
4	Rest/ XT	5 miles	Rest/ XT	6 miles total, with 4 miles @ HMP	4 miles	Rest/ XT	9 miles LSD or 10k race	24 miles
5	Rest/ XT	5 miles	3 miles	4 miles	4 miles	Rest/ XT	5 miles LSD	21 miles
6	Rest/ XT	4 miles	Rest/ XT	Mile repeats 7 miles with 3 × 1 mile	4 miles	Rest/ XT	10 miles LSD	25 miles
7	Rest/ XT	3 miles	3 miles	6 miles total, with 4 miles @ HMP	3 miles	Rest/ XT	11 miles LSD	26 miles
8	Rest/ XT	3 miles	3 miles	7 miles total, with 5 miles @ HMP	4 miles	Rest/ XT	13 miles LSD	30 miles
9	Rest/ XT	3 miles	3 miles	Mile repeats 8 miles with 4 × 1 mile	3 miles	Rest/ XT	11 miles LSD	28 miles
10	Rest/ XT	3 miles	3 miles	5 miles total, with 3 miles @ HMP	4 miles	Rest/ XT	Race Day	27.1 miles

Note: On days with speedwork, the total mileage has been rounded up to the nearest mile.

Key

All miles should be run at a comfortable, conversational pace unless otherwise noted. To figure out your half-marathon and 10-K paces, use the training calculator at runnersworld.com/tools.

REST/XT: Take a rest day, or do moderate cross-training with a no-impact activity like yoga or swimming.

LSD: This is a long slow distance run to build endurance. It should be done at an easy pace, 1 to 2 minutes slower than your goal race pace.

HMP: Half-marathon pace. This is the pace that you hope to maintain during the race. Run 1 mile easy for a warmup and 1 mile easy for a cooldown.

MILE REPEATS: After a 1-mile warmup, run 1 mile at your 10-K pace, jog two laps around the track, (or a half mile) for recovery. Repeat that cycle as directed. Cool down with 1 mile of easy running.

Advanced Half-Marathon Plan

This 10-week plan is ideal for those who have been running for at least 6 months, who have finished at least one half-marathon and average more than 35 miles per week. Each week of training includes 5 to 6 days of running and 1 to 2 days of rest. The weekly mileage starts at 31 miles and peaks at 43 miles. The long runs start at 10 miles and peak at 13 miles a few weeks before the race.

WEEK	MON	TUES	WED	THURS	FRI	SAT	SUN	TOTAL
1	Rest/ XT	5 miles	5 miles	6 miles total, with 4 miles @ HMP	5 miles	Rest/ XT	10 miles LSD	**31 miles**
2	Rest/ XT	6 miles	5 miles	Mile repeats 7 miles with 3 × 1 mile	5 miles	Rest/ XT	10 miles LSD	**33 miles**
3	Rest/ XT	6 miles	6 miles	6 miles total, with 4 miles @ HMP	6 miles	Rest/ XT	11 miles LSD	**35 miles**
4	Rest/ XT	7 miles	6 miles	7 miles total, with 5 miles @ HMP	6 miles	Rest/ XT	11 miles LSD or 10k race	**37 miles**
5	Rest/ XT	6 miles	6 miles	6 miles	5 miles	Rest/ XT	6 miles LSD	**29 miles**
6	Rest/ XT	7 miles	6 miles	Mile repeats 8 miles with 4 × 1 mile	6 miles	Rest/ XT	12 miles LSD	**39 miles**

(continued)

Advanced Half-Marathon Plan (cont.)

WEEK	MON	TUES	WED	THURS	FRI	SAT	SUN	TOTAL
7	Rest/XT	6 miles	6 miles	7 miles total, with 5 miles @ HMP	5 miles	5 miles	12 miles LSD	41 miles
8	Rest/XT	6 miles	6 miles	8 miles total, with 6 miles @ HMP	5 miles	5 miles	13 miles LSD	43 miles
9	Rest/XT	6 miles	6 miles	Mile repeats 10 miles with 5 × 1 mile	Rest/XT	5 miles	11 miles LSD	38 miles
10	Rest/XT	4 miles	4 miles	6 miles total, with 4 miles @ HMP	4 miles	Rest/XT	Race Day	30.1 miles

Note: On days with speedwork, the total mileage has been rounded up to the nearest mile.

Key

All miles should be run at a comfortable, conversational pace unless otherwise noted. To figure out your half-marathon and 10-K paces, use the training calculator at runnersworld.com/tools.

REST/XT: Take a rest day, or do moderate cross-training with a no-impact activity like yoga or swimming.

LSD: This is a long slow distance run to build endurance. It should be done at an easy pace, 1 to 2 minutes slower than your goal race pace.

HMP: Half-marathon pace. This is the pace that you hope to maintain during the race. Run 1 mile easy for a warmup and 1 mile easy for a cooldown.

MILE REPEATS: After a 1-mile warmup, run 1 mile at your 10-K pace, jog two laps around the track, (or a half mile) for recovery. Repeat that cycle as directed. Cool down with 1 mile of easy running.

Beginner Marathon Plan

This 16-week plan is ideal for first-timers. Before starting this plan it's best to have at least 1 year of experience, and run, on average, 3 to 4 times per week. Each week of training includes 4 days of running and 3 days of rest. The weekly mileage starts at 15 miles and peaks at 40 miles. The long runs start at 5 miles and peak at 20 miles a few weeks before the race.

WEEK	MON	TUES	WED	THURS	FRI	SAT	SUN	TOTAL
1	Rest	3 miles	Rest	4 miles	Rest	3 miles	5 miles LSD	**15 miles**
2	Rest	3 miles	Rest	3 miles	Rest	4 miles	7 miles LSD	**17 miles**
3	Rest	3 miles	Rest	4 miles	Rest	4 miles	9 miles LSD	**20 miles**
4	Rest	4 miles	Time Trial (1 mile)	3 miles	Rest	4 miles	7 miles LSD	**19 miles**
5	Rest	4 miles	Rest	3 miles	Rest	5 miles	10 miles LSD	**22 miles**
6	Rest	4 miles	Rest	3 miles	Rest	5 miles	12 miles LSD	**24 miles**
7	Rest	4 miles	Rest	4 miles	Rest	4 miles	15 miles LSD	**27 miles**
8	Rest	4 miles	Time Trial (1 mile)	4 miles	Rest	4 miles	12 miles LSD or ½ marathon	**25 miles**
9	Rest	4 miles with 4 strides	Rest	6 miles	Rest	4 miles	16 miles LSD	**30 miles**
10	Rest	4 miles with 4 strides	Rest	6 miles	Rest	4 miles	18 miles LSD	**32 miles**
11	Rest	6 miles with 6 strides	Rest	5 miles	Rest	5 miles	20 miles LSD	**36 miles**
12	Rest	7 miles with 7 strides	Time Trial (1 mile)	7 miles	Rest	7 miles	14 miles LSD	**36 miles**
13	Rest	6 miles with 6 strides	Rest	7 miles	Rest	7 miles	20 miles LSD	**40 miles**
14	Rest	7 miles with 7 strides	Rest	7 miles	Rest	7 miles	13 miles LSD	**34 miles**

(continued)

Beginner Marathon Plan (cont.)

WEEK	MON	TUES	WED	THURS	FRI	SAT	SUN	TOTAL
15	Rest	5 miles with 5 strides	Rest	4 miles	Rest	5 miles	10 miles LSD	24 miles
16	Rest	3 miles	Time Trial (1 mile)	4 miles	Rest	3 miles	Race Day	37.2 miles

Key

REST: Take a rest day, or do moderate cross-training with a no-impact activity like yoga or swimming.

LSD: This is a long slow distance run to build endurance and help get you accustomed to spending time on your feet. Don't worry about your pace during these runs. Just focus on finishing.

TIME TRIAL: A 1-mile time trial can help you track your fitness and set realistic race goals. Go to a 400-meter track or any 1-mile stretch of road. After a 10-minute warmup, time yourself while running four laps (or 1 mile) as fast as you can. Note your finish time, then cool down with 10 minutes of walking and jogging. Over the course of training, your fitness gains will be reflected in your time-trial results.

STRIDES: Adding strides to any easy run activates fast-twitch muscle fibers, improves coordination and leg turnover, and preps your body for the race. Near the end of your run, gradually accelerate over 100 meters until you reach 90 percent of all-out effort. Hold that effort for 5 seconds, then smoothly decelerate. Walk to recover between each stride. The exact distance of each stride is not critical.

Intermediate Marathon Plan

This 16-week plan is for runners who have 2 to 3 years of experience, who have finished a few half-marathons and at least one marathon, and who regularly log up to 30 miles per week. Each week of training includes 5 days of running and 2 days of rest. The weekly mileage starts at 25 miles and peaks at 50 miles. The long runs start at 9 miles and peak at 22 miles a few weeks before the race.

WEEK	MON	TUES	WED	THURS	FRI	SAT	SUN	TOTAL
1	Rest	4 miles easy	4 miles hills	Rest	4 miles easy	4 miles easy	9 miles LSD	25 miles
2	Rest	4 miles easy	5 miles hills	Rest	5 miles easy	5 miles easy	9 miles LSD	28 miles
3	Rest	3 miles easy	5 miles hills	Rest	5 miles easy	5 miles easy	12 miles LSD	30 miles
4	Rest	4 miles easy	5 miles hills	Time Trial (1 mile)	Rest	4 miles easy	10 miles LSD	28 miles
5	Rest	4 miles easy with 4 strides	7 miles hills	Rest	4 miles total, with 2 miles @ MP	4 miles easy	13 miles LSD	32 miles
6	Rest	5 miles easy with 5 strides	6 miles hills	Rest	4 miles total, with 2 miles @ MP	6 miles easy	15 miles LSD	36 miles
7	Rest	6 miles easy with 6 strides	7 miles hills	Rest	5 miles total, with 3 miles @ MP	5 miles easy	16 miles LSD	39 miles
8	Rest	5 miles easy with 5 strides	Hill repeats 8 miles with 8 hill repeats	Rest	Time Trial	4 miles easy	14 miles LSD or ½ marathon	32 miles
9	Rest	3 miles easy with 3 strides	Mile repeats 8 miles with 3 × 1 mile	Rest	9 miles total, with 7 miles @ MP	3 miles easy	18 miles LSD, fast finish	41 miles

(continued)

Intermediate Marathon Plan (cont.)

WEEK	MON	TUES	WED	THURS	FRI	SAT	SUN	TOTAL
10	Rest	4 miles easy with 4 strides	Yasso 800s 9 miles with 6 × 800	Rest	10 miles total, with 8 miles @ MP	Rest	20 miles LSD, fast finish	43 miles
11	Rest	4 miles easy with 4 strides	7 miles easy	Rest	10 miles total, with 8 miles @ MP	4 miles easy	20 miles LSD, fast finish	45 miles
12	Rest	Time Trial	Mile repeats 9 miles with 4 × 1 mile	6 miles easy	7 miles total, with 5 miles @ MP	8 miles easy	15 miles LSD	46 miles
13	Rest	6 miles easy with 6 strides	Yasso 800s 10 miles with 8 × 800	Rest	6 miles easy	6 miles easy	22 miles LSD	50 miles
14	Rest	8 miles easy with 8 strides	Mile Repeats 8 miles with 3 × 1 mile	Rest	7 miles easy	7 miles easy	15 miles LSD or 1/2 marathon	45 miles
15	Rest	5 miles easy with 5 strides	4 miles easy	Rest	6 miles easy	5 miles easy	12 miles LSD	32 miles
16	Rest	Time Trial	Rest	5 miles easy	Rest	3 miles very easy	Race Day	35.2 miles

Note: On days with speedwork, the total mileage has been rounded up to the nearest mile.

Key

REST: Take a rest day, or do moderate cross-training with a no-impact activity like yoga or swimming.

EASY: Run at a comfortable, conversational pace. These are interchangeable with rest days. You can cross-train on an easy day instead with a sustained aerobic effort on a bike or the elliptical trainer.

HILLS: Run the mileage for the day on the hilliest course you can find. Hills build a base of strength during the first 7 weeks of the program.

LSD: This is a long slow distance run to build endurance. LSDs should be done at an easy, conversational pace, 1 to 2 minutes slower than your goal race pace. Later in the program, you can practice a fast finish by picking up the pace during the last 2 to 3 miles.

TIME TRIAL: A 1-mile time trial can help you track your fitness and set realistic race goals. Go to a 400-meter track or any 1-mile stretch of road. After a 10-minute warmup, time yourself while running 4 laps (or 1 mile) as fast as you can. Note your finish time, then cool down with 10 minutes of walking and jogging. Over the course of training, your fitness gains will be reflected in your time-trial results.

STRIDES: Adding strides to any easy run activates fast-twitch muscle fibers, improves coordination and leg turnover, and preps your body for the race. Near the finish of your run, gradually accelerate over 100 meters until you reach 90 percent of all-out effort. Hold that effort for 5 seconds, then smoothly decelerate. Walk to recover between each stride. The exact distance of each stride is not critical.

HILL REPEATS: Find a hill that will take you at least 2 minutes to climb, and mark off a "short" repeat halfway from the bottom and a "long" repeat at the top. After a 2-mile warmup, run up to the short mark three or four times, jogging back down to recover in between. Then run up to the top three or four times, jogging back down to the short mark and then sprinting to the bottom. (Try to maintain smooth form, without slapping your feet.) Finish with three or four sprints up to the short mark. Cool down with 2 miles of easy running. The total mileage for the day will amount to about 8 miles.

MP: Marathon goal pace. Practice the speed you're hoping to maintain in the race. Run 1 mile easy for a warmup and 1 mile easy for a cooldown.

MILE REPEATS: Warm up with 2 miles of easy running. Run 1 mile at your 10-K pace, jog a lap for recovery, and repeat that cycle as directed. Cool down with 2 miles of easy running.

YASSO 800s: Warm up with 2 miles of easy running, then run 800 meters at a time that's "equal" to your marathon time. That is, if you're shooting for a 4:10 marathon, try to run each 800-meter repeat in 4 minutes and 10 seconds. Jog 400 meters in between the 800s. Cool down with 2 miles of easy running.

Advanced Marathon Plan

This 16-week plan is for runners who have at least 3 years of experience, those who have comfortably completed other marathons and shorter races, and who regularly log 35 to 40 miles per week. Each week of training includes 6 days of running and 1 day of rest. The weekly mileage starts at 33 miles and peaks at 60 miles. The long runs start at 10 miles and peak at 23 miles a few weeks before the race.

WEEK	MON	TUES	WED	THURS	FRI	SAT	SUN	TOTAL
1	4 miles easy	4 miles easy	6 miles hills	4 miles easy	Rest	5 miles easy	10 miles LSD	33 miles
2	5 miles easy	6 miles hills	4 miles easy	6 miles total, with 4 miles @ MP	Rest	5 miles easy	12 miles LSD	38 miles
3	4 miles easy	6 miles hills	4 miles easy	8 miles total, with 6 miles @ MP	Rest	5 miles easy	14 miles LSD	41 miles
4	4 miles easy	5 miles hills	5 miles easy	4 miles total, with 2 miles @ MP	Rest	5 miles easy	10 miles LSD	33 miles
5	3 miles easy with 3 strides	8 miles hills	5 miles easy	8 miles total, with 6 miles @ MP	Rest	4 miles easy	14 miles LSD	42 miles
6	6 miles easy with 6 strides	7 miles easy	5 miles easy	8 miles total, with 6 miles @ MP	Rest	4 miles easy	16 miles LSD	46 miles
7	5 miles easy with 5 strides	8 miles hills	5 miles easy	8 miles total, with 6 miles @ MP	Rest	4 miles easy	18 miles LSD	48 miles
8	5 miles easy with 5 strides	Hill repeats 8 miles with 8 hill repeats	4 miles easy	9 miles total, with 7 miles @ MP	Rest	3 miles easy	13 miles LSD or ½ marathon	42 miles

WEEK	MON	TUES	WED	THURS	FRI	SAT	SUN	TOTAL
9	Rest	5 miles easy with 5 strides	Mile repeats 8 miles with 3 × 1 miles	4 miles easy	9 miles with 7 miles @ MP	5 miles easy	20 miles LSD, fast finish	**51 miles**
10	Rest	6 miles easy with 6 strides	Yasso 800s 9 miles with 6 × 800	6 miles easy	10 miles with 8 miles @ MP	6 miles easy	22 miles LSD, fast finish	**59 miles**
11	Rest	8 miles easy with 8 strides	Yasso 800s 9 miles with 6 × 800	7 miles easy	8 miles with 6 miles @ MP	6 miles easy	22 miles LSD, fast finish	**60 miles**
12	Rest	6 miles easy with 6 strides	Mile repeats 9 miles with 4 × 1 mile	7 miles easy	10 miles with 8 miles @ MP	8 miles easy	14 miles LSD, fast finish	**54 miles**
13	Rest	6 miles easy with 6 strides	Yasso 800s 10 miles with 8 × 800	7 miles easy	8 miles hills	6 miles easy	23 miles LSD, fast finish	**60 miles**
14	Rest	7 miles easy with 7 strides	Mile repeats 8 miles with 3 × 1 mile	6 miles easy	10 miles with 8 miles @ MP	6 miles easy	16 miles LSD, fast finish	**53 miles**
15	Rest	4 miles easy with 4 strides	7 miles hills	4 miles easy	8 miles with 6 miles @ MP	4 miles easy	13 miles LSD	**40 miles**
16	Rest	5 miles easy with 5 strides	Rest	3 miles easy	Rest	3 miles very easy	Race Day	**37.2 miles**

Note: On days with speedwork, the total mileage has been rounded up to the nearest mile.

Key

REST: Take a rest day, or do moderate cross-training with a no-impact activity like yoga or swimming.

EASY: Run at a comfortable, conversational pace. These are interchangeable with rest days. You can cross-train on an easy day instead with a sustained aerobic effort on a bike or the elliptical trainer.

HILLS: Run the mileage for the day on the hilliest course you can find. Hills build a base of strength during the first 7 weeks of the program.

LSD: This is a long slow distance run to build endurance. LSDs should be done at an easy, conversational pace, 1 to 2 minutes slower than your goal marathon pace. Later in the program you can practice a fast finish by picking up the pace for the last 2 to 3 miles.

MP: Marathon goal pace. Practice the speed you're hoping to hit in the race. Run 1 mile easy for a warmup and 1 mile easy for a cooldown.

STRIDES: Adding strides to any easy run activates fast-twitch muscle fibers, improves coordination and leg turnover, and preps your body for the race. Near the end of your run, gradually accelerate over 100 meters until you reach 90 percent of all-out effort. Hold that effort for 5 seconds, then smoothly decelerate. Walk to recover between each stride. The exact distance of each stride is not critical.

HILL REPEATS: Find a hill that will take you at least 2 minutes to climb, and mark off a "short" repeat halfway from the bottom and a "long" repeat at the top. After a 2-mile warmup, run up to the short mark three or four times, jogging back down to recover in between. Then run up to the top three or four times, jogging back down to the short mark and then sprinting to the bottom. (Try to maintain smooth form, without slapping your feet.) Finish with three or four sprints up to the short mark. Cool down with 2 miles of easy running. The total mileage for the day will amount to about 8 miles.

MILE REPEATS: Warm up with 2 miles of easy running. Run a mile at your 10-K pace, jog 400 meters for recovery, and repeat that cycle as directed. Cool down with 2 two miles of easy running.

YASSO 800s: Warm up with 2 miles of easy running, then run 800 meters at a time that's "equal" to your marathon time. That is, if you're shooting for a 4:10 marathon, try to run each 800-meter repeat in 4 minutes and 10 seconds. Jog 400 meters in between the 800s. Cool down with 2 miles of easy running.

Endnotes

Chapter 1 Getting Started

1 Matthew R. Ely, Samuel N. Cheuvront, William O. Roberts, and Scott J. Montain. "Impact of Weather on Marathon-Running Performance," *Medicine and Science in Sports and Exercise, 2007:* 487–93.

2 Darci Smith, "Wash Out," *Runner's World,* May 2012: 98.

3 Amby Burfoot, "Grave Concerns," *Runner's World,* December 2008: 92–99.

Chapter 2 Training Basics

1 Erin Strout, "Get on Track." *Runner's World,* June 2009: 65–69.

2 Nicholas Luden, Erik Hayes, Andrew Galpin, Kiril Minchev, Bozena Jemiolo, Ulrika Raue, Todd A. Trappe, Matthew P. Harber, Ted Bowers, and Scott Trappe, "Myocellular basis for tapering in competitive distance runners," *Journal of Applied Physiology* 108, no. 6 (2010): 1501–9.

3 Martha Gulati, L. J. Shaw, R. A. Thisted, H. R. Black, C. N. Bairey Merz, and M. F. Arnsdorf, "Heart rate response to exercise stress testing in asymptomatic women: the St. James Women take heart project," *Circulation* 122, no. 2 (July 2010): 130–37.

4 Michell A. Cleary, Ronald K. Hetzler, Jennifer J. Wages, Melissa A. Lentz, Christopher D. Stickley, Iris F. Kimura, "Comparisons of age-predicted maximum heart rate equations in college-aged subjects," *Journal of Strength and Conditioning Research* 25, no. 9 (September 2011): 2591–97.

5 Elizabeth A. Jeans, Carl Foster, John P. Porcari, Mark Gibson, Scott Doberstein, "Translation of Exercise Testing to Exercise Prescription Using the Talk Test," *Journal of Strength and Conditioning Research* 25, no. 3 (March 2011): 590–96.

6 Bob Cooper, "Runner's World Challenge," *Runner's World,* November 2010, 40.

7 ———. "*Runner's World* Challenge," *Runner's World,* September 2010, 44.

8 Ibid.

Chapter 3 Integrated Training into Your Everyday Life

1 Jim McKenna, Jo Coulson, "How does exercising at work influence work productivity? A randomized crossover trial," *Medicine and Science in Sports and Exercise* 37, no. 5 (May 2005): S323.

2 Matt Fitzgerald, "Take a Shortcut," *Runner's World,* April 2009, 27–28.

3 Ed Eyestone, "Double Duty," *Runner's World,* July 2009, 34.

4 Bob Cooper, "*Runner's World* Challenge," *Runner's World,* October 2010, 44.

5 ———. "*Runner's World* Challenge," *Runner's World,* November 2010, 40.

6 ———. "*Runner's World* Challenge," *Runner's World,* May 2010, 42.

7 ———. "*Runner's World* Challenge," *Runner's World,* June 2010, 38.

8 Ibid.

9 Ibid.

Chapter 4 Everyday Eating

1 A. E. Jeukendrup, "Carbohydrate intake during exercise and performance," *Nutrition* 20, no. 7–8 (July–August 2004): 669–77.

2 Whole Grains Council, "Identifying Whole Grains," http://www .wholegrainscouncil.org/whole-grains-101 /identifying-whole-grain-products.

3 Kristen E. Gerlach, Harold W. Burton, Joan M. Dorn, John J. Leddy, and Peter J Horvath, "Fat intake and injury in female runners," *Journal of International Society of Sports Nutrition* 5 (2008): 1.

4 J. A. Paniagua, A. Gallego de la Sacristana, I. Romero, A. Vidal-Puig, J. M. Latre, E. Sanchez, P. Perez-Martinez, J. Lopez-Miranda, and F. Perez-Jiminez, "Monoun-saturated fat-rich diet prevents central body fat distribution and decreases postproandial adiponectin expression induced by a carbohydrate-rich diet in insulin-resistant subjects," *Diabetes Care* 30, no. 7 (July 2007): 1717–23.

5 American Heart Association, *Fat,* http: //www.americanheart.org/presenter .jhtml?identifier=4582 (March 8, 2011).

6 Winston J. Craig, PhD, MPH, RD, Ann Reed Mangels, PhD, RD, LDN, FADA, "Position of the American Dietetic Associa-tion: Vegetarian Diets," *Journal of the American Dietetic Association* 109 (2009): 1266–82.

Chapter 5 Eating Before You Run, On the Road, and After You're Done

1 Michael N. Sawka, Luise M. Burke, E. Randy Eichner, Ronald J. Maughan, Soctt J. Montain, and Nina S. Stachenfeld, "Exercise and Fluid replacement. Position statement," *Medicine and Science in Sports and Exercise* 39, no. 2 (2007): 377–90.

2 Timothy David Noakes, "Is drinking to thirst optimum"? *Annals of Nutrition and Metabolism* 57 (sup. 2) February 2011: 9–17.

3 Sawka et al., "Exercise and fluid replace-ments" *Medicine and Science in Sports and Exercise* (2007): 377–90.

4 Ibid.

5 Stephen M. Simons and Gregory G. Shaskan, "Gastrointestinal problems in

distance running," *International Journal of Sports Medicine* 6, no. 3 (2005): 162–70.

6 Kristin Bjornsen, "Runner's Digest," *Runner's World,* September 2006, 53.

7. Armstrong L. E., Pumerantz A. C., Roti M. W., Judelson D. A., Watson G., Dias J. C., Sökmen B., Casa D. J., Maresh C. M. "Fluid, electrolyte, and renal indices of hydration during 11 days of controlled caffeine consumption." *International Journal of Sport Nutrition and Exercise Metabolism* 15. (2005) 252–65.

8 Bulent Sokmen, Lawrence E. Armstrong, William J. Kraemer, Douglas J. Casa, Joao C. Dias, Daniel A. Judelson, and Carl M. Maresh, "Caffeine Use in Sports: Considerations for the Athlete," *Journal of Strength and Conditioning Research* 22, iss. 3 (May 2008): 978–86.

9 Center for Science in the Public Interest, www.cspinet.org/reports/caffeine.pdf.

10. http://www.starbucks.com/menu/drinks /espresso/caffe-latte

11. Center for Science in the Public Interest. www.cspinet.org/reports/caffeine.pdf

12. http://www.pepsicobeveragefacts.com /infobyproduct.php

13. http://www.redbullusa.com/cs /Satellite/en_US/red-bull-energy-drink /001242989766321?pcs_c=PCS_Product&pcs _cid=1242989299257&pcs_pvt =ingredient&pcs_iid=1242989298306

14. http://productnutrition.thecoca -colacompany.com/products/coca- cola#ingredients

15. http://www.thehersheycompany.com /nutrition-and-wellness/chocolate-101 /caffeine.aspx

16. Ibid.

17 L. Perry Kozir, PhD, "Alcohol and athletic performance." (ASCM position statement.)

18 Kristen Wolfe Bieler, "What Are You Drinking"? *Runner's World,* August 2004, www.runnersworld.com/article/1,7124,s6 -242-302-7908-0,00.html.

19 David Stensel, "Exercise, appetite, and appetite-regulating hormones: implications for food intake and weight control," *Annals of Nutrition and Metabolism* 57 (2010): 36–42.

Chapter 6 Weight Management

1 M. A. Kennedy, J. M. Sacheck, R. Houser, S. A. Folta, M. E. Nelson, "Impact of marathon training on body weight in recreational runners," *Medicine and Science in Sports and Exercise* 42, no. 5 (2010): S441.

2 FDA, "Definitions of Nutrient Content Claims," www.fda.gov/Food /GuidanceComplianceRegulatoryInformation /GuidanceDocuments/FoodLabelingNutrition /FoodLabelingGuide/ucm064911.htm.

3 Bidisha Mandal, "Use of food labels as a

weight-loss behavior," *Journal of Consumer Affairs* 44, no. 3 (September 2010): 516–27.

4 Brian Wansink and Pierre Chandon, "Can 'low-fat' nutrition labels lead to obesity"? *Journal of Marketing Research* 43, no. 4 (2006): 605–17.

5 American Heart Association, "Sugars and Carbohydrates," www.heart.org /HEARTORG/GettingHealthy /NutritionCenter/HealthyDietGoals /Sugars-and-Carbohydrates_UCM_303296 _Article.jsp.

6 Cherina Kelly, Angus Burnett, and Michael Newton, "The effect of strength training on three-kilometer performance in recreational women endurance runners," *Journal of Strength and Conditioning Research* 22, no. 2 (2008): 396–403.

7 Jack Hollis, Christina Gullion, Victor Stevens, Phillip J. Brantley, Lawrence Appel, et. al, "Weight loss during the intensive intervention phase of the weight-loss maintenance trial," *American Journal of Preventive Medicine* 35, iss. 2 (August 2008): 118–26.

8 A. V. Nedeltcheva, J. M. Kilkus, J. Imperial, K. Kasza, D. A. Schoeller, P. D. Penev, "Sleep curtailment is accompanied by increased intake of calories from snacks," *American Journal of Clinical Nutrition* 89, no. 1 (January 2009): 126–33.

9 T. A. Hagobian, C. G. Sharoff, B. R. Stephens, G. N. Wade, J. E. Silva, S. R. Chipkin,

B. Braun, "Effects of exercise on energy-regulating hormones and appetite in men and women," *Am J Physiol Regul Integr Comp Physiol*, 296 (2009): R233–42.

10 Matthew G. Kadey, MSc, RD, "Weight Loss Myths Exposed!" *Runner's World,* April 2010: 57–66.

11 Paul Vanderburgh and Lloyd Laubach, "Validation of 5-K age and weight run handicap model," *Journal of Exercise Physiology* 9, no. 3 (December 2006): 33–40.

12 Cameron Hall Arturo Figueroa, Bo Fernall, and Jill A. Kanaley, "Energy expenditure of walking and running: comparison with prediction equations," *Medicine and Science in Sport and Exercise*, 36, iss. 12 (December 2004): 2128–34.

13. Amby Burfoot, "How many calories are you really burning?" *Runner's World*, http://www.runnersworld.com/article /0,7120,s6-242-304-311-8402-0,00.html September 2005.

14. Ibid.

15 Darlene A. Sedlock, Jean A. Fissinger, and Christopher L. Melby, "Effect of exercise intensity and duration on post-exercise energy expenditure," *Medicine and Science in Sports and Exercise* 21, no. 6 (December 1989): 662–66.

16. Matthew G. Kadey, MSc, RD, "Weight Loss Myths Exposed!" *Runner's World*, April 2010: 57–66

Chapter 7 Staying Healthy

1 Amby Burfoot, "The Laws of Perpetual Motion," *Runner's World*, March 2010, 50–58.

2 Liz Plosser, "Cold Call," *Runner's World,* December 2009, 48.

3 D. M. Bailey, S. J. Erith, P. J. Griffin, A. Dowson, D. S. Brewer, N. Gant, C. Williams, "Influence of cold-water immersion on indices of muscle damage following prolonged intermittent shuttle running," *Journal of Sports Science* 25, no. 11 (September 2007): 1163–70.

4 Lisa Jhung, "Vision Quest," *Runner's World,* January 2010, 91.

5 Liz Robbins, "Collision Course," *Runner's World,* January 2010: 86–91.

6 Liz Robbins, "Collision Course," *Runner's World,* January 2010, 86–91.

7 US Department of Transportation, "Statistics and Facts about Distracted Driving," www.distraction.gov/stats-and -facts/.

8 Amby Burfoot, "Turning Up the Heat," *Runner's World,* August 2009: 62–65.

9 M. R. Ely, S. N. Cheuvront, W. O. Roberts, and S. J. Montain, "Impact of weather on marathon-running performance," *Medicine and Science in Sports and Exercise* 39, no. 3 (March 2007): 487–93.

10 L. E. Armstrong, D. J. Casa, M. Millard-Stafford, D. S. Moran, S. W. Pyne, W. O. Roberts, "ACSM Statement: Exertional Heat Illness During Training and Competition," *Medicine and Science in Sports and Exercise* 39, no. 3 (2007 March): 556–72.

11 John W. Castellani, Andrew J. Young, Michel B. Ducharme, Gordon G. Giesbrecht, Ellen Glickman, and Robert E. Sallis, "ACSM Statement: Prevention of Cold Injuries During Exercise," *Medicine and Science in Sports and Exercise* (2006): 2014–29.

12 Christina Ambros-Rudolph, Rainer Hofmann-Wellenhof, Erka Richtig, Manuela Muller-Furstner, Peter Soyer, and Helmut Kerl, "Malignant Melanoma in Marathon Runners," *Archives of Dermatology* 142 (2006): 1471–74.

13 Nikki Kimball, "A Dynamic Routine," *Runner's World,* March 2010, 44.

14 Sage Rountree, "Flexible Routine," *Runner's World,* October 2009, 52.

Chapter 8 Getting Hurt and Getting Over It

1 Erin Strout, "The Backup Plan," *Runner's World,* August 2009, 88–89.

2 Christie Aschwanden, "Mistaken Identity," *Runner's World,* September 2008, 47–48.

3 Adam Bean, "Cramping Out," *Runner's World,* April 2011, 56.

4 Christie Aschwanden, "Know Your Limits," *Runner's World,* October 2007, 52.

5 Meghan Rabbitt, "The Bright Side," *Runner's World,* May 2010, 54.

6 Ed Eyestone, "Come Back Strong," *Runner's World,* February 2010, 30.

7 Liz Plosser, "Damage Control," *Runner's World,* December 2010, 48–49.

8 Adam Bean, "Cramping Out," *Runner's World,* April 2011, 56.

Chapter 9 Before the Race

1 Nicholas Luden, Erik Hayes, Andrew Galpin, Kiril Minchev, Bozena Jemiolo, Ulrika Raue, Todd A. Trappe, Matthew P. Harber, Ted Bowers, and Scott Trappe, "Myocellular basis for tapering in competitive distance runners," *Journal of Applied Physiology* 108 (June 2010): 1501–9.

2 D. C. Nieman, "Upper respiratory tract infections and exercise" *Thorax* 50, no. 12 (1995 Dec): 1229–31.

3 David Nieman, "Risk of Upper Respiratory Tract Infection in Athletes: An epidemiologic and Immunologic Perspective," *Journal of Athletic Training,* 32, no. 4 (December 1997): 344–49.

Chapter 10 The Big Day

1 Katie Neitz, "Midrun Mishaps," *Runner's World,* June 2009, 46.

Chapter 11 Beyond the Finish Line

1 Sage Rountree, "Race Recovery," *Runner's World,* November 2008, 52.

2 Kelly Pate Dwyer, "Second Chances," *Runner's World,* November 2008, 31.

Index

Boldfaced page references indicate photographs. Underscored references indicate boxed text.